W0018319

Dr. Almonroeder is uniquely qualified to author a text on applied research as it relates to the rehabilitation professions. As a practicing clinician, researcher, and faculty member, he has the rare ability to describe the complexities of research and statistics in a relevant and understandable way to bridge the gap between research and clinical practice.

Nathan Short, *PhD, OTD, OTR/L, CHT, Huntington University, USA*

Advanced Statistics for Physical and Occupational Therapy

Advanced Statistics for Physical and Occupational Therapy explains the basis for statistical analyses that are commonly used to answer clinical research questions related to physical and occupational therapy. This textbook provides a resource to help students and faculty in physical and occupational therapy graduate programs understand the basis for common statistical analyses and be able to apply these techniques in their own research. This textbook provides readers with the basis for common statistical analyses, including *t*-tests, analysis of variance, regression, and nonparametric tests. Each chapter includes step-by-step tutorials with corresponding example data sets explaining how to conduct these statistical analyses using Statistical Package for the Social Sciences (SPSS) software and the Excel Analysis ToolPak, as well as how to identify and interpret relevant output and report results.

Advanced Statistics for Physical and Occupational Therapy is key reading for students in physical therapy, occupational therapy, sport performance, and sport rehabilitation graduate programs as well as students in athletic training courses, applied statistics in sport, and research methods in sport modules.

This new text will also be of interest to practicing clinicians who hope to better understand the research they are reading and/or are interested in starting to conduct their own clinical research.

Thomas Gus Almonroeder, PT, DPT, PhD, is an assistant professor in the Department of Health Professions at the University of Wisconsin – La Crosse, USA.

Advanced Statistics for Physical and Occupational Therapy

Thomas Gus Almonroeder

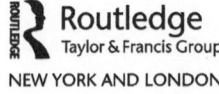
Routledge
Taylor & Francis Group

NEW YORK AND LONDON

Cover image: © kali9 / Getty images

First published 2022
by Routledge
605 Third Avenue, New York, NY 10158

and by Routledge
4 Park Square, Milton Park, Abingdon, Oxon, OX14 4RN

Routledge is an imprint of the Taylor & Francis Group, an informa business

© 2022 Thomas Gus Almonroeder

The right of Thomas Gus Almonroeder to be identified as author of this work has been asserted by him in accordance with sections 77 and 78 of the Copyright, Designs and Patents Act 1988.

All rights reserved. No part of this book may be reprinted or reproduced or utilised in any form or by any electronic, mechanical, or other means, now known or hereafter invented, including photocopying and recording, or in any information storage or retrieval system, without permission in writing from the publishers.

Trademark notice: Product or corporate names may be trademarks or registered trademarks, and are used only for identification and explanation without intent to infringe.

Library of Congress Cataloging-in-Publication Data
Names: Almonroeder, Thomas Gus, author.
Title: Advanced statistics for physical and occupational therapy / Thomas
    Gus Almonroeder.
Description: First edition. | New York, NY : Routledge, 2022. | Includes bibliographical
    references and index.
Identifiers: LCCN 2021061866 (print) | LCCN 2021061867 (ebook) |
    ISBN 9781032017129 (hardback) | ISBN 9781032017112 (paperback) |
    ISBN 9781003179757 (ebook)
Subjects: LCSH: Physical therapy—Statistical aspects. | Occupational therapy. | Statistics.
Classification: LCC RM695 .A36 2022 (print) | LCC RM695 (ebook) |
    DDC 615.8/2—dc23/eng/20211220
LC record available at https://lccn.loc.gov/2021061866
LC ebook record available at https://lccn.loc.gov/2021061867

ISBN: 978-1-032-01712-9 (hbk)
ISBN: 978-1-032-01711-2 (pbk)
ISBN: 978-1-003-17975-7 (ebk)

DOI: 10.4324/9781003179757

Typeset in Times New Roman
by Apex CoVantage, LLC

Access the Support Material: www.routledge.com/9781032017112

Contents

Figures

Tables

Boxes

Preface

My reason for writing this book is simple: I strongly believe in the importance of developing clinicians who have the knowledge and skills needed to be critical consumers of research and to contribute to the development of new knowledge in their field. I also appreciate that many clinicians feel that their limited understanding of statistics hinders their ability to understand, critically evaluate, and conduct research. Therefore, my goal in developing this book was to provide clinicians, aspiring clinicians, and clinician-educators with a resource that could help to explain the theoretical basis for commonly used statistical analyses and provide step-by-step tutorials for how to conduct, interpret, and report the results of these analyses. My hope is that this book strikes a nice balance between explaining underlying theory and providing 'real-world' examples and application opportunities.

While this book certainly isn't all-encompassing, it covers the core analyses that are most commonly used in rehabilitation research, based on a survey of the literature conducted by Schwartz et al. (1996). Therefore, it's a good starting point for those in the fields of physical and occupational therapy, as well as those in other health-related fields, such as athletic training, chiropractic, and speech-language pathology.

How this book is organized

This book is generally organized into four sections: Chapters 1–4 introduce foundational concepts, Chapters 5–7 discuss analyses that are used to compare means, Chapters 8–11 discuss analyses that are used to examine relationships and/or make predictions, and Chapters 12–16 introduce more advanced topics. Each chapter includes examples related to health, medicine, or rehabilitation. My goal in providing these examples is to show how the concepts can be applied to address clinical research questions.

Many of the chapters also include data sets* and step-by-step video tutorials that demonstrate how to perform different statistical analyses using the popular statistical analysis software package SPSS (IBM Corp., IBM SPSS Statistics for Windows, Version 27.0. Armonk, NY, USA). In addition, the videos also show how to conduct many of these analyses using the Microsoft Excel Analysis ToolPak. I encourage you to work through the examples provided, since it's a good way to apply the concepts discussed in the chapters.

*Note: the examples provided in this book are for the sole purpose of helping you learn how to analyze data, interpret statistical tests, and so on. You shouldn't use the examples from this book to guide your clinical practice.

Here are some video tutorials that can help you get started:

SPSS_intro.mp4 – provides an overview of the basic layout of SPSS and describes how
   to import data.
ExcelToolPak.mp4 – shows how to activate the Microsoft Excel Analysis ToolPak.

Acknowledgments

This is the first textbook I've written. While I've enjoyed the process, writing a book certainly requires a tremendous amount of support and encouragement. Therefore, I'd like to thank some of the people who helped make this work possible.

First and foremost, I'd like to thank my wife Sarah, daughter Grace, and son Jack. This book wouldn't have happened without their love and support. I'm a lucky man to have such a great family.

I'd also like to thank Kelsey Redman and Jillian Hebert. Kelsey is a student of mine who provided excellent feedback for many of the chapters in this book. Her perspective as a student physical therapist was tremendously helpful in making this book 'user-friendly'. Jillian is a data analyst at the University of California, San Francisco. She served as a content reviewer for this book and provided me with excellent ideas and feedback. I learned a lot from working with her.

Finally, I'd like to thank those who reviewed my book proposal and helped to move this project along. It's always been a goal of mine to write a book. I'm excited to see it come to fruition.

Glossary

Alpha level: the probability of falsely rejecting the null hypothesis when it is actually true. (Chapter 4)

Alternative hypothesis: hypothesis stating that an observed effect (e.g. mean difference, correlation) is due to a true effect in the population; a directional alternative hypothesis specifies the nature of the anticipated effect, while a nondirectional alternative hypothesis does not. (Chapter 4)

Analysis of covariance: a family of statistical analyses that are generally used to examine the effects of an independent variable on a dependent variable while accounting for the influence of another variable referred to as a covariate. (Chapter 15)

Analysis of variance: a family of statistical analyses that are generally used to analyze differences among means. (Chapter 6)

Box plot: a graph that displays the first quartile (Q1), median (Q2), third quartile (Q3), interquartile range (Q3–Q1), and lowest and highest scores ('whiskers') for a variable. (Chapter 2)

Central tendency: the location where a frequency distribution tends to be centered; the mean, median, and mode are measures of central tendency. (Chapter 2)

Change score: a value that reflects the difference in performance across two time points (e.g. post–pre) or conditions. (Chapter 5)

Coefficient of determination(R^2): the proportion of variance in a variable that is explained by another variable or set of variables. (Chapter 8)

Confidence interval: a range of values that is likely to include the population parameter of interest. (Chapter 4)

Continuous variable: a variable that can take on any value within the range of possible values. (Chapter 1)

Correlation: a family of statistical procedures that involve examining relationships among variables. (Chapter 8)

*Correlation coefficient:*a metric that captures the direction and strength of the relationship between variables. (Chapter 8)

Covariance: the extent to which two variables vary together. (Chapter 8)

Covariate: a continuous variable that can influence the dependent variable but is not the independent variable of interest in a study. (Chapter 15)

Cross-validation: process in which a regression model is applied to a new data set to see how well its accuracy is maintained. (Chapter 10)

Degrees of freedom: the number of values that are free to vary when estimating a parameter. (Chapter 5)

Dependent variable: a variable that has the potential to be influenced by an independent variable; typically the outcome of interest in a study. (Chapter 1)

Descriptive statistics: procedures used to summarize data from a sample or population. (Chapter 1)

Discrete variable: a variable that can only take on a limited number of values. (Chapter 1)

Effect size: a metric that represents the extent to which the results of a study deviate from what is expected if the null hypothesis were true. (Chapter 13)

Familywise error rate: the probability of committing at least one Type I error when performing multiple tests of statistical significance. (Chapter 6)

Frequency distribution: a count of the number of times each score, or range of scores, was observed for a given data set. (Chapter 2)

Histogram: a specific type of frequency distribution graph where the number of observations is plotted for the various scores or ranges of scores. (Chapter 2)

Independent variable: a variable that has the potential to influence, or cause a change in, a dependent variable. (Chapter 1)

Inferential statistics: procedures used to make inferences about a population or populations, based on sample data. (Chapter 1)

Interaction effect: when the effect of an independent variable on a dependent variable is influenced by the level of another independent variable in the statistical model. (Chapter 7)

Interaction plot: a specific type of plot where separate lines are used to differentiate the levels of one independent variable, while the levels of another independent variable are plotted along the *x*-axis and the dependent variable is plotted along the *y*-axis. (Chapter 7)

Interquartile range: the range for the middle 50% of scores (Q1 to Q3). (Chapter 2)

Interval variable: a variable that is rank ordered, with equal intervals between consecutive values, but does not have a true zero. (Chapter 1)

Kurtosis: the characteristic of a frequency distribution that describes the concentration of scores in the tails; distributions with a prominent peak and a relatively high concentration of scores in the tails are described as *leptokurtic*, while distributions with a flatter peak and a relatively low concentration of scores in the tails are described as *platykurtic*. (Chapter 2)

Linear regression: a family of statistical procedures that generally involve predicting the value of an outcome variable based on a predictor variable or set of predictor variables. (Chapter 9)

Logistic regression: statistical procedures that generally involve predicting a categorical outcome based on a set of predictor variables. (Chapter 11)

Main effect: the effect of an independent variable on a dependent variable, regardless of the other independent variables in the statistical model. (Chapter 7)

Marginal mean: the average for one level of an independent variable across all levels of another independent variable. (Chapter 7)

Mean: a common measure of central tendency that is calculated by dividing the sum of a set of values by the number of values. (Chapter 2)

Median: the midpoint of a set of rank-ordered values. (Chapter 2)

Modality: the number of prominent peaks in a frequency distribution. (Chapter 2)

Mode: the most frequently observed value in a data set. (Chapter 2)

Multivariate analysis of variance: an extension of analysis of variance, where multiple dependent variables are combined and examined together. (Chapter 16)

Nominal variable: a variable that has categories with no inherent rank ordering. (Chapter 1)

Normality test: a null hypothesis significance test that tests whether an observed distribution of scores deviates significantly from the normal distribution. (Appendix A)

Null hypothesis: hypothesis stating that an observed effect (e.g. mean difference, correlation) is simply due to chance. (Chapter 4)

Odds: the ratio of the probability of an event occurring, relative to the probability of the event not occurring. (Chapter 4)

Omnibus test: a statistical test that examines an overall effect, such as the difference among three or more sample means. (Chapter 6)

Ordinal variable: a variable that has categories which are logically rank ordered. (Chapter 1)

Outcome variable: the variable that is being predicted in a regression analysis. (Chapter 9)

Population: all individuals for a specific group. (Chapter 1)

Population parameter: a value that describes a characteristic of a population. (Chapter 1)

Post-hoc tests: tests that are generally conducted as a follow-up to a significant omnibus test to compare pairs of groups, conditions, time points, and so on. (Chapter 6)

Predictor variable: a variable that is used to predict an outcome variable in a regression analysis. (Chapter 9)

Probability: how likely an event is to occur, given all possible outcomes. (Chapter 3)

Probability-probability plot (P-P plot): a plot where the cumulative probabilities associated with two distributions are plotted against one another; probability-probability plots are commonly used to examine how a distribution of scores deviates from the normal distribution. (Appendix A)

p-value: a value that reflects the probability of observing a given effect if the null hypothesis were true. (Chapter 4)

Quantile-quantile plot (Q-Q plot): a plot where the quantiles of two distributions are plotted against one another; quantile-quantile plots are commonly used to examine how a distribution of scores deviates from the normal distribution. (Appendix A)

Range: the difference between the highest and lowest scores in a data set. (Chapter 2)

Ratio variable: a variable that is rank ordered, has equal intervals between consecutive values, and has a true zero. (Chapter 1)

Regression equation: the equation used in regression to predict an outcome based on a predictor variable or set of predictor variables. (Chapter 9)

Residual: the difference between the actual and predicted values of the outcome variable in a regression analysis. (Chapter 9)

Sample: a subset of individuals from the entire population. (Chapter 1)

Sample size estimation: process used to derive the minimum number of subjects needed for a study based on the desired level of statistical power, alpha level, and anticipated effect size. (Chapter 14)

Sample statistic: a value that describes a characteristic of a sample. (Chapter 1)

Sampling: the selection of a subset of individuals from a population. (Chapter 1)

Sampling error: the difference between a sample statistic and its corresponding population parameter. (Chapter 1)

Sampling distribution: a distribution of statistics derived from samples taken from a population. (Chapter 3)

Scales of measurement: classification scheme where variables are classified as nominal, ordinal, interval, or ratio, depending on their characteristics. (Chapter 1)

Scatter plot: a plot used to display the relationship between two variables; the points on a scatter plot represent the values for a pair of variables. (Chapter 8)

Skewness: the degree of asymmetry in a frequency distribution. (Chapter 2)

Standard deviation: a measure of variability that captures how scores tend to deviate about the mean; calculated by finding the square root of the variance. (Chapter 2)

Standard error: the standard deviation of a sampling distribution. (Chapter 4)

Standard error of the estimate: a metric that represents the average degree of error when predicting the values of an outcome variable based on a regression equation. (Chapter 9)

Standard normal distribution: normal distribution where scores have been standardized by converting to *z*-scores; has a mean of 0 and a standard deviation of 1. (Chapter 3)

Statistical inference: the process of making inferences about a population based on observations from sample data. (Chapter 1)

Statistical power: the probability of rejecting the null hypothesis when it is false. (Chapter 4)

Stem-and-leaf plot: a specific type of frequency distribution graph where the leading digit(s) represent the 'stem' and the trailing digit represents the 'leaves'; displays the general shape of a frequency distribution while also presenting the values of the observed scores. (Chapter 2)

Sum of squares: the sum of the squared differences between each score and the mean. (Chapter 2)

t-test: a type of null hypothesis significance test that can be used to test whether there is a statistically significant difference between two sample means (independent *t*-test) or a statistically significant change/difference between two time points or conditions (paired *t*-test). (Chapter 5)

Type I error: error that occurs when the null hypothesis is rejected when it is actually true. (Chapter 4)

Type II error: error that occurs when the null hypothesis is not rejected when it is actually false. (Chapter 4)

Variability: the extent to which the scores in a data set vary about the average. (Chapter 2)

Variable: a characteristic that can take on different values. (Chapter 1)

Variable selection methods: procedures used in regression to identify a subset of predictor variables from a larger set of possible predictor variables. (Chapter 10)

Variance: a measure of variability that captures how scores tend to deviate about the mean; calculated by dividing the sum of squares by the number of observations (*n* or $n - 1$). (Chapter 2)

z-score: value that reflects how far a score is from the mean in terms of standard deviations. (Chapter 2)

Note: the chapter listed (Chapter -) is the chapter in which the term was first introduced.

1 Introduction to fundamental concepts

Chapter Objectives

The objectives of this chapter are to . . .

1) differentiate between populations and samples
2) introduce the general concept of statistical inference
3) discuss the difference between population parameters and sample statistics
4) describe, and provide examples of, sampling error
5) differentiate between independent variables and dependent variables
6) differentiate between discrete variables and continuous variables
7) describe the different scales of measurement
8) discuss the difference between descriptive statistics and inferential statistics
9) differentiate between parametric statistical tests and non-parametric statistical tests

Introduction

The purpose of this chapter is to introduce a few of the fundamental concepts in statistics and to establish some basic terminology. Don't expect to see the 'big picture' after reading this chapter; we're just getting started. Each of the basic concepts introduced in this chapter will be revisited at some point in the remainder of this book.

Populations vs. samples

A research study typically begins with a question about a group of individuals. The entire collection of individuals who make up this group of interest is referred to as the *population*.* For example, imagine that we wanted to examine the effects of a new cartilage regeneration procedure on cartilage thickness in individuals with knee osteoarthritis. In this case, our population of interest would be everyone with knee osteoarthritis.

* Note: populations don't need to be composed of individuals. For instance, we may be interested in the mechanical properties of a new type of medical implant (population = all medical implants of this type) or the amount of money hospitals spend on medical malpractice insurance (population = all hospitals). That said, I'll continue to refer to samples/populations as being composed of individuals, since that's most often the case in clinical research.

DOI: 10.4324/9781003179757-1

In most cases, the purpose of a study is to learn something about a population; however, we rarely have access to the entire population. Therefore, we must rely on *sampling*. A *sample* is a subset of individuals from the population of interest. We can use observations from samples to approximate the characteristics, treatment effects, and so on in the corresponding population. This process of drawing conclusions about a population, based on observations made from a sample, is referred to as *statistical inference.*

As an example, let's revisit our study examining the effects of the new cartilage regeneration procedure. The optimal way to assess the effectiveness of this new procedure would be to treat and evaluate the entire population of individuals with knee osteoarthritis; however, this certainly isn't feasible given the large number of people with knee osteoarthritis. Therefore, we would need to sample a subset of individuals with knee osteoarthritis, treat these individuals with the cartilage regeneration procedure, and then examine the changes in cartilage thickness for our sample. Assuming that the individuals in the sample adequately represent the population, we would expect the changes in cartilage thickness for our sample to reflect the changes that would occur in the population (at least to some extent). In this case, we're making inferences about the effects of a treatment in the population based on the observed effects of the treatment in our sample, which is a common application of statistical inference in medical research.

Defining the population

Defining the population of interest isn't always as straightforward as it would seem. In some cases, the same groups of individuals could be defined as a sample or a population, depending on whom we plan to generalize our results to.

For example, imagine that you work as part of a quality assurance team for a large healthcare system and that you're tasked with determining the average wait time for patients who visit your healthcare system's emergency departments. In this case, you're not interested in generalizing your findings to patients who visit emergency departments outside of your organization, since your job is just to determine how long patients are waiting when they visit one of your healthcare system's emergency departments. Therefore, your population would be all visitors to the emergency departments associated with your organization. Now, imagine a different scenario where you're conducting a study to estimate the average wait time for patients who visit any emergency department across the country. In other words, your goal is to generalize your findings to all emergency department visits. In this case, visits to a single healthcare system would represent a sample from the larger population of visits to all emergency departments. Again, defining the population requires us to consider how we plan to generalize our results.

We also have control over how broadly we define our population(s) of interest. For instance, imagine that we're conducting a study to examine the effects of a new medication on motor performance in individuals with Parkinson's disease. As investigators, it would be important for us to clearly identify whom we would like to generalize our results to. In this case, we may decide to target a relatively narrow population of individuals with Parkinson's disease by establishing a strict list of eligibility requirements. For instance, we could decide to only enroll individuals who are in the early stages of Parkinson's disease, who are younger than a certain age, and who don't already take medication to manage their symptoms. In contrast, we may decide to be more broad in how we define our population and include anyone with a medical diagnosis of Parkinson's disease, regardless of the stage of their disease, their age, or whether they already take medication. A benefit of strictly defining the population of interest is that it helps to limit extraneous factors that may inadvertently influence the results of a study; however, the drawback is that the study findings generalize to fewer people.

Note: establishing eligibility criteria that appropriately define the population (or populations) of interest is more of a study design consideration. However, I think it's important to highlight whenever discussing populations and samples.

Population parameters vs. sample statistics

A *parameter* is a value that describes a characteristic of a population, while a *statistic* is a value that describes a characteristic of a sample. For instance, let's consider the variable body mass index (BMI) for the population of adult males in the United States. BMI is a metric that reflects an individual's mass relative to their height squared (kg/m^2). The average BMI for all adult males in the United States would be an example of a *parameter* since it's derived from all individuals in the population of interest. However, if we found the average BMI for a sample of individuals from the population, this would be a *statistic*.

In most cases, we work with sample statistics, not population parameters, since we rarely have access to data from the entire population. However, we're typically interested in the corresponding population parameter, and therefore, we often use sample statistics to estimate unknown population parameters. In other words, we make inferences about population parameters based on observed sample statistics. For instance, we may use the average from a sample to estimate the average for the population.

Sampling error

While we typically use sample statistics to estimate population parameters, there will almost always be some degree of error in our estimate, since the individuals in a sample don't perfectly represent all individuals in the population. The difference between a sample statistic and its corresponding population parameter is referred to as *sampling error*. Figure 1.1 depicts the concept of sampling error.

It's important to note that sampling 'error' isn't due to a mistake made by investigators, sloppy data entry, negligence, misconduct, and so on. It's simply the result of a sample not including every member of the corresponding population. While the extent may vary, all sample statistics include some degree of sampling error.

Throughout this book, you'll see references made to certain observations occurring 'by chance alone'. In general, what this means is that the observed effects are simply due to sampling error. For example, imagine that we wanted to compare the reaction times of the populations of men and women. We can't measure the reaction times of all men and women, so we rely on sampling. Let's assume that there's no difference in the reaction times for the populations of men and women. However, imagine that we just happened to sample men with atypically slow reaction times and women with atypically fast reaction times. In this case, we would observe a difference in the average reaction times of the samples of men and women, even though there's no difference in the populations. This observed difference in the samples is a result of sampling error, not a true difference in the reaction times of the populations. In other words, the observed difference in reaction times between the samples of men and women simply occurred by chance alone.

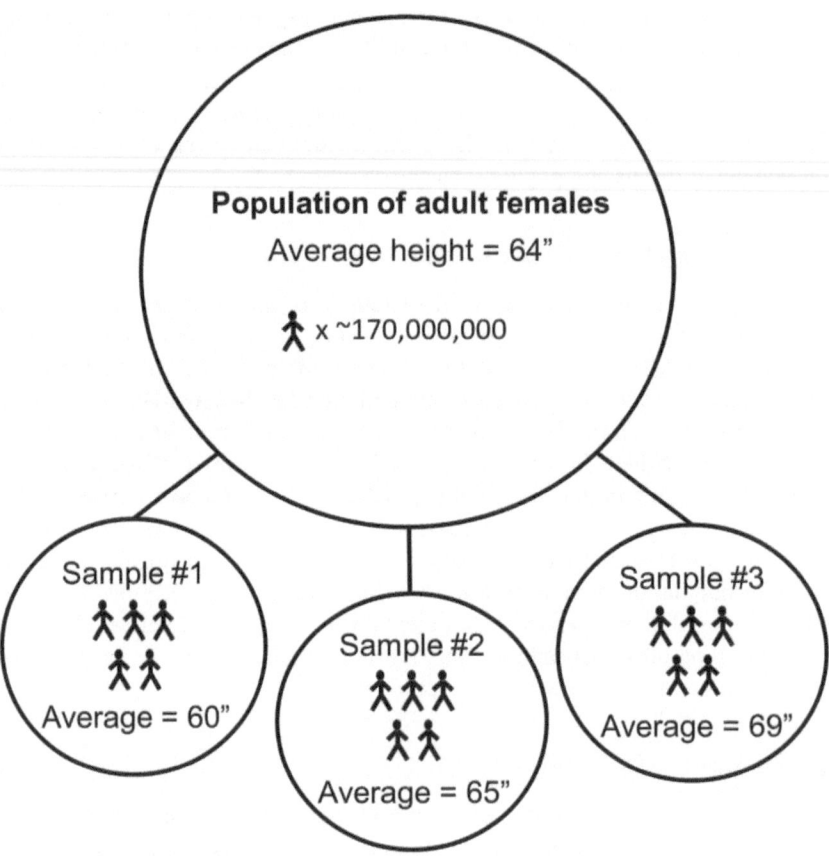

Figure 1.1 Diagram depicting sampling error. For this example, the population is composed of all adult females in the United States (~170,000,000 individuals). The average height for adult females in the population is 64 inches ("). Three different samples of five women are taken from the population. Notice that the average height for each sample differs from the average height of the population because of sampling error. Sample #1 underestimates the height of the population by 4 inches, Sample #2 overestimates the height of the population by 1 inch, and Sample #3 overestimates the height of the population by 5 inches. Also notice that the sample statistics vary from sample to sample, since the samples are composed of different individuals. This is generally referred to as *sampling variance*.

The concept of sampling error is fundamental to inferential statistics. As a result, we'll revisit this concept in almost every chapter of this book. The context will change, but the general principle will remain the same. Much of the discussion will involve examining how we can account for sampling error when making statistical inferences.

The influence of sample size on sampling error

In general, statistics derived from relatively large samples will more closely approximate the corresponding population parameter compared to statistics derived from relatively small samples.* In other words, large samples tend to result in less sampling error compared to small samples. This should be fairly intuitive. Basically, the more individuals we include in our sample, the more closely the characteristics of the sample will reflect those of the population. This is why we generally want our samples to be as large as feasibly possible when conducting a study.

* **Note:** this general phenomenon is explained by a rule known as the *law of large numbers*.

Independent variables vs. dependent variables

A *variable* is a characteristic that can take on different values. In other words, a variable can *vary*. Attributes such as weight, age, sex, disease status, treatment received, and so on are examples of variables since they can vary.

We often delineate between two distinct types of variables: *independent variables* and *dependent variables*. An independent variable is a variable that has the potential to influence, or cause a change in, the dependent variable. In the case of an experimental study, the independent variable is the variable that is manipulated by the investigators. In contrast, the dependent variable is the variable that may be influenced by the independent variable. In most cases, the dependent variable is our outcome of interest, since we typically analyze the dependent variable in order to determine whether it was influenced by the independent variable. Basically, the purpose of a study is related to the independent variable(s), while the results of the study are based on the dependent variable.

Note: independent variables are also commonly referred to as 'factors'.

Now, let's consider an example. Imagine that we conduct a study to compare the pain levels of patients who were prescribed two different pain medications (Medication A, Medication B). In this case, the independent variable could be described as 'medication type', which varies based on whether the patient was prescribed Medication A or Medication B, and the dependent variable is the subjects' pain level, since this may be *dependent* upon the medication prescribed. We would compare the pain levels (dependent variable – outcome of interest) in order to determine if they differed based on the type of medication prescribed (Medication A vs. Medication B).

Levels of an independent variable

An independent variable will often have corresponding levels, which represent discrete subcategories of the variable. For example, consider our hypothetical study comparing pain levels in patients who received two different types of pain medications (Medication A, Medication B). In this case, our independent variable 'medication type' would have two levels, since there are two subcategories of the variable: 1) Medication A, 2) Medication B.

Now imagine that we expanded our study to also include a control group that receives a placebo pill, so that the study now includes three groups: 1) patients prescribed Medication A, 2) patients prescribed Medication B, and 3) patients prescribed a placebo pill ('control group'). In this case, our independent variable 'medication type' would include three levels (Medication A, Medication B, placebo).

Cause and effect

Independent and dependent variables are often assumed to have what is described as a 'cause-and-effect relationship', as the independent variable is typically thought of as being the cause of an observed change in the dependent variable ('effect'). As an example, consider our study comparing pain medications. In this case, the different pain medications are expected to be the cause of differences in pain levels among the groups.

In some instances, it's impossible to determine the direction of the effect. In other words, the variables appear to be related to one another, but we don't know which variable is responsible for causing the change. This is essentially the classic 'chicken or the egg dilemma'. In this case, we typically consider both variables dependent. Chapter 8 ('Correlation') includes additional discussion on this topic.

Discrete variables vs. continuous variables

We can also distinguish between *discrete variables* and *continuous variables*. Discrete variables can only take on a limited number of values and, as a result, cannot be broken down into smaller increments. For example, the number of patient visits in a day is a discrete variable (8, 9, 10 . . .). Notice that this value can't be broken down into smaller increments (i.e. you can't treat 8.2 patients in a given day). Heart rate is another example of a discrete variable, since it's recorded as the number of beats (whole integer) per minute. A patient's heart rate could be 79 or 80, but not 79.5, 79.51, and so on.

In contrast, continuous variables can take on any value within the range of possible values. As a result, continuous variables can be broken down into infinitely smaller increments. Examples of continuous variables include age, time, and weight. Consider the variable weight. Someone's weight could fall anywhere along a continuum from 0 to infinity and could be expressed in infinitely smaller units (pounds, ounces, grams . . .).

One way to distinguish between discrete and continuous variables is to consider how the values are obtained. The values of a discrete variable are obtained by counting, while the values of a continuous variable are generally obtained by measurement.

Scales of measurement

Variables can also be classified into distinct scales, or levels, which are referred to as the *scales of measurement* or the *levels of measurement*. This classification scheme was described in a paper by Stanley Smith Stevens in 1946 and has become quite popular. The four fundamental scales of measurement are nominal scales, ordinal scales, interval scales, and ratio scales.

Nominal scales

Nominal variables, which are also referred to as 'categorical variables', have categories that can be labeled, but these categories aren't naturally ordered in any logical way. In other words, a nominal variable has categories with no inherent rank ordering. Examples of nominal variables include sex (male, female), injury status (injured, uninjured), and blood type (A, B, AB, O). Consider the variable blood type. Individuals can be categorized as either having blood type A, B, AB, or O; however, these are just labels, without a logical ordering.* While we can assign values to the categories of a nominal variable (e.g. blood type A = 1, B = 2, AB = 3, O = 4), these are still just numeric labels associated with the different categories.

All we can really do with nominal variables is count the number of observations in each category, such as the number of individuals with each different blood type.

* **Note**: the Latin root word 'nom' means name, which refers to the fact that nominal variables are simply labels (i.e. 'names') assigned to the variables.

Ordinal scales

An ordinal variable has categories which are rank ordered; however, the intervals between the categories aren't necessarily equivalent. In other words, the categories are ordered from least to greatest, but the differences between the categorical levels aren't necessarily the same.

Many clinical measures incorporate ordinal scales, where constructs such as function, quality of life, or independence are classified into discrete, rank-ordered categories. For instance, clinicians often describe the level of assistance a patient requires as 'independent', 'supervision', 'minimal assistance', 'moderate assistance', or 'maximal assistance'. Notice that there's a natural rank ordering to the levels of this variable (assistance needed: independent < supervision < minimal assistance < moderate assistance < maximal assistance). For instance, a patient who requires supervision requires less assistance than a patient who requires minimal assistance but more assistance than a patient who is independent. However, the points along the scale may not be evenly spaced. For example, the difference between requiring supervision vs. being independent isn't necessarily the same as the difference between requiring maximal assistance and moderate assistance.

Interval scales

Interval variables are rank ordered and have equal intervals between consecutive values along the scale. Temperature on a Fahrenheit or Celsius scale is a classic example of an interval variable since the increments between the intervals are consistent. For instance, the difference between 2° and 3° is the same as the difference between 3° and 4°.

A feature that distinguishes interval variables from ratio variables (discussed next) is that interval variables don't have a 'true' zero point. By a true zero, I mean a zero value that reflects the complete absence of whatever is being measured. Consider the variable temperature; 0° Fahrenheit is an artificial zero point that doesn't represent a complete lack of thermal energy. This is also true of 0° Celsius. The lack of a true zero is readily apparent when you consider that negative temperatures are possible (and quite common if you live in Wisconsin like I do) on both the Fahrenheit and Celsius scales. If 0 truly reflected a complete absence of temperature, negative values wouldn't be possible.

The lack of a true zero affects our ability to create meaningful ratios. For instance, consider the temperatures 100° and 50° on the Fahrenheit scale. While it's tempting to say that 100° is twice as warm as 50°, this wouldn't hold true if these temperatures were converted to the Celsius scale (100°F = 37.8°C; 50°F = 10.0°C), where the ratio between the temperatures would be closer to 4 to 1 (37.8°C vs. 10.0°C). This highlights the arbitrary nature of ratios when dealing with an interval variable.

Ratio scales

Ratio scales are the same as interval scales, except there's a true zero. As an example, let's consider the variable grip strength, measured via a handgrip dynamometer. Grip strength is

	Nominal	Ordinal	Interval	Ratio
Categories	✓	✓	✓	✓
Rank ordered		✓	✓	✓
Equal intervals			✓	✓
True zero				✓

Figure 1.2 Table highlighting the attributes of nominal, ordinal, interval, and ratio variables.

an example of a variable that's measured on a ratio scale, since there are equal intervals along the scale and a true zero (i.e. 0 represents the complete absence of grip force).

Since grip strength is measured on a ratio scale, we can create meaningful ratios. For instance, imagine that Patient A produces a maximal grip force of 25 kg, while Patient B produces a maximal grip force of 50 kg. Since grip strength is measured on a ratio scale, we could reasonably conclude that Patient B produced two times more force than Patient A. Notice that if we converted these values to pounds (25 kg = 55.1 pounds; 50 kg = 110.2 pounds), the ratio would still be 2 to 1. Essentially, Patient B is twice as strong as Patient A, regardless of how we express the data.

Many of the variables we work with as clinicians are on a ratio scale (e.g. gait speed, range of motion, walk distance).

Figure 1.2 highlights the unique features of nominal, ordinal, interval, and ratio scales, and Learning Activity 1.1 provides you with the opportunity to practice differentiating between the different scales of measurement.

Learning Activity 1.1

Examples of five different variables are given in the following. Identify the scale of measurement associated with each variable (nominal, ordinal, interval, or ratio).

1) Manual muscle testing grades
2) Vaccination status
3) Blood glucose levels
4) Modified Ashworth scale scores
5) Medical specialty

The answers are included at the end of the chapter.

Why does it matter?

It's good to have a general appreciation for the scales of measurement, since there are different ways to summarize, graphically represent, and analyze the different types of variables. Although I've differentiated between the four scales, we typically only need to determine whether our variable of interest is measured on a nominal, ordinal, or interval/ratio scale, since we tend to treat interval and ratio data in much the same way.

It's also important to note that some variables don't fit neatly into one of the four scales of measurement, and there will often be disagreement about whether a variable is ordinal or interval/ratio. In general, it's important to use common sense when deciding how to best summarize, present, and analyze data. You can use the scales of measurement as a guide, but don't let the scale of a variable completely dictate your decisions.

Descriptive statistics vs. inferential statistics

There are essentially two broad categories of statistics: descriptive statistics and inferential statistics. *Descriptive statistics* are used to *describe*, or summarize, data from a sample or population. For example, we may create graphs to display general features of a data set or generate metrics that capture some general characteristics, such as the 'average'. Essentially, descriptive statistics help us make sense of an unorganized collection of raw data. You're likely familiar with the general nature of descriptive statistics, since we're bombarded with them daily. For example, after an exam, your instructor may report the class average, describe the spread of the scores among the class (i.e. did students tend to receive similar scores or did scores vary widely among students?), and/or show a graph of the scores. In this case, your instructor is using descriptive statistics to convey your class's overall exam performance.

Inferential statistics involve using data from a sample to make inferences about the population. In other words, we attempt to learn something about a population based on what we observe from our sample data. In general, inferential statistics involve defining the population of interest, selecting a representative sample from this population, collecting data from the sample, and then using procedures to account for sampling error.

Chapter 2 provides an overview of descriptive statistics, while the rest of this book focuses on inferential statistics. While inferential statistics are typically used to address our research questions, most research papers will include a combination of descriptive and inferential statistics.

Parametric vs. non-parametric statistical tests

Most of this book focuses on what are generally referred to as *parametric tests*. You're probably already familiar with some common types of parametric tests, such as *t*-tests, analysis of variance (ANOVA), and so on. However, I'll also introduce some non-parametric alternatives throughout this book and discuss the basis for common non-parametric tests in Chapter 12.

In general, the difference between parametric and non-parametric tests is related to the number of assumptions made about the population data, with parametric tests making more assumptions than non-parametric tests.

Throughout this book, I'll discuss the key assumptions associated with each parametric test described, ways to test these assumptions, and options for how to proceed if your data fails to satisfy these assumptions.

Final thoughts

Before moving forward, I want to reiterate that the purpose of this chapter is just to serve as a primer for subsequent chapters. Each of the concepts introduced in this chapter will be revisited multiple times throughout the remainder of this book. At this point, don't worry if you're unsure of how these concepts are applied or their relevance. This should become clearer as you move forward.

Answers to Learning Activity 1.1

1) Manual muscle testing grades

   Answer – ordinal

2) Vaccination status

   Answer – nominal

3) Blood glucose levels

   Answer – ratio

4) Modified Ashworth scale scores

   Answer – ordinal

5) Medical specialty

   Answer – nominal

2   Descriptive statistics

Chapter Objectives

The objectives of this chapter are to . . .

1) highlight the general purpose of descriptive statistics
2) describe how data can be organized into a frequency distribution table
3) explain how continuous data can be organized into a grouped frequency distribution
4) describe the general layout of common frequency distribution graphs
5) discuss how the shape of a distribution can be described in terms of its modality, symmetry, and kurtosis
6) describe common measures of central tendency and variability
7) highlight the advantages and drawbacks of different measures of central tendency and variability
8) explain how raw scores can be standardized by converting to z-scores
9) demonstrate how to generate descriptive statistics using SPSS and Excel software

Introduction

Descriptive statistics are used to summarize, or *describe*, a set of data. In most cases, the data has been collected from a sample of individuals from a population.* For instance, we may use descriptive statistics to summarize the general characteristics of individuals who participated in a study (e.g. average age, proportions of males and females, disease severity) or to describe their performance on a certain outcome measure of interest. It's important to note that descriptive statistics aren't used to make inferences about a population or to test hypotheses. Instead, they simply describe some general features of the data that was collected. More specifically, descriptive statistics are used to summarize the *shape*, *central tendency*, and *variability* of a distribution of data. We'll discuss each of these features (shape, central tendency, variability) in this chapter.

* **Note:** remember that a *sample* is a subset of individuals from the entire *population* (Chapter 1). Descriptive statistics can also be used to summarize population data; however, in most cases, we don't have access to data from the entire population.

While most of this book is devoted to inferential statistics, it's important to have a solid understanding of the fundamental concepts discussed in this chapter, since almost every research paper you read will report some type of descriptive statistic. In addition, many of the basic concepts introduced in this chapter will be revisited in subsequent chapters.

DOI: 10.4324/9781003179757-2

Examining frequency distributions

Most clinical research questions involve collection of some type of quantitative data from a sample. Initially, this data exists in 'raw' form, with no meaningful organization or structure, which makes it difficult to gain any useful insights. Therefore, we typically start by sorting data in a manner that will make them more understandable. We may also create graphs to help us visually observe some of the general features or tendencies from a data set.

Frequency distribution tables

As a first step, we typically sort data into a more useful format, referred to as a *frequency distribution*. As an example, let's consider the hypothetical data set included in Table 2.1A. The table includes Berg Balance Scale scores for a sample of 25 older adults. The Berg Balance Scale is a 14-item standardized performance-based measure that's commonly used to assess an individual's balance (Berg et al., 1989). Scores on the Berg Balance Scale can range from 0 to 56, with higher scores reflecting better balance. The first column in Table 2.1A ('Subject') includes the assigned subject number (1–25) for each of the individuals in the study, while the second column ('BBS Score') includes each subject's Berg Balance Scale score.

Table 2.1 Hypothetical data set of Berg Balance Scale (BBS) scores for a sample of 25 older adults. Table 2.1A includes the entire set of scores, and Table 2.1B includes a frequency distribution based on the scores.

Table 2.1A			Table 2.1B		
Subject	BBS score		BBS score	Frequency	Percent
1	46		<39	0	0
2	51		39	1	4
3	44		40	0	0
4	48		41	1	4
5	47		42	1	4
6	47		43	1	4
7	46		44	3	12
8	42		45	3	12
9	49		46	3	12
10	44		47	4	16
11	46		48	3	12
12	45		49	2	8
13	49		50	2	8
14	41		51	1	4
15	48		52	0	0
16	43		53	0	0
17	48		54	0	0
18	45		Total	25	100%
19	45				
20	47				
21	39				
22	50				
23	47				
24	50				
25	44				

Our objective is to get a general idea of how the subjects in the sample performed on the Berg Balance Scale. Notice that it's virtually impossible for us to gain any useful insights by looking at the raw data included in Table 2.1A. In its current format, it's just an unorganized set of random values. To address this, we can re-organize our data into a frequency distribution. In a frequency distribution, the possible scores are rank ordered, and the number of observations is recorded for each potential outcome. In other words, a frequency distribution represents the number of times (i.e. the *frequency*) each score was observed. Table 2.1B includes a frequency distribution table based on the Berg Balance Scale scores reported in Table 2.1A. The first column ('Score') represents the different possible Berg Balance Scale scores, while the second column ('Frequency') represents the number of times each score was observed. For instance, four subjects (frequency = 4) had a Berg Balance Scale score of 47, while none of the subjects had a score of less than 39 (frequency = 0).

Notice that simply reorganizing the data into a frequency distribution allows us to more easily appreciate some of the general features of the data set. For instance, we can readily determine the highest and lowest scores, as well as the most common score. We can also see where most of the scores tended to cluster in the distribution. For example, based on Table 2.1B, we can see that the highest and lowest Berg Balance Scale scores were 51 and 39, respectively, while the most commonly observed score was 47. We can also see that most scores tended to cluster between values of 44 and 50. Again, these types of observations are difficult to make when simply examining the original distribution of scores (Table 2.1A).

Frequency distributions are often reported as a table, such as in Table 2.1B. These tables also commonly report the number of observations for each specific score as a percentage of the total number of observations in the data set. For example, column 3 ('Percent') in Table 2.1B represents the percentage of subjects who received each of the different Berg Balance Scale scores. For instance, 16% of subjects (4/25 = 16%) had a Berg Balance Scale score of 47, while 8% of subjects (2/25 = 8%) had a score of 50. Percentages are useful when analyzing and reporting frequencies since they are independent of the number of observations in the data set. For instance, imagine that a certain score was observed 10 times (frequency = 10). It would be difficult to determine how common this score was without knowing the total number of observations in the data set. If the sample were composed of 50 subjects, a frequency of 10 would make up 20% of the observed scores; however, if the sample were composed of 1000 subjects, a frequency of 10 would only make up 1% of the observed scores. Again, reporting frequencies as a percentage allows us to more easily appreciate how common or rare a certain score was in the context of the total number of observations.

Grouped frequency distributions

Many times we are working with continuous data instead of discrete values such as Berg Balance Scale scores. In this case, it's likely that very few subjects, if any, will have the same exact value for our variable of interest. For instance, imagine that we collected 6 Minute Walk Test distances for 50 subjects as a measure of their aerobic endurance. For the 6 Minute Walk Test, subjects walk as far as they can in 6 minutes and their distance walked is recorded in meters (American Thoracic Society, 2002). With a sample size of 50, it's unlikely that any subjects would walk the exact same distance over a 6-minute period. Therefore, it wouldn't be very helpful to create a frequency distribution based on the individual walk distances, since almost every observed distance would likely have a frequency of 1. In these situations, we can create *grouped frequency distributions*, where the observed values are grouped into intervals, or ranges of values. For instance, in the case of our 6 Minute Walk

Test example, we could create intervals of 50 meters and classify the subjects within these intervals. Table 2.2 includes a grouped frequency distribution based on 6 Minute Walk Test distances from our hypothetical sample of 50 subjects. Notice that 10 of the subjects (20%) walked between 500 and 549 meters, while only 1 subject walked at least 800 meters (2%).

It's important to note that, although necessary in many cases, grouping data into intervals results in a loss of information. For instance, consider our 6 Minute Walk Test example. By classifying subjects into 50-meter intervals, we lose the ability to discern their precise 6 Minute Walk Test distance, since we only know which 50-meter interval their walk distance was located within. We can increase precision by narrowing the intervals (e.g. 25-meter intervals instead of 50-meter intervals); however, this reduces the number of observations in each grouping. As you can see, it's important to carefully consider how to best group your data so that notable features can be recognized. In the end, our primary objective is to organize the data in a manner that will convey the greatest amount of information possible.

Graphing frequency distributions

So far, we've discussed how we can examine frequency distributions that are in a tabular format. However, we can also graph frequency distributions. In most cases, graphically displaying a frequency distribution makes it easier to observe some of the general characteristics of the data set.

While there are several different ways to graph frequency distributions, two commonly used types of graphs are the histogram and the stem-and-leaf plot.

Histograms

A histogram is a specific type of frequency distribution graph where the different data values or intervals are plotted along the x-axis, while the frequency is plotted along the y-axis. Figure 2.1 includes a histogram based on the 6 Minute Walk Test distances from Table 2.2.

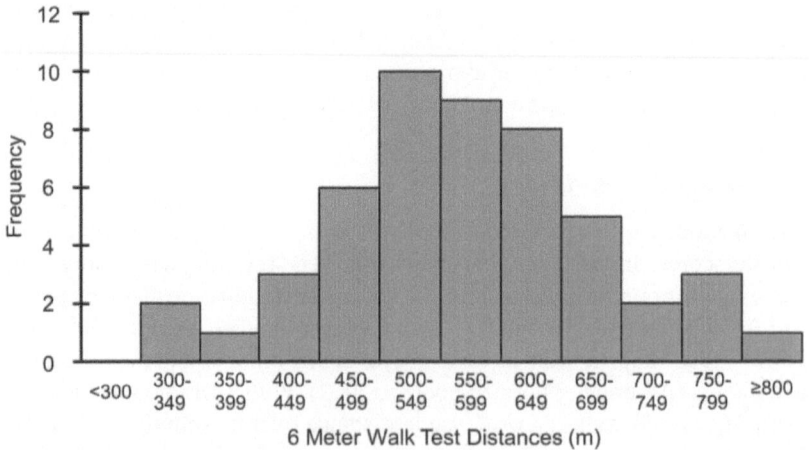

Figure 2.1 Histogram of 6 Minute Walk Test distances for a hypothetical sample of 50 subjects. The walk distance intervals are plotted along the x-axis, while the y-axis includes the number of subjects (frequency) included in each interval.

Table 2.2 Grouped frequency distribution of 6 Minute Walk Test (6MWT) distances based on our hypothetical data set of 50 subjects. 6MWT distances are divided into intervals of 50 meters.

6MWT distances (m)	Frequency	Percent
<300	0	0
300–349	2	4
350–399	1	2
400–449	3	6
450–499	6	12
500–549	10	20
550–599	9	18
600–649	8	16
650–699	5	10
700–749	2	4
750–799	3	6
≥800	1	2
Total	50	100%

Notice that the *x*-axis includes the different intervals, while the *y*-axis includes a count (i.e. frequency) of the number of subjects who were categorized into each interval.

By looking at the histogram in Figure 2.1, it's easy to see that most subjects' 6 Minute Walk Test distance tended to fall within the 500–549 (20%), 550–599 (18%), or 600–649 (16%) meter intervals. In other words, most walk distances tended to cluster within a range of 500–649 meters. Walk distances that fell above or below these intervals were much less common. You can also see that no subjects walked less than 300 meters (frequency = 0), and only one subject walked at least 800 meters.

Notice that a histogram graphically displays the same information that was included in a frequency distribution table.

Note: histograms are typically used with continuous data that's been grouped into intervals, such as in the case of our 6 Minute Walk Test example. However, they can also be used with discrete data, such as Berg Balance Scale scores.

Stem-and-leaf plots

Another common way of graphically displaying a frequency distribution is with a *stem-and-leaf plot*. Like histograms, stem-and-leaf plots display the general shape of a frequency distribution; however, unlike histograms, they also include the individual values within the display.

As an example, imagine that we recorded resting heart rates for a sample of 40 subjects. The raw data is included on the left side of Figure 2.2. Notice that 3 subjects had a resting heart rate in the 50s, 8 subjects had a resting heart rate in the 60s, 12 subjects had a resting heart rate in the 70s, 9 subjects had a resting heart rate in the 80s, 6 subjects had a resting heart rate in the 90s, and 2 subjects had a resting heart rate in the 100s.

In a stem-and-leaf plot, the leading digits form the stem of the plot, while the trailing digits form the leaves. In the case of our resting heart rate example, the digits in the tens place and above ('leading digits' – 5, 6, 7, 8, 9, 10) would serve as the stem, while the digits in the ones place ('trailing digits') would serve as the leaves. An example of a

Raw Data	Stem	Leaf
56, 57, 59	5	6 7 9
64, 64, 64, 65, 65, 67, 68, 69	6	4 4 4 5 5 7 8 9
70, 70, 71, 72, 72, 74, 76, 76, 77, 78, 78, 79	7	0 0 1 2 2 4 6 6 7 8 8 9
80, 82, 84, 85, 85, 87, 88, 88, 89	8	0 2 4 5 5 7 8 8 9
91, 93, 93, 94, 94, 94	9	1 3 3 4 4 4
100, 102	10	0 2

Figure 2.2 Stem-and-leaf plot of resting heart rate values for a hypothetical sample of 40 subjects. The left side of the figure includes the original resting heart rate values ('Raw Data'), while the stem-and-leaf plot is shown on the right.

stem-and-leaf plot is included on the right side of Figure 2.2. Notice that the stem of 5 is aligned with the trailing digits 6, 7, and 9, since subjects demonstrated resting heart rates of 56, 57, and 59 beats per minute (stem = 5; leaves = 6, 7, 9), while stem 10 is aligned with the trailing digits 0 and 2, since subjects demonstrated resting heart rates of 100 and 102 (stem = 10; leaves = 0, 2).

If you look carefully at the stem-and-leaf plot in Figure 2.2, you'll see that it's essentially a histogram turned onto its side. Notice that this stem-and-leaf plot allows us to easily see that most subjects had a resting heart rate within the 70 beats per minute range (70–79 beats per minute) and that resting heart rates above (80s, 90s, 100s) and below (60s, 50s) this range became progressively less common.

Again, an advantage of stem-and-leaf plots is that they not only display the general shape of a frequency distribution but also include the individual values within the display. In fact, you could completely regenerate the original raw data set if provided with a stem-and-leaf plot.

Distribution shape

Now that we've discussed ways to organize and graphically display data, let's discuss terms used to describe the general shape of a distribution.

Modality

The first feature we can appreciate is the number of prominent peaks in a frequency distribution, which is generally referred to as the *modality*. A distribution with one prominent peak is described as *unimodal*, while a distribution with two prominent peaks is described as *bimodal*. The more general term *multimodal* is typically used when a frequency distribution has more than two prominent peaks. Figure 2.3 includes examples of both a unimodal distribution and a bimodal distribution.

Most distributions exhibit a single prominent peak, with scores clustered around one area of the distribution (i.e. unimodal) (Figure 2.3, subplot A). However, there are instances where distributions will exhibit multiple peaks. Let's consider an example. For a few years, I had the opportunity to teach a functional anatomy course. The course primarily included undergraduate students; however, there was also a cohort of students from a master's-level occupational therapy program. Most of the undergraduate students had never taken an anatomy

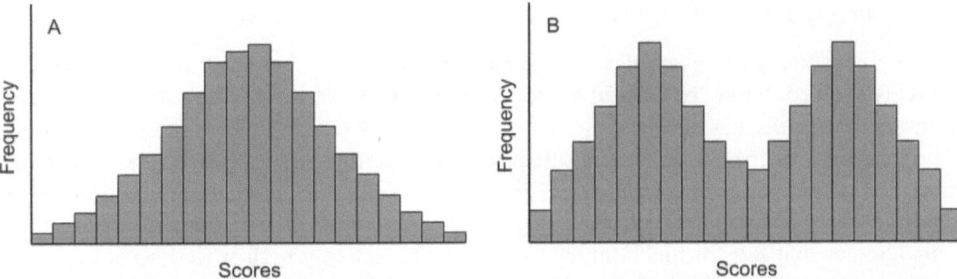

Figure 2.3 Subplot A includes an example of a unimodal distribution (one peak), while subplot B includes an example of a bimodal distribution (two peaks). Notice that both distributions are symmetrical. Note: the peaks don't need to be the same height for a distribution to be described as bimodal.

course before, while the occupational therapy students had all completed an anatomy course as part of their prerequisites for graduate school. Not surprisingly, the occupational therapy students tended to outperform the undergraduate students by a wide margin (it's amazing how much easier anatomy is the second time around). After each exam, I would create a histogram and look at the distribution of scores for the entire class. Without fail, the distribution of scores would exhibit a bimodal pattern (similar to Figure 2.3, subplot B), with a cluster of scores from the occupational therapy students in the 'A' range and a separate cluster of scores from the undergraduate students in the 'B–BC' range. It was as if two different distributions of scores had been squeezed together on the same histogram.

Symmetry

In addition to the modality of a frequency distribution, we can also describe a distribution's degree of symmetry. A symmetric distribution is one in which the upper and lower halves exhibit approximately the same shape. Essentially, the areas above and below the center of the distribution are mirror images of one another. In other words, the data is evenly divided by the center of the distribution. The frequency distributions shown in Figure 2.3 are both examples of symmetric distributions. Imagine folding these distributions along a line that divides them down the middle of their *x*-axis. In each case, the left and right sides of the distribution would be approximately the same shape. Notice that I've used the term *approximately*; the sides of a distribution don't need to perfectly match in order for a distribution to be described as symmetrical.

When the sides of a distribution differ, we describe the distribution as being *skewed*. More specifically, when the tail of a distribution extends (or 'tails off') to the right, the distribution is described as being *positively skewed*, whereas when the tail extends to the left, the distribution is described as being *negatively skewed*.* Figure 2.4 includes examples of positively skewed (subplot A) and negatively skewed (subplot B) frequency distributions.

* **Note:** the area of a distribution where most scores tend to be located is often referred to as the 'body', while areas where there are fewer scores are often referred to as the 'tails'. The 'upper tail' contains the higher values (right side of the distribution), and the 'lower tail' contains the lower values (left side of the distribution).

Examples of positively and negatively skewed frequency distributions

Now let's consider some examples of frequency distributions that tend to be positively or negatively skewed. It may be helpful to draw out the general shape of these frequency distributions as they're discussed.

The frequency distribution of home sale prices is an example of a positively skewed distribution. The vast majority of homes in the United States sell for somewhere between $100,000 and $500,000, making up the bulk of all sale prices (body of the distribution). However, there are also homes that sell for much, much more. These relatively high-priced homes result in the upper tail of the distribution extending well beyond the price where most homes tend to be sold (positive skew). For a more clinically relevant example, consider the number of days patients spend in the hospital following a routine joint replacement procedure. While most patients tend to be discharged within a couple days, some patients may need more time to recover. If we examined a frequency distribution of the number of days spent in the hospital, we would likely see that most patients tend to be discharged within a range of 2–3 days, with almost none discharged earlier. However, the patients who spend an atypically long time in the hospital would cause the upper tail of the distribution to extend well beyond the body of the distribution (positive skew).

The lifespan frequency distribution is an example of a distribution that tends to be negatively skewed. While most individuals live well into their late 70s and beyond, some, unfortunately, die at a much younger age, which results in a negatively skewed distribution.

Quantifying skewness

While we can visually inspect the degree of skewness in a distribution, it's also possible to quantify skewness with what are generally referred to as 'skewness coefficients'. If a distribution is perfectly symmetrical (i.e. no skew), the skewness coefficient will be 0. Deviations from 0 indicate that the distribution exhibits some degree of asymmetry or skew. A negative skewness coefficient indicates that the distribution is negatively skewed, while a positive skewness coefficient indicates that the distribution is positively skewed. The magnitude of the skewness coefficient reflects the degree of asymmetry in the distribution; the more the skewness coefficient deviates from the 0, the greater the asymmetry.

Most statistical analysis software packages, such as SPSS, provide you with the option to generate some type of skewness coefficient. These metrics are also fairly easy to calculate

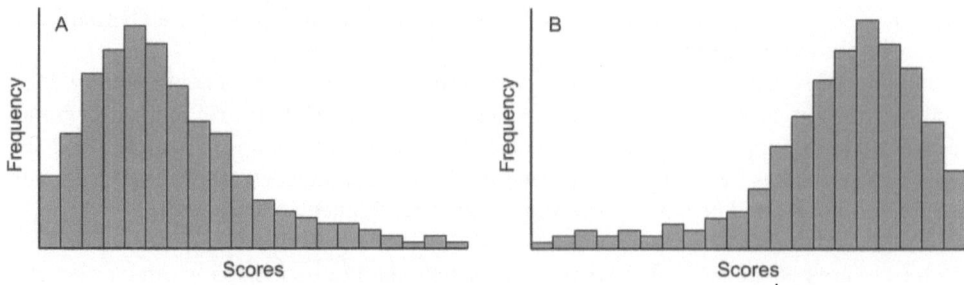

Figure 2.4 Subplot A includes an example of a positively skewed distribution ('tails off' to the right), while subplot B includes an example of a negatively skewed distribution ('tails off' to the left). Notice that both of these distributions are asymmetrical.

by hand once you're familiar with the measures used to quantify central tendency and variability (discussed in subsequent sections of this chapter).

Kurtosis

The last shape-related characteristic I'll introduce is *kurtosis*. Kurtosis describes how scores are concentrated in the center and tails of a distribution. Distributions with high kurtosis have a relatively high concentration of scores in their outer tails ('heavier tails'). They also tend to be relatively narrow in the center, with a distinct peak. In contrast, distributions with low kurtosis have fewer scores in their outer tails ('lighter tails') and tend to be flatter in the center (i.e. 'less peaked'). Distributions with relatively high kurtosis are referred to as *leptokurtic* distributions, while distributions with relatively low kurtosis are referred to as *platykurtic* distributions (Figure 2.5). The determination of whether a distribution is leptokurtic or platykurtic is based on comparison to the *normal distribution*, which is discussed in Chapter 3.

There's a lot more to be said about kurtosis. What I've presented here is a gross oversimplification. That said, considering the scope of this book, I don't think there's much to be gained from discussing the nuances of kurtosis, since kurtosis tends to receive less attention than other descriptors, such as skewness, central tendency, and variability. Being generally familiar with the concept of kurtosis is a good starting point.

Note: most statistical software packages, including SPSS, have options for quantifying the degree of kurtosis.

Normally distributed

The normal distribution is a specific type of distribution that serves many key purposes in inferential statistics. In the normal distribution, scores cluster in the center and then progressively taper off equally in both directions (note: the normal distribution is unimodal and perfectly symmetric). The normal distribution is commonly referred to as the 'bell curve' since its shape is similar to that of a bell (Figure 2.6).

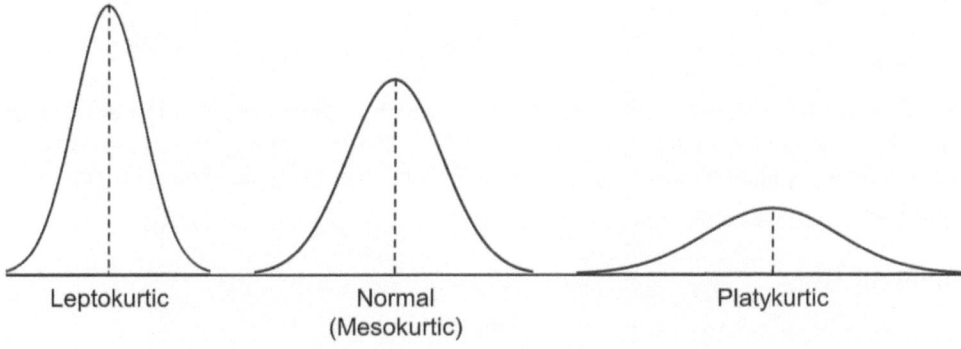

Figure 2.5 Examples of a leptokurtic distribution and a platykurtic distribution. For reference, the figure also includes the normal distribution, which is described as being mesokurtic.

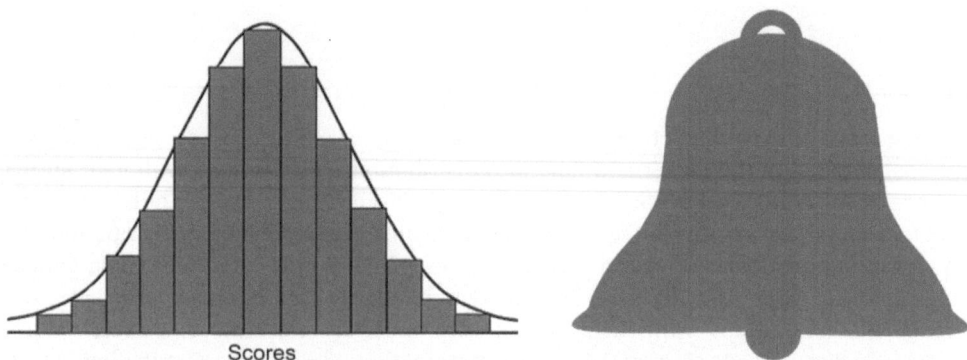

Figure 2.6 Example of a frequency distribution with the normal distribution curve superimposed (left side of the figure). Notice how the normal distribution curve resembles the shape of a bell (right side of the figure), hence the term 'bell curve'.

A distribution of scores will be described as being 'normally distributed' when the shape resembles that of the normal distribution. Many inferential procedures assume that the distribution of scores approximates the shape of the normal distribution. In most cases, this is a reasonable assumption, as long as the sample size is sufficiently large, since many variables tend to naturally be normally distributed. For instance, consider variables such as height, weight, blood pressure, and so on. In each case, most individuals tend to cluster within a certain range of values, with progressively fewer individuals exhibiting values that are well above or below average.

Chapter 3 includes a more in-depth discussion of the normal distribution.

Measures of central tendency

In addition to describing the shape of a frequency distribution, we also need to be able to describe where the distribution tends to be centered or, in other words, where most scores tend to cluster. This is referred to as a distribution's *central tendency*. Three different metrics can be used to describe where the center of a distribution lies: 1) the mean, 2) the median, and 3) the mode.

The mean

You're probably already familiar with the *mean*, which is simply the sum (Σ) of all scores, divided by the number of scores (n) (Equation 2.1). The symbol μ ('mu') is typically used to represent a population mean, while the symbol $\bar{X}$ ('x-bar') is typically used to represent a sample mean.

Equation 2.1

$$\text{Mean} = \frac{\sum X}{n}$$

* Note: while the mean is commonly referred to as the 'average', technically, 'average' refers to any measure of central tendency (mean, median, or mode). Regardless, when I use the term 'average' in this book, I'm generally referring to the mean.

The median

The *median* is the middle score when the data is rank ordered. To find the median, we can simply arrange the data in ascending order and then find the score located at the midpoint of the list of scores. When there are an even number of observations, two values will constitute the middle of this rank-ordered list of scores. In this case, the median is the average of these two numbers.

The mode

The mode is simply the most frequently observed value in a data set. In other words, the score or interval with the highest count in a frequency distribution.

Table 2.3 includes an example data set along with the mean, median, and mode associated with the set of observed scores.

Note: when a distribution is perfectly symmetric, the mean and median will be equal. The mean, median, and mode will all be equal in the case of a perfectly symmetric, unimodal distribution, such as the normal distribution.

Comparing the measures of central tendency

The mean is the most commonly reported measure of central tendency when dealing with continuous data (interval or ratio scale). The mean is popular because it's the only measure of central tendency that incorporates the value of each observed score in the calculation. In other words, all scores are represented when calculating the mean. In addition, the mean is easy to work with mathematically since it can be written in the form of an equation (Equation 2.1), which isn't true for the median and mode. Finally, the mean also tends to fluctuate less from sample to sample compared to the median and mode (i.e. the mean is more 'stable').

However, the mean has its drawbacks. For one, it's more greatly influenced by relatively extreme scores in a data set (often referred to as 'outliers') compared to the median and mode, especially when there are a small number of observations. Also, the mean doesn't represent central tendency very well for skewed distributions, since it tends to be pulled into the upper tail of a positively skewed distribution and into the lower tail of a negatively skewed distribution (depicted in Figure 2.7).

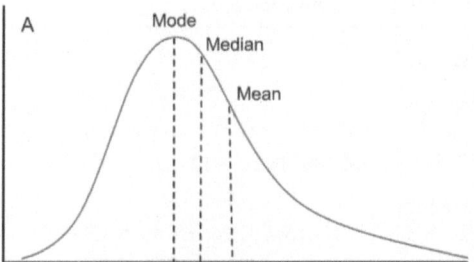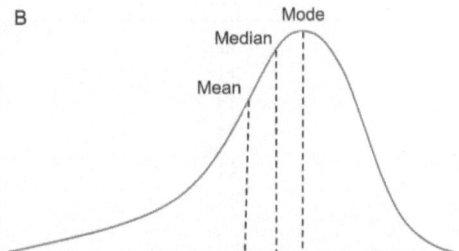

Figure 2.7 Examples of how the locations of the mean, median, and mode differ for positively (subplot A) and negatively (subplot B) skewed distributions. Notice that the scores in the tail of the distribution tend to draw the mean, and the median to a lesser extent, away from where most of the scores tend to cluster.

The median is less affected by extreme scores* and better represents the central location of a skewed distribution. The median is also commonly used when working with ordinal data, which has an inherent ordering. That said, a disadvantage of the median is that it essentially ignores the value of most scores (i.e. the rank order is considered, but not the value). The median is also harder to work with mathematically, since it can't really be expressed as an equation.

* **Note:** as an example, look at the squat test data in Table 2.3. Notice that one score is quite a bit lower than the rest of scores in the data set (Subject 7 = 1 repetition). This relatively low score has no influence on the median or mode but has the effect of lowering the mean.

The mode is by far the least commonly reported measure of central tendency. It's really only useful when working with nominal data, as a way to describe which category was most frequently observed. Otherwise, it's rare to report the mode.

In most cases, we're essentially deciding between the mean and the median to approximate the central tendency of a distribution. In general, it's a good idea to examine a frequency distribution table or graph to guide your decision. It can also be informative to compare the mean and median to see if they're similar. If not, the distribution is skewed in some way.

Measures of variability

Measures of *variability* describe how scores are dispersed about the center of the distribution. In other words, they quantify how the scores *vary* relative to one another. If all scores tend to cluster close to the average, there's little variability in the data set. Conversely, if the scores are more spread out, there's greater variability (depicted in Figure 2.8).

Table 2.3 The 'squat test' is commonly used to assess lower extremity strength in children with cerebral palsy (Eken et al., 2017, 2020). For the squat test, the child completes double-leg bodyweight squats until exhaustion (or until they perform 20 squats). A therapist observes the child during squat performance and records the number of squats they complete. This table includes a hypothetical data set of squat test repetitions for a sample of 10 children with cerebral palsy. The table also includes the mean, median, and mode for the data set. Notice that the relatively low score of 1 repetition for subject 7 has no influence on the median or mode but lowers the mean.

Subject	Repetitions	Measures of central tendency
1	12	**Mean**
2	11	
3	15	$\dfrac{\sum X}{n} = (12 + 11 + 15 + 13 + 11 + 13 + 1 + 17$
4	13	$+ 14 + 13)/10 = \mathbf{12}$
5	11	
6	13	**Median**
7	1	~~1~~, ~~11~~, ~~11~~, ~~12~~, 13, 13, ~~13~~, ~~14~~, ~~15~~, ~~17~~ = 13
8	17	**Mode = 13** (observed 3 times)
9	14	
10	13	

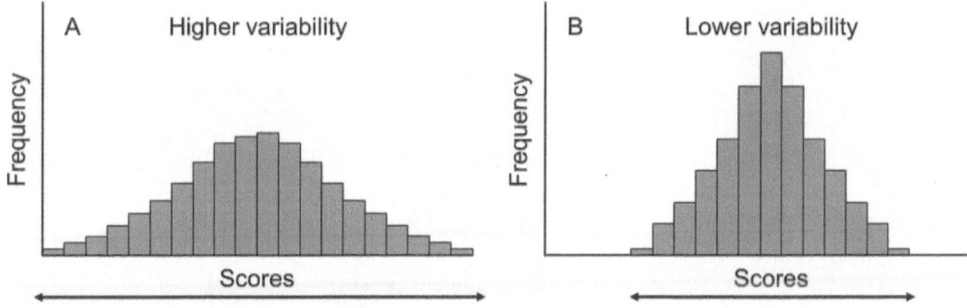

Figure 2.8 Examples of two distributions of scores with the same means but different degrees of variability. Notice how the scores are more spread out in subplot A (greater variability) vs. subplot B (less variability).

It's important to note that two sets of scores can have the same central tendency but different variability. As a result, any report of a measure of central tendency, such as the mean, should be accompanied by some indication of the degree of variability.

While there are many different ways to quantify variability, we'll focus on four common metrics: 1) the range, 2) the interquartile range, 3) the variance, and 4) the standard deviation.

Range

The *range* is simply the difference between the highest and lowest scores in a data set. For instance, let's consider the resting heart rate values from the hypothetical data set included in Figure 2.2. The highest recorded resting heart rate was 102 beats per minute, while the lowest recorded resting heart rate was 56 beats per minute. The range would be the difference between these two values: range = 102 – 56 = 46 beats per minute.

The major limitation of the range as a measure of variability is that it only incorporates two scores from the data set. Therefore, one or two extreme scores can cause the range to drastically overestimate the variability associated with a set of scores (depicted in Figure 2.9). In other words, the scores will seem to be more dispersed, or spread out, than they actually are. As a result, the range is not a commonly reported measure of variability, at least on its own, unless the objective is to provide an indication of the full range of observed scores.

Interquartile range

As discussed, a limitation of the range as a measure of variability is that it's heavily influenced by extreme scores. One way to address this problem is to neglect the scores in the upper and lower 25% of the distribution and to find the range for the middle 50% of scores, which is referred to as the *interquartile range*.

To find the interquartile range, we first rank order the values and find the scores that divide the distribution into four equal parts, or *quartiles*. The first quartile (Q1) is the score that separates the lowest 25% of scores from the rest of the distribution; the second quartile (Q2) is the median, which divides the distribution into upper and lower halves (50% of scores below Q2, 50% of scores above Q2); and the third quartile (Q3) is the score that separates

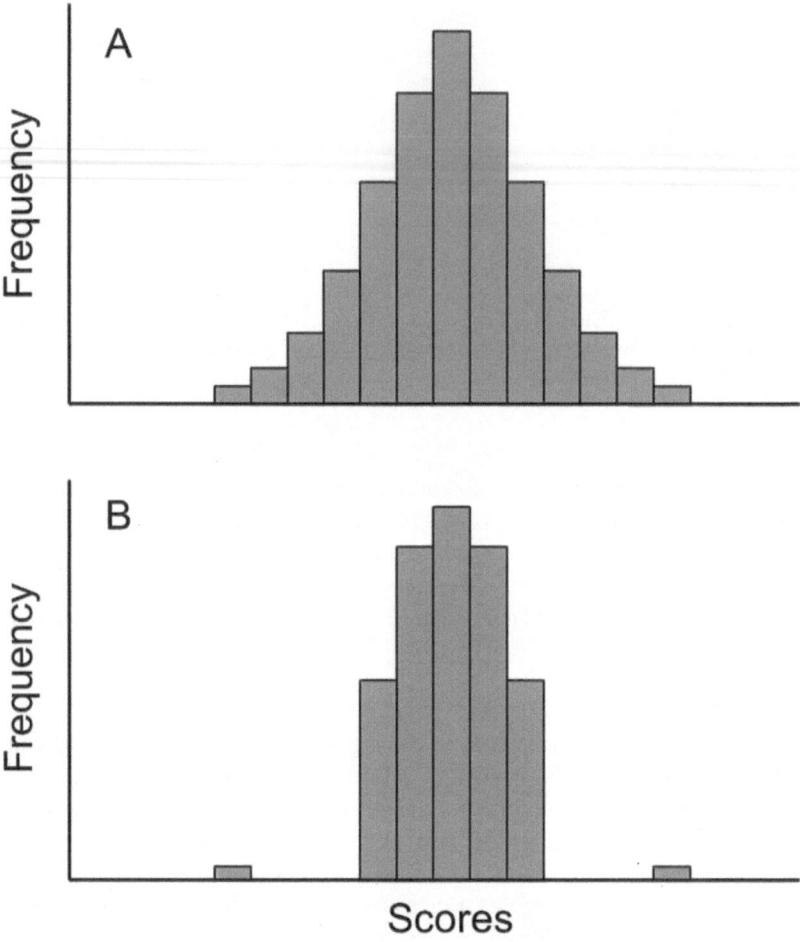

Figure 2.9 Examples of two different distributions of scores. While the scores in subplot A are clearly more dispersed about the center of the distribution compared to those in subplot B, both distributions have the same range (range = highest score – lowest score). Notice that the extreme scores at the upper end and lower end of the distribution in subplot B cause the range to be relatively high, even though most scores are concentrated in the center of the distribution.

the highest 25% of scores from the rest of the distribution. The interquartile range (IQR) is the difference between Q3 and Q1 (IQR = Q3 – Q1) (Figure 2.10). Again, this represents the middle 50% of the distribution.

A *box plot* is a useful way of graphically displaying the variability associated with a set of scores by highlighting the quartiles and interquartile range. The box represents the interquartile range and is bounded by Q1 and Q3. A line in the center of the box represents the median (Q2). Box plots also typically include 'whiskers' that reflect the values associated with the highest and lowest scores (note: box plots are also commonly referred to as *box-and-whisker plots*). Figure 2.11 includes an example of a box plot.

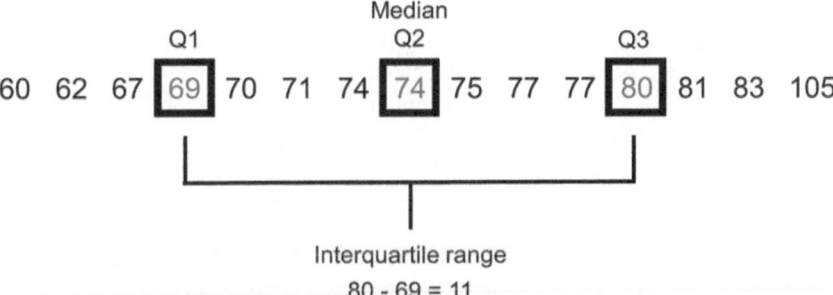

Figure 2.10 Resting heart rates for 15 individuals. The values are rank ordered from lowest (leftmost – 60 beats per minute) to highest (rightmost – 105 beats per minute). The median (Q2) separates the distribution of values into an upper half and a lower half (7 scores above and 7 scores below the median of 74). The first quartile (Q1) is the median for the lower half of the scores, while the third quartile (Q3) is the median for the upper half of the scores. Notice that the quartiles (Q1, Q2, Q3) divide the distribution into four equal parts. The interquartile range (IQR) is the difference between Q3 and Q1 (IQR = 80 – 69 = 11). Note that the relatively extreme value of 105 beats per minute distorts the range but doesn't influence the interquartile range.

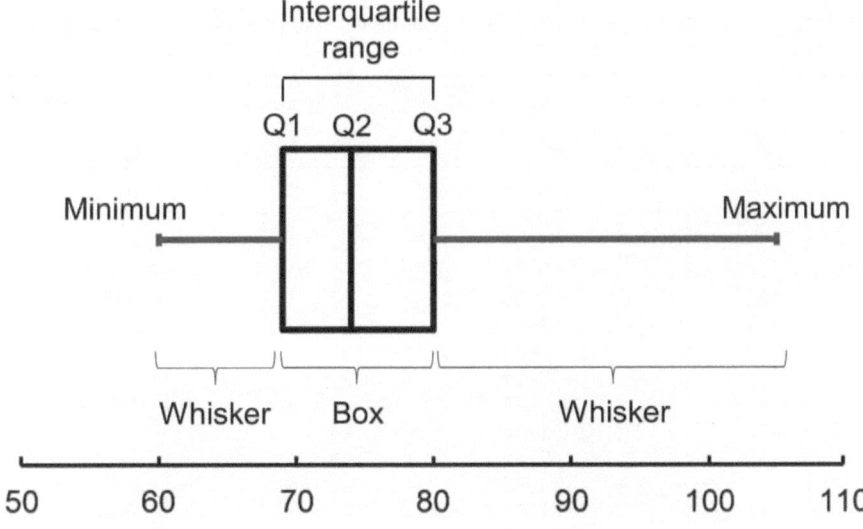

Figure 2.11 Box plot based on the resting heart rate data from *Figure 2.10*. The left and right sides of the box are located at Q1 and Q3, respectively. The vertical line in the center of the box represents the median (Q2). The whiskers extend off the box to represent the minimum and maximum values.

Variance

Measures of range are limited in that they don't incorporate all of the scores in a data set. In contrast, the *variance* is a measure of variability that's based on the entire set of scores. The variance essentially captures how the individual scores tend to deviate, or are dispersed, about the mean. If the scores tend to cluster close to the mean, the variance will be relatively low. In fact, if all scores are equal, the variance will be 0. If the scores tend to be more spread out about the mean, the variance will be relatively high.

The first step in calculating the variance is to find the *sum of squares*, which is the sum (Σ) of the squared differences, or deviations, between each individual score (X) and the mean ($\bar{X}$ if working with sample data, μ if working with population data) (Equation 2.2). This may sound complex, but all we're doing is finding the difference between each individual score and the mean, squaring these differences, and adding the squared differences together [$\Sigma(X-\bar{X})^2$].

Equation 2.2

$$\text{Sum of squares} = \sum\left(X-\bar{X}\right)^2$$

You're probably wondering why we square the differences. First, it's important to note that some scores will be lower than the mean ($X < \bar{X}$), while other scores will be higher than the mean ($X > \bar{X}$). Scores below the mean will produce negative differences, whereas scores above the mean will produce positive differences. If we added these differences together without squaring, the positives and negatives would cancel each other out and sum to 0. We square the differences so that they all become positive values, and therefore the sum of squares is positive.* Table 2.4 shows an example of how the sum of squares is calculated.

Table 2.4 Table showing the steps involved in calculating the sum of squares, variance, and standard deviation based on resting heart rates for a sample of 15 subjects.

Subject	Heart rates	Differences	Differences	Squared differences
	X	$(X-\bar{X})$	$(X-\bar{X})$	$(X-\bar{X})^2$
1	69	69–75	−6	36
2	105	105–75	30	900
3	77	77–75	2	4
4	70	70–75	−5	25
5	62	62–75	−13	169
6	83	83–75	8	64
7	80	80–75	5	25
8	77	77–75	2	4
9	60	60–75	−15	225
10	71	71–75	−4	16
11	67	67–75	−8	64
12	74	74–75	−1	1
13	81	81–75	6	36
14	74	74–75	−1	1
15	75	75–75	0	0
	$\bar{X} = 75$		Sum = 0	SS = 1570

X = individual heart rates, $\bar{X}$ = mean heart rate; SS = sum of squares
Notice that the sum of the differences ('Sum') is 0, since the positive and negative values cancel each other out. By squaring the differences, all values become positive or zero, so the sum of squares (SS) is positive.
Calculating the variance (s^2) involves dividing the sum of squares by the number of subjects (n), minus 1 ($n-1$). Note: $n-1$, since we're working with sample data.

$$s^2 = \frac{\text{sum of squares}}{n-1} = \frac{1570}{15-1} = 112.1 \text{ beats/min}^2$$

The square root of the variance is the standard deviation (s).

$$s = \sqrt{s^2} = \sqrt{112.1} = 10.6 \text{ beats/min}$$

* **Note:** the sum of squares is positive, unless all scores are equal (i.e. no variance). If all scores are equal, the sum of squares will be 0 (all values of X equal $\bar{X}$).

The sum of squares represents the total dispersion of all of the scores relative to the mean. What we want is a value that represents, on average, how the scores tend to be dispersed about the mean. Therefore, we divide the sum of squares by the number of observations (n). More specifically, we divide by n when calculating the variance for a population (Equation 2.2) and by $n - 1$ when calculating the variance for a sample (Equation 2.3). We're almost always working with sample data, so in most cases we'll use Equation 2.3 to calculate a variance. Note that σ^2 (lowercase sigma, squared) is typically used to represent a population variance, while s^2 is typically used to represent a sample variance.

Equation 2.2

$$\text{Population variance} \left(\sigma^2\right) = \frac{\sum(X - \mu)^2}{n}$$

or

$$\text{Population variance} \left(\sigma^2\right) = \frac{\text{Sum of squares}}{n}$$

Equation 2.3

$$\text{Sample variance} \left(s^2\right) = \frac{\sum\left(X - \bar{X}\right)^2}{n - 1}$$

or

$$\text{Sample variance} \left(s^2\right) = \frac{\text{Sum of squares}}{n - 1}$$

So why $n - 1$ when calculating a sample variance? The reason is that the variance from a sample will tend to underrepresent the variance for a population. Subtracting 1 from the denominator increases the sample variance so that it's likely to better represent the population variance.

Note: it's important to have a good understanding of what the sum of squares and the variance represent, since these metrics will be incorporated in many of the analyses discussed in subsequent chapters.

Standard deviation

Although the variance is a very useful measure of variability, it's a bit odd to consider on its own, since the units are squared. For instance, the variance for the resting heart rate data included in Table 2.4 is 112.1 beats per minute squared (beats/min²). We can revert the variance back to the original units of the measure by simply finding the square root of the variance. Essentially, we square the differences so we can calculate the variance and then take the square root so that our measure of variability is back into the original units. This square root of the variance is the *standard deviation*. For example, the standard deviation for the resting heart rate data is 10.6 beats/min ($s = \sqrt{s^2} = \sqrt{112.1} = 10.6$). Notice that the units for the standard deviation are back into their original form (beats/min, instead of beats/min²). Equation 2.4 can be used to calculate the standard deviation for a population (σ), while Equation 2.5 can be used to calculate the standard deviation for a sample (s).

Equation 2.4

$$\text{Population standard deviation} \left(\sigma \right) = \sqrt{\frac{\sum \left(X - \mu \right)^2}{n}}$$

Equation 2.5

$$\text{Sample standard deviation} \left(s \right) = \sqrt{\frac{\sum \left(X - \bar{X} \right)^2}{n - 1}}$$

Note: the symbol SD is also commonly used to represent the standard deviation for a sample.

In most cases, the standard deviation is reported along with the mean in order to show both the central tendency and the variability associated with a set of scores. For instance, the mean (±standard deviation) for the resting heart rate data included in Table 2.4 is 75 ± 10.6 beats/min. This tells us that the mean resting heart rate was 75 beats/min and that the average deviation from the mean was 10.6 beats/min.

It's important to remember that simply reporting the mean doesn't provide the entire story, since we also need to know how the scores tended to vary. For example, if our sample had a mean of 75 beats/min but a standard deviation of 2 beats/min (instead of 10 beats/minute), it would indicate that most subjects' resting heart rates tended to be clustered very closely to the mean of 75 beats/min.

Standardized scores

In some cases, we'll 'standardize' raw scores so that their deviation from the mean is expressed in units of standard deviations. These standard scores are typically referred to as *z-scores*. Equation 2.6 includes the general form of the equation for calculating a *z*-score. Notice that the numerator of the equation is the difference between the raw score (X) and the mean (μ or $\bar{X}$), while the denominator is the standard deviation (σ or s).

Equation 2.6

$$z\text{-score} \left(\text{population} \right) = \frac{X - \mu}{\sigma}$$

or

$$z\text{-score} \left(\text{sample} \right) = \frac{X - \bar{X}}{s}$$

Standardizing raw scores has many advantages, some of which will become clearer in Chapter 3. One advantage is that it provides an indication of how extreme an individual score is in relation to the rest of scores in the distribution by accounting for how scores typically tend to deviate about the mean.

Let's consider an example. Imagine that the mean birth weight for babies born in the United States is approximately 7.5 pounds, with a standard deviation of 1.3 pounds (7.5 ± 1.3 pounds) (note: it's pretty close to these values). Now, let's say that a baby is born weighing 7.0 pounds. The z-score associated with this 7.0-pound birth weight is -0.38 (z-score $= \frac{7.0 - 7.5}{1.3} = -0.38$). In other words, the child's birth weight is 0.38 standard deviations below the mean birth weight.

We'll continue to add context to z-scores in the next chapter. For now, just trust that a score located 0.38 standard deviations below the mean (z-score $= -0.38$) wouldn't be considered 'extreme'. It's slightly below average but certainly within a range of what's commonly observed (i.e. close to the center of the distribution of birth weights).

Learning Activity 2.1 provides an opportunity for you to work with the equation for calculating a z-score.

Learning Activity 2.1

Continue to assume that the mean ($\pm$standard deviation) birth weight is 7.5 ± 1.3 pounds. If the z-score associated with a specific child's birth weight was $+2.3$, what was this child's actual birth weight?

The answer is included at the end of the chapter.

Assessing normality

As I alluded to earlier in this chapter, most of the statistical tests discussed in the remainder of this book are based on the assumption that the distribution of scores approximates the shape of the normal distribution. Therefore, we should check to see whether this assumption is reasonable before running any of these analyses. Examining a histogram is a good starting point; however, there are other ways to assess the assumption of normality. Appendix A ('Assessing Normality') includes a supplementary discussion of various ways to check whether the assumption of normality is satisfied.

Application opportunity

Example data set

This example data set includes reaction times for 30 subjects. The subjects were asked to respond as quickly as possible by pressing a button when a visual stimulus appeared on a computer screen in front of them (simple reaction time). The reaction time values reflect the time (units – milliseconds) between the appearance of the visual stimulus and the button press.

Data files

RT_data.xlsx – Excel file that includes the subjects' reaction times. The first column ('Subject') includes the subject number (1–30), while the second column ('RT') includes the reaction time values.

RT_data.sav – SPSS file that includes the subjects' reaction times in the first column ('RT').

Video

Descriptives – video that includes a demonstration of how to generate descriptive statistics using SPSS and the Excel Analysis ToolPak.

Answers to learning activity

Learning Activity 2.1

Answer

$$z\text{-score} = \frac{X - 7.5}{1.3} = +2.3; X = ?$$

The child's birth weight was approximately 10.5 pounds, which is 2.3 standard deviations above the mean birth weight of 7.5 pounds (z-score = +2.3). Note that this birth weight would be considered more atypical, or 'extreme', than the birth weight of 7.0 pounds, discussed in the chapter (z-score = –0.38).

3 The normal distribution

Chapter Objectives

The objectives of this chapter are to . . .

1) introduce the basis for the normal distribution
2) highlight the characteristics of the normal distribution
3) discuss the importance of the normal distribution in the context of inferential statistics
4) describe the standard normal distribution
5) explain how the areas under the normal distribution curve represent the proportion of scores within a range of values
6) provide examples of how the probability of observing a value within any area of the normal distribution can be derived

Introduction

Even if you haven't taken a statistics course, you've probably heard of the *normal distribution*, which is also commonly referred to as the 'bell curve', since its shape resembles that of a bell, or the 'Gaussian distribution', since it was described by mathematician Carl Friedrich Gauss. The normal distribution serves many important purposes in inferential statistics and will be referenced frequently throughout the remaining chapters of this book, which is why I've devoted this entire chapter to introducing it.

The normal distribution is based on a specific mathematical function defined by two parameters: the mean (μ) and the standard deviation (σ) (Equation 3.1). μ specifies the location of the center of the distribution (central tendency), and σ specifies the width of the distribution (variability). When plotted, the normal distribution is a smooth continuous curve, with a vertical axis that represents the frequency of observations* and a horizontal axis that includes the possible values for the dependent variable of interest (Figure 3.1).

* **Note:** although you can think of the normal distribution curve as a frequency distribution, it's technically a continuous distribution of probabilities (referred to as a *continuous probability distribution*). The link between frequencies (or proportions) and probabilities is discussed later in this chapter.

DOI: 10.4324/9781003179757-3

Equation 3.1

$$f(X) = \frac{1}{\sigma\sqrt{2\pi}} e^{-\frac{1}{2}\left(\frac{X-\mu}{\sigma}\right)^2}$$

π and e are mathematical constants; X represents all possible values for the dependent variable; μ is the population mean; σ is the standard deviation; f(X) represents the height of the curve for each possible value of the dependent variable X. Don't worry about the specifics of this function. You'll probably never need to work with it directly. Just appreciate that its two inputs are the mean and standard deviation.

The normal distribution is perfectly symmetrical and unimodal, with most scores clustering in the center of the distribution and then the number of scores tapering off equally in both directions (Figure 3.1). The tails of the normal distribution curve extend out indefinitely in the positive and negative directions, never reaching 0 (X limits = ±infinity). Note that the normal distribution is not an empirical distribution based on sample data. It's more of a theoretical concept, which represents how many variables naturally tend to be distributed.

Importance of the normal distribution

There are many reasons the normal distribution is one of the most important distributions in statistics. For one, many variables tend to be normally distributed in the population. For instance, consider variables such as height, weight, blood pressure, and so on. In each case, most individuals cluster close to the center, or body, of the distribution, with progressively fewer individuals in the tails of the distribution. As an example, consider height. The average height of males in the United States is approximately 69 inches (5 feet, 9 inches) (Fryar et al., 2021). Most men are within a few inches of this height (body of distribution); however, there are men who are quite a bit taller than average and other men who are quite

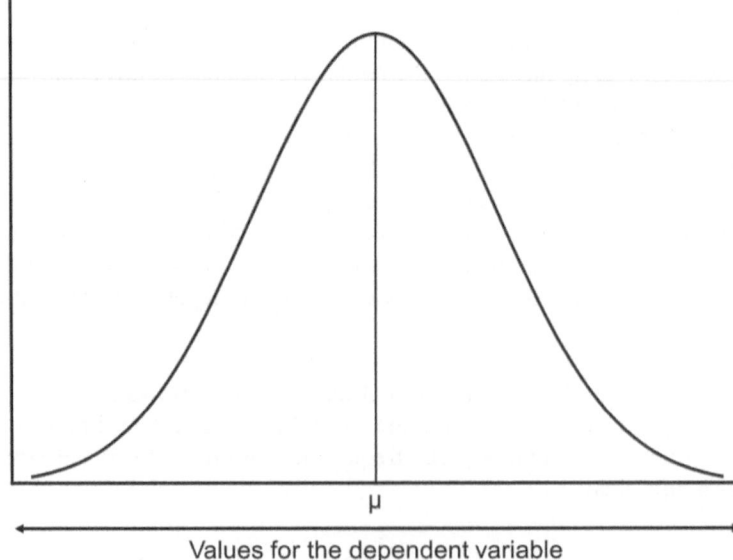

μ

Values for the dependent variable

Figure 3.1 Graph of the normal distribution curve. Notice that most scores are clustered around the mean (μ), with progressively fewer scores located in the upper and lower tails of the distribution. Note that since the normal distribution is unimodal and perfectly symmetrical, the mean, median, and mode are all equivalent (mean = median = mode).

a bit shorter than average. These relatively tall and short men make up the outer tails of the height distribution.

In addition, statistics derived from multiple samples taken from a population tend to be normally distributed about the corresponding population parameter.* For example, imagine that we repeatedly took samples of a certain size from the population, found the mean for each sample ($\bar{X}$), and then examined a frequency distribution of the sample means (generally referred to as a *sampling distribution*). The sample means would tend to be normally distributed around the population mean (μ), with most sample means located in the body of the distribution and progressively fewer sample means extending into the tails of the distribution. In other words, sampling errors tend to be normally distributed about the true population parameter. Sometimes we overestimate the population parameter, and other times we underestimate the population parameter, but over a large number of samples, most statistics will fall relatively close to the population parameter of interest (center of the distribution). If it's unclear to you why we'd ever care about the characteristics of these types of sampling distributions, don't worry; we'll discuss sampling distributions in greater detail in subsequent chapters. For now, just know that statistics derived from multiple samples tend to be normally distributed about the corresponding population parameter and that this has relevance to many inferential statistical procedures.

* **Note:** this is true as long as the population distribution is normal or the sample size is sufficiently large (number of subjects $\geq \sim 30$). The characteristics of sampling distributions are described by the central limit theorem. Sampling distributions will be discussed in greater detail in Chapter 4.

It's also important to note that the general features of the normal distribution are constant and therefore predictable. This makes it very appealing from a statistical perspective, since we can use the characteristics of the normal distribution to make inferences based on sample data, which is the essence of inferential statistics. We'll continue to discuss how we can make use of the properties of the normal distribution throughout the rest of this chapter and in the chapters that follow.

The standard normal (z) distribution

The normal distribution can be standardized by transforming the values for the dependent variable of interest into z-scores. Remember that a z-score quantifies the extent to which an individual score (X) deviates from the mean (μ), in terms of standard deviations (σ) (Equation 3.2) (note: z-scores were introduced in Chapter 2). The sign of a z-score reflects its relation to the mean; scores above the mean ($X > \mu$) have a positive z-score ($z > 0$), scores below the mean ($X < \mu$) have a negative z-score ($z < 0$), and scores equal to the mean ($X = \mu$) have a z-score of 0 ($z = 0$). The magnitude of a z-score reflects the extent of its deviation from the mean; the farther the score is from the mean, the greater the magnitude of its z-score. The standardized version of the normal distribution is referred to as the standard normal distribution, or the z distribution. The standard normal distribution has a mean of 0 ($\mu = 0$) and a standard deviation of 1 ($\sigma = 1$).

Equation 3.2

$$z\text{-score} = \frac{X - \mu}{\sigma}$$

A key benefit of working with the standard normal distribution is that we can readily determine the proportion of scores located in any area of a normal distribution, regardless of its mean and standard deviation. To find the proportion of scores located in a certain area of a

Table 3.1 Example of a standard normal (*z*) distribution table. *z* represents the various *z*-scores. The values in the cells of columns 2–4 represent the proportion of scores in different areas of the distribution (multiply by 100 to express as a percentage). Appendix C includes a more complete standard normal distribution table. Note: since the normal distribution is perfectly symmetrical, the areas are the same regardless of whether *z* is positive or negative.

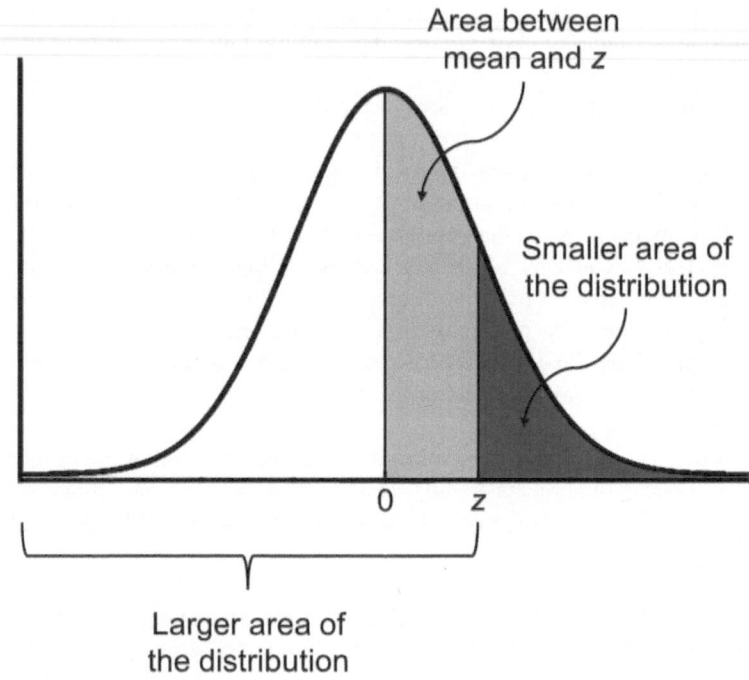

z (±)	Area between mean and z	Larger area of the distribution	Smaller area of the distribution
0.00	0.0000	0.5000	0.5000
0.01	0.0040	0.5040	0.4960
0.02	0.0080	0.5080	0.4920
0.03	0.0120	0.5120	0.4880
0.04	0.0160	0.5160	0.4840
0.05	0.0199	0.5199	0.4801
...	...	...	...
0.98	0.3365	0.8365	0.1635
0.99	0.3389	0.8389	0.1611
1.00	0.3413	0.8413	0.1587
1.01	0.3438	0.8438	0.1562
1.02	0.3461	0.8461	0.1539
...	...	...	...
1.98	0.4761	0.9761	0.0239
1.99	0.4767	0.9767	0.0233
2.00	0.4772	0.9772	0.0228
2.01	0.4778	0.9778	0.0222
2.02	0.4783	0.9783	0.0217
...	...	...	...
2.98	0.4986	0.9986	0.0014
2.99	0.4986	0.9986	0.0014
3.00	0.4987	0.9987	0.0013
...	...	...	...

normal distribution, we must calculate the area under the curve defined by a *z*-score or a pair of *z*-scores through the process of integration (note: integration is the mathematical process of finding the area under a curve). Fortunately, this work of integrating the areas under different portions of the standard normal curve has been done for us and is commonly reported in tabular form. A sample of a standard normal distribution table is included in Table 3.1, and a more complete version of this table is included in Appendix C ['Standard Normal (*z*) Distribution Table']. Notice that the table includes different *z* values, as well as the proportions of scores in different areas of the normal distribution curve.

For instance, the proportion of scores beyond a *z* value of +1.00 is 0.1587 (smaller area of the distribution) (Figure 3.2, subplot A). In other words, 15.87% of scores are more than one standard deviation above the mean (*z*-score > +1.00) in a normal distribution. Of course, this also means that 84.13% of scores are below this value, since this makes up the remaining area under the curve (note: the entire area under the curve sums to 1.0 or 100%). As another example, only 2.28% of scores are more than two standard deviations below the mean (*z*-score < –2.00) (Figure 3.2, subplot B).

We can also find the areas that extend beyond two *z* values or the area between two *z* values. For instance, 4.56% of all scores are beyond two standard deviations from the mean (*z* < –2.00 and *z* > +2.00) (Figure 3.2, subplot C), while 95.44% of scores are located within two standard deviations of the mean (–2.00 < *z* < +2.00) (Figure 3.2, subplot D). Note that these proportions are consistent across all normal distributions, regardless of μ and σ.

Note: there are many different versions of the standard normal table available online and in other textbooks. There are also a lot of freely available programs that allow you to find the proportion of scores located in different areas of a normal distribution.

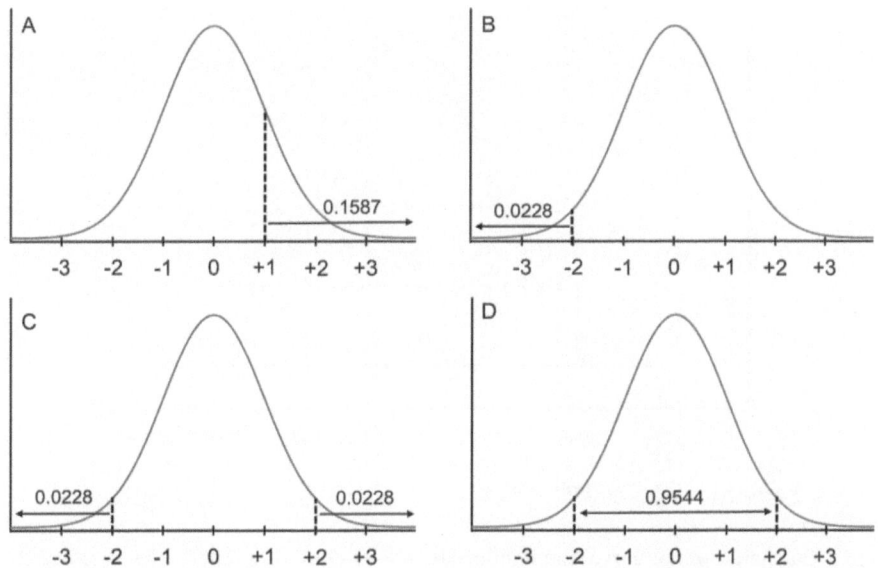

Figure 3.2 Standard normal curves with different areas designated. The arrows highlight the relevant areas of the distributions. The proportion of scores located in the given area(s) are included on the figures. Multiplying these proportions by 100 reflects the percentage of the total number of scores located in the relevant area(s) of the distribution. Note: the values of *z* are denoted along the *x*-axis.

68–95–99.7 rule

The 68–95–99.7 rule, which is also commonly referred to as the *empirical rule*, is a simple way of remembering approximately what proportion of scores are located within one, two, and three standard deviations from the mean. The rule specifies that in the case of a normal distribution, approximately 68% of scores fall within one standard deviation of the mean ($-1.00 < z < +1.00$), approximately 95% of scores fall within two standard deviations of the mean ($-2.00 < z < +2.00$),* and approximately 99.7% of scores fall within three standard deviations of the mean ($-3.00 < z < +3.00$) (Figure 3.3).

* **Note:** the z values that bound exactly 95% of a normal distribution are $z = \pm 1.96$. You'll see this 1.96 z value frequently in the upcoming chapters, since we often attempt to precisely define the area that makes up the middle 95% of a normal distribution. For reference, the precise z values that bound the middle 90%, 95%, and 99% of a normal distribution are 1.645, 1.96, and 2.576, respectively. These z values have been bolded in the standard normal distribution table in Appendix C since they're commonly referenced.

Birth weight example

Now, let's consider an example. Let's assume that the mean birth weight for babies born in the United States is 7.5 pounds, with a standard deviation of 1.3 pounds ($\mu = 7.5$ pounds, $\sigma = 1.3$ pounds) and that birth weights are normally distributed. Now, imagine that a baby is born weighing 6.8 pounds ($X = 6.8$ pounds). We know that this birth weight is below the average of 7.5 pounds, but it's difficult to get an appreciation for how rare or 'extreme' this birth weight of 6.8 pounds is without considering the variability in birth weights. The z-score that

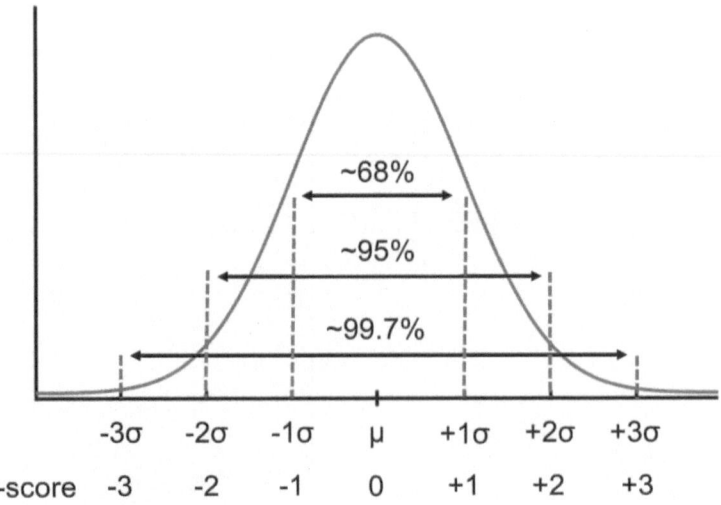

Figure 3.3 Standard normal curve highlighting the 68–95–99.7 rule. The dashed vertical lines and arrows signify the different areas of the distribution. Notice that approximately 68% of scores are located within one standard deviation ($\pm 1\sigma$) of the mean, approximately 95% of scores are located within two standard deviations ($\pm 2\sigma$) of the mean, and approximately 99.7% of scores are located within three standard deviations ($\pm 3\sigma$) of the mean.

corresponds with our observed 6.8-pound birth weight is -0.54 ($z = \dfrac{X-\mu}{\sigma} = \dfrac{6.8-7.5}{1.3} = -0.54$) (Figure 3.4, subplot A). In other words, the 6.8-pound birth weight is a little over 0.5 standard deviations below the mean. If you reference the standard normal distribution table in Appendix C, you'll find that 29.46% of values fall beyond a z-score of 0.54 (*smaller area of the distribution*), which, in this case, indicates that almost 30% of babies are born weighing less than 6.8 pounds. This should put us at ease that our observed birth weight of 6.8 pounds isn't that extreme; it's below average but not uncommon to observe.

Now, let's say that another baby is born weighing 5.3 pounds ($X = 5.3$ pounds). The z-score that corresponds with this 5.3-pound birth weight is -1.69 ($z = \dfrac{X-\mu}{\sigma} = \dfrac{5.3-7.5}{1.3} = -1.69$) (Figure 3.4, subplot B). Again, you can reference Appendix C to find the proportion of babies born weighing less (or more than) than 5.3 pounds. In this case, you'll find that only 4.55% of babies are born weighing less than 5.3 pounds (*smaller area of the distribution*). In other words, 95.45% of babies are born weighing more than 5.3 pounds. Regardless, the 5.3-pound birth weight appears to be somewhat rare, or 'extreme', at least in comparison to the 6.8-pound birth weight.

Learning Activity 3.1 provides opportunities for you to practice using the standard normal distribution table.

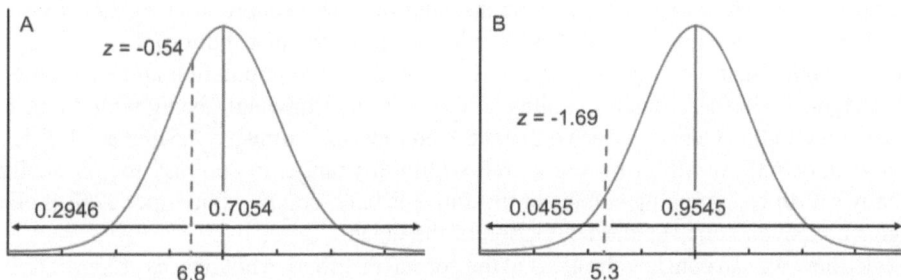

Figure 3.4 Normal distribution curves for birth weights of babies born in the United States ($\mu = 7.5$ pounds, $\sigma = 1.3$ pounds). The dashed vertical lines represent the location of the 6.8-pound (subplot A) and 5.3-pound (subplot B) birth weights in the distribution. The z-scores associated with the 6.8- and 5.3-pound birth weights are -0.54 and -1.69, respectively. Notice that 29.46% of babies are born weighing less than 6.8 pounds (area below $z = -0.54$), while only 4.55% of babies are born weighing less than 5.3 pounds (area below $z = -1.69$). As you can see, a birth weight of 5.3 pounds would be considered more extreme than a birth weight of 6.8 pounds. Note: the μ and σ values were derived for this example; they may not be exactly accurate.

Learning Activity 3.1

Continue to assume that the mean (±standard deviation) birth weight for the population is 7.5 ± 1.3 pounds and that birth weights are normally distributed. Use the standard normal distribution table in Appendix C to determine:

1) the percentage of babies born weighing more than 11 pounds
2) the percentage of babies born weighing between 6 pounds and 9 pounds

3) the percentage of babies born weighing beyond 1.5 standard deviations from the mean
4) the percentage of babies born within 1.5 standard deviations of the mean

The answers are included at the end of the chapter.

Thinking in terms of probabilities

So far, we've discussed the areas of the normal distribution in terms of proportions or frequencies; however, we can also consider these areas in terms of probabilities. We'll discuss probability in greater detail in Chapter 4, but in general, a probability (p) is the likelihood that an event will occur, given all possible outcomes. For instance, if a medication is associated with an adverse reaction 1% of the time it's taken, we would say that the probability of experiencing an adverse reaction is 0.01, or 1% ($p = \dfrac{\text{number of adverse reactions}}{\text{all instances where the medication is taken}}$).

To demonstrate this concept, let's revisit our birth weight example. As discussed earlier in this chapter, approximately 68% of all values are within ± 1 standard deviation of the mean for a normal distribution. In other words, 68% of the area under the normal distribution curve is between the z values of ± 1 (body of the distribution), while approximately 32% of the area under the curve is located beyond these z values (tails of the distribution).

Now imagine that we randomly selected a baby from the population and examined their birth weight. In this case, the probability of this baby's birth weight being within one standard deviation of the mean (between 6.2 and 8.8 pounds, assuming $\mu = 7.5$ and $\sigma = 1.3$) is 0.68, or 68%, since 68% of all birth weights fall within this range. In contrast, the probability of the baby's birth weight being outside of this range is 0.32, or 32%, since only 32% of all birth weights are beyond one standard deviation of the mean.

Notice how we can consider the areas of the normal distribution not only as proportions or frequencies but also as probabilities. We'll continue to build on this concept in subsequent chapters.

Final thoughts

As I explained at the beginning of this chapter, the normal distribution is fundamental to inferential statistics. While at this point you may not fully comprehend its importance, you'll come to appreciate the different ways we make use of the properties of the normal distribution as you progress through the remaining chapters.

Answers to learning activity

Learning Activity 3.1

Answers

1) $z > +2.69$; **0.36%**
2) z within ± 1.15; **74.98%**
3) $z < -1.50$ and $z > +1.50$; **13.36%**
4) z within ± 1.50; **86.64%**

Figure 3.5 depicts the relevant areas of the distributions for questions 1–4.

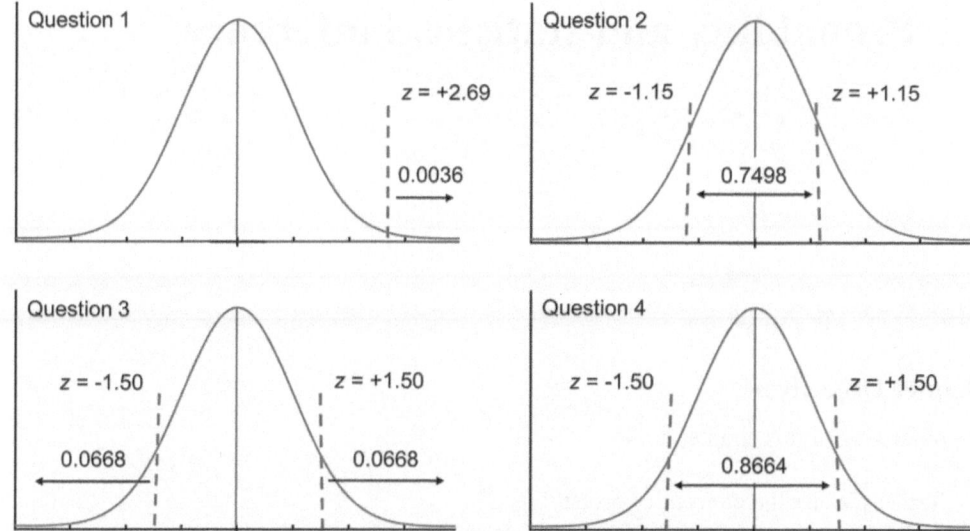

Figure 3.5 Relevant areas of the distributions for Learning Activity 3.1. The vertical lines represent the locations of the *z* value(s) within the distribution, while the arrows highlight the relevant areas of the distributions.

4 Probability and statistical inference

Chapter Objectives

The objectives of this chapter are to . . .

1) further discuss the concept of probability
2) discuss sampling error in the context of parameter estimation and hypothesis testing
3) describe what a sampling distribution is and discuss typical characteristics of sampling distributions
4) define the standard error and describe how it's estimated
5) explain the conceptual basis for a confidence interval and provide an example of how a confidence interval is constructed
6) introduce the general logic of null hypothesis significance testing
7) differentiate between the null hypothesis and alternative hypothesis
8) distinguish between Type I and Type II errors
9) explain what a p-value represents and discuss its role in hypothesis testing
10) describe how the alpha level is used to determine whether to reject the null hypothesis
11) explain how the alpha level influences the risk of Type I and Type II errors
12) highlight some of the main criticisms of null hypothesis significance testing
13) introduce the concept of statistical power and discuss influential factors

Introduction

Inferential statistics involves using observations from sample data to make inferences about a population. The concept of *probability* is fundamental to inferential statistics, as the relationship between samples and populations is usually defined in terms of probabilities. This chapter will provide a general overview of the procedures used to estimate population parameters and test hypotheses. At this point, we won't go into the details of different types of statistical tests. Instead, we'll focus on the foundational concepts of statistical inference. These concepts will be built upon in subsequent chapters.

Probability

Let's start by defining probability using a simple example. Imagine a jar containing 100 marbles; 75 of the marbles are red, and 25 of the marbles are blue. You can think of this jar of 100 marbles as the population in this example. *Probability*, which is typically denoted p, can be defined as the likelihood that an event will occur, given all possible outcomes. Therefore, in this case, the probability of selecting a red marble from the jar is 0.75 ($p = \dfrac{75}{25 + 75} = 0.75$),

DOI: 10.4324/9781003179757-4

while the probability of selecting a blue marble from the jar is 0.25 ($p = \dfrac{25}{25 + 75} = 0.25$).
While we can't know for sure whether a single marble selected from the jar will be red or blue, we can consider the different outcomes in terms of their probabilities.

Clinicians often speak in terms of probability. For instance, if a surgeon tells a patient that surgery has a 90% chance of success, they're referencing the probability of a successful outcome ($p = \dfrac{\text{successful surgeries}}{\text{all surgeries performed}}$). While the surgeon doesn't know whether surgery will be successful for a specific patient, they do know how often the surgery is successful for patients in general. In this case, a 90% probability of success indicates that surgery is successful 90 out of every 100 times it's performed.

Using probability as a basis for inference

Up to this point in the chapter, the examples have involved known population characteristics, as we knew how many red and blue marbles were in the jar and how often surgery was successful overall. However, statistical inference works in the other direction. We have information about a sample (or samples) and use this information to infer something about the population(s). Let's explore this concept with another simple example. Imagine there are two jars (jar A and jar B), each containing 100 marbles. Some of the marbles are colored red, and some are colored blue. Our objective is to determine if there's a difference in the jars with respect to the proportions of red marbles they contain. We take separate samples of 20 marbles from each jar. The sample from jar A includes 16 red marbles and 4 blue marbles, while the sample from jar B includes 5 red marbles and 15 blue marbles. Although there appears to be a difference in the jar proportions, these differences may simply be due to chance. In other words, we may have just happened to sample an uncharacteristically large proportion of red marbles from jar A and/or an uncharacteristically small proportion of red marbles from jar B.

While we won't know for sure whether the observed difference in sample proportions is a result of a true difference in the contents of the jars, we could determine the probability of observing such a large difference in samples, if there wasn't actually a difference in the jar proportions. If the probability is low, we may decide to conclude that the jar proportions differ, even though we only examined 20% of their total contents, since it would be very unlikely to observe such a large difference in sample proportions by chance. This is just one example of how probability can be used to make inferences based on sample data. We'll continue to explore this concept throughout the remainder of the chapter.

Probability vs. odds

In our everyday language, the terms probability and *odds* are often used interchangeably. While these concepts are certainly related, they're not the same. Odds are defined as the ratio of the probability of an event occurring relative to the probability of an event not occurring. For example, the odds of selecting a red marble from a jar with 75 red marbles and 25 blue marbles are 3 $\left(\dfrac{0.75}{0.25} = 3 \right)$. In other words, the odds of selecting a red marble from the jar are 3 to 1. If a surgery is successful 90% of the time, then the odds of a successful outcome are 9 $\left(\dfrac{0.90}{0.10} = 9 \right)$, or 9 to 1. Investigators will often report the odds of an event, such as an injury or fall, or the odds of achieving a certain outcome (e.g. successful surgery). Odds will be revisited later in this book; however, I've introduced the concept here since it's so closely related to probability.

Probability in the context of a distribution

Now, let's apply the concept of probability to a distribution. Chapter 3 introduced the normal distribution. Remember that for a normal distribution, the proportion of scores in each area of the distribution are known. For instance, 68% of scores fall within one standard deviation of the mean, 95% of scores fall within two standard deviations of the mean, and over 99% of scores fall within three standard deviations of the mean (remember the 68–95–99.7 rule).

While we can consider the areas under the normal distribution curve in terms of proportions, we can also think of these areas in terms of probabilities. For example, imagine that we were able to record the body mass index of all adults in the population of the United States and that these values are normally distributed around a mean of 28.0 kg/m² and that the distribution had a standard deviation of 4.5 kg/m² ($\mu = 28.0$ kg/m²; $\sigma = 4.5$ kg/m²). Now, let's say that we were to randomly select an individual from this population. Based on the characteristics of the normal distribution, we could determine the probability that this individual's BMI would fall in any area of the distribution. For instance, the probability of their BMI being two standard deviations or more above the mean is only 0.025 ($p = 0.025$), since only 2.5% of all observations fall within this area of a normal distribution (Figure 4.1). Notice how distributions essentially map out the probabilities associated with observing a value in any range.

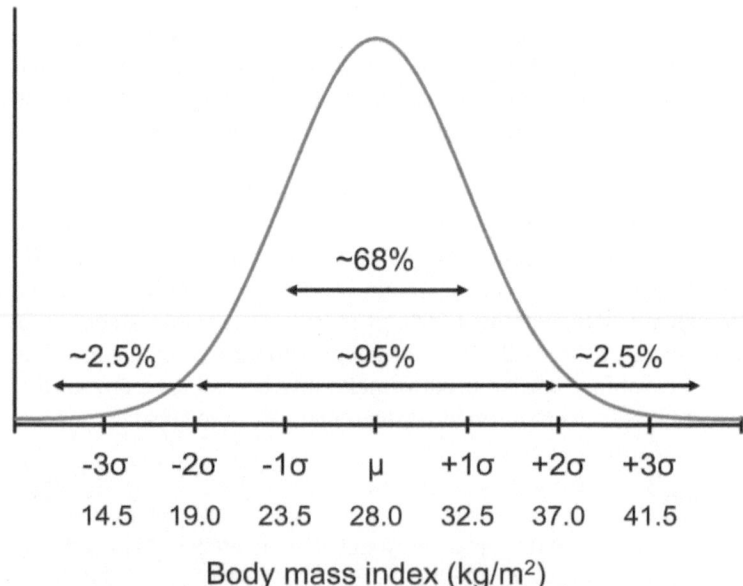

Figure 4.1 Hypothetical distribution of body mass index (BMI) values for adults in the United States population. The distribution has a mean (μ) of 28.0 kg/m² and a standard deviation (σ) of 4.5 kg/m². The percentages shown on the distribution correspond with the proportion of individuals whose BMI falls within different areas of the distribution. For instance, only approximately 2.5% of all individuals in the population have a BMI greater than 37.0 kg/m² (two standard deviations above the mean). Therefore, if we randomly selected one individual from the population, the probability of this individual's BMI being greater than 37.0 kg/m² is approximately 0.025 ($p = 0.025$).

Sampling error

As discussed in Chapter 1, a statistic derived from a sample will differ from the true population parameter. This discrepancy between sample statistics and the population parameters they're intended to represent is referred to as *sampling error*. For example, if we selected a sample of individuals from the population and recorded their BMI, the sample mean ($\bar{X}$) would likely differ from the population mean (μ), since the sample is only composed of a subset of individuals from the population. If we took another sample of individuals from the population, we would likely observe a different sample mean. In the end, no two samples will be exactly the same, even if they are from the same population, since they include different individuals.

Sampling error tends to be random, as sometimes the sample statistic will overestimate the population parameter, and other times the sample statistic will underestimate the population parameter. This presents a challenge, since in practice, we typically only rely on a single sample to estimate a population parameter. However, we can estimate the amount of sample-to-sample variability in sampling error, which proves very useful when estimating population parameters and conducting hypothesis tests.

Sampling distributions

Chapter 2 discussed how individual scores can be organized into a distribution. *Sampling distributions* are similar, except they're composed of statistics derived from multiple samples taken from the population instead of individual scores. Sampling distributions play a critical role in inferential statistics. Therefore, it's important to understand what these distributions represent. Let's begin by discussing a relatively simple type of sampling distribution, the *distribution of sample means*.

The distribution of sample means

Imagine that we repeatedly took samples of a certain size (n) from a population, recorded some variable (e.g. BMI), and calculated the mean for each of these samples ($\bar{X}_1$ to $\bar{X}_k$, where k represents the number of samples). As we've already discussed, some of these sample means would overestimate the population mean, and others would underestimate the population mean because of sampling error. Much like individual scores, we could organize these sample means into a distribution. This distribution is the distribution of sample means.

If we took a really large number of samples, the distribution of sample means would exhibit some predictable characteristics.* First, it would be centered around the population mean. In fact, the average of the sample means would equal the population mean. In addition, the sample means would tend to be normally distributed, as long as the population from which the samples were taken was normally distributed or the samples were relatively large ($n \geq \sim 30$). In other words, most sample means would tend to be clustered around the population mean (body of the sampling distribution), with fewer sample means drastically overestimating or underestimating the population mean (tails of the sampling distribution).

* **Note:** the *central limit theorem* describes key characteristics of sampling distributions.

The standard error

Chapter 2 introduced the standard deviation as a common measure of variability for a distribution of scores. Remember, the standard deviation captures how the individual scores in a distribution vary about the mean, with a greater standard deviation reflecting more spread in the scores. The *standard error* is analogous to the standard deviation; however, it captures how statistics derived from multiple samples tend to vary about the population parameter. In other words, the variability of a sampling distribution. As a result, the standard error represents the degree of sample-to-sample variability due to sampling error. A relatively low standard error indicates that most sample statistics closely match the population parameter (i.e. minimal sampling error).

The standard error for the distribution of sample means (commonly referred to as the *standard error of the mean*) captures how sample means vary about the population mean. The more spread out the sample means about the population mean, the greater the standard error. The spread of the distribution of sample means depends on the size of the samples (n) taken from the population. The distribution of sample means will become narrower (lower standard error) as the sample size becomes larger, since samples composed of a large number of individuals generally produce sample means that more closely approximate the population mean. Figure 4.2 demonstrates how sample size influences the variability of the distribution of sample means. This relationship between sample size and variability is also true for other sampling distributions.

Technically, the standard error of the mean is calculated by dividing the population standard deviation (σ) by the square root of the sample size ($\sqrt{n}$) ; however, the population standard deviation is seldom known. To address this, we typically estimate the standard error by substituting the sample standard deviation (s) in place of the population standard deviation, since the sample standard deviation is probably our 'best guess' of the population standard

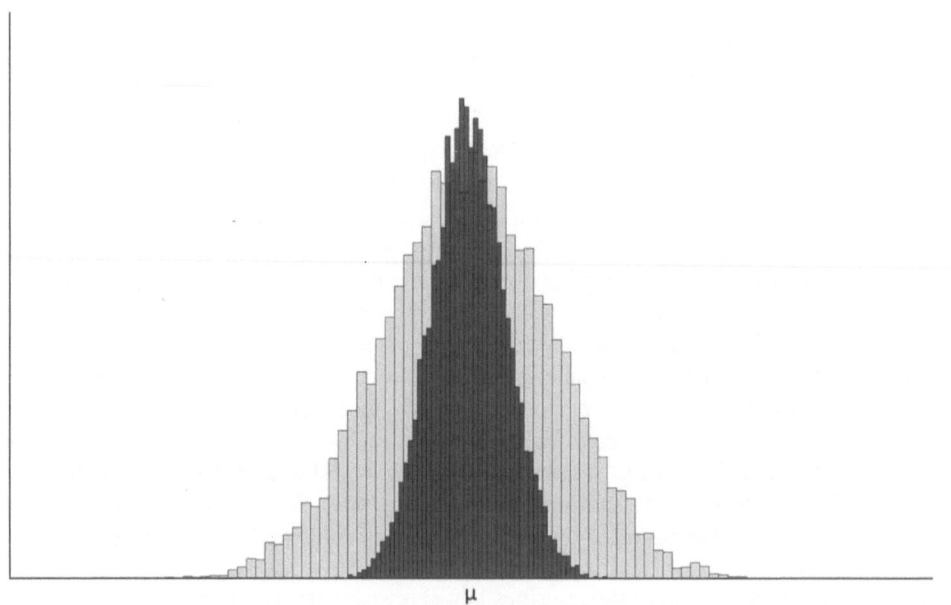

μ

Figure 4.2 Two superimposed distributions of sample means. Both distributions are based on 10,000 samples taken from a population of random numbers. The light gray distribution is based on random samples of size 10 ($n = 10$), while the dark gray distribution is based on random samples of size 50 ($n = 50$). Notice that both samples are normally distributed about the population mean (μ); however, the distribution is wider (i.e. larger standard error) when $n = 10$ compared to when $n = 50$.

deviation. Equation 4.1 includes the general form of the equation for the estimated standard error of the mean $\left(s_{\bar{x}}\right)$.

Equation 4.1

$$\text{standard error } (s_{\bar{x}}) = \frac{s}{\sqrt{n}}$$

The standard error is a key component of many aspects of inferential statistics, since it essentially captures the average degree of sampling error. Once we have an idea of the typical amount of error from sample to sample, we can start to determine how likely it would be to observe different sample statistics.

Largely theoretical, not empirical

It's important to realize that sampling distributions are almost always theoretical, not empirical. In other words, we don't really go through the process of repeatedly sampling and constructing these distributions. Instead, we contrive these sampling distributions based on sample data and our knowledge of how these distributions tend to behave with respect to their shape, central tendency, and variability.

Sampling distributions and probability

Earlier in this chapter, we discussed how the area under the curve of a distribution can be considered in terms of probability and how this allows us to determine the probability of observing different values. The same concept applies to sampling distributions, except we are thinking in terms of sample statistics, not individual scores.

For example, the probability of observing a sample mean that falls within two standard errors of the population mean is 0.95 ($p = 0.95$), since 95% of all sample means are expected to fall within this region of the distribution of sample means (notice that we're talking in terms of *standard errors* now instead of *standard deviations*, since we're discussing a sampling distribution). Of course, this also means that the probability of observing a sample mean that falls beyond two standard errors from the population mean is 0.05 ($p = 0.05$).

Confidence intervals

We're often interested in estimating a parameter, such as the population mean. While a sample statistic can be used to estimate a population parameter, there will be some discrepancy because of sampling error. To address this, we can generate an interval, or range of values, that's likely to include the population parameter. This range of values is referred to as a *confidence interval* (CI). While a confidence interval can be generated for any parameter of interest, we'll start by discussing confidence intervals in the context of estimating a population mean.

When estimating a population mean, the boundaries of a confidence interval are dependent on the sample mean ($\bar{X}$) and the standard error ($s_{\bar{x}}$). Equation 4.2 includes the general form of the equation for constructing a confidence interval around the population mean. As you can see from the $\pm$ in the equation, the result will be a lower boundary ($\bar{X} - (z) \times s_{\bar{x}}$) and an upper boundary ($\bar{X} + (z) \times s_{\bar{x}}$) of the interval. The variable z will determine our level of confidence. Remember that a z value (or 'z-score') allows us to define any area of a standard normal distribution (Chapter 3). In Equation 4.2, z is the z value that bounds a certain area of the normal distribution.

Equation 4.2

$$CI = \overline{X} \pm (z) \times s_{\bar{X}}$$

Let's start by discussing a 95% confidence interval, since these are most commonly reported. If you examine the standard normal (z) distribution table in Appendix C, you'll find that 95% of all values fall within precisely ± 1.96 z-scores of the mean. Therefore, when constructing a 95% confidence interval, z is 1.96 $[CI = \overline{X} \pm (1.96) \times s_{\bar{X}}]$.

So what does this 95% confidence interval represent? If we repeatedly sampled from the population and generated confidence intervals, 95% of these intervals would likely contain the population parameter of interest (Figure 4.3). In other words, the probability that the population parameter falls within the interval is 0.95 $(p = \dfrac{\text{intervals containing parameter}}{\text{all intervals}})$.

Example

Now, let's consider an example. Imagine that we want to estimate the average hemoglobin level of adult males. Obviously, we can't test every adult male in the population, so we rely on sampling. We select a large sample of males from the population and record their hemoglobin levels. The sample mean is 15.0 g/dl, and the estimated standard error $(\frac{s}{\sqrt{n}})$ is 1.3 g/dl. In this case, the lower and upper boundaries of a 95% confidence interval are 12.5 [15.0 − (1.96 × 1.3)] and 17.5 [15.0 + (1.96 × 1.3)] g/dl, respectively. This indicates that the mean hemoglobin level for males in the population likely falls within a range from 12.5 to 17.5 g/dl. Notice that by reporting a range, we account for the fact that our sample mean will not exactly match the population mean. You can think of this as adding some 'room for error' in the estimate. If we repeated this process 100 times, 95 of the 100 confidence intervals generated would be expected to include the population mean. Therefore, we can be fairly confident that the average hemoglobin level of the population falls within the range of 12.5 to 17.5 g/dl.

Adjusting our level of confidence

While 95% confidence intervals are most commonly reported, we can generate other confidence intervals, such as 90% or 99% confidence intervals, by adjusting z. When generating a 90% confidence interval, z is 1.645, since 90% of all values fall within 1.645 z-scores of the mean in a normal distribution. For the hemoglobin example, the lower and upper boundaries of a 90% confidence interval are 12.9 g/dl and 17.1 g/dl. Notice that the boundaries of the 90% confidence interval are narrower than those of a 95% confidence interval, and thus our estimate is more precise; however, we're less confident that the interval includes the population mean.

In the case of a 99% confidence interval, z is 2.576, since 99% of all values fall within 2.576 z-scores of the mean in a normal distribution. The lower and upper boundaries of the 99% confidence are 11.7 g/dl and 18.3 g/dl for the hemoglobin example. Notice that the boundaries of a 99% confidence interval are relatively wide, giving us greater confidence that the population mean falls within this interval; however, our estimate is less precise. When generating confidence intervals, there's always a tradeoff between confidence and precision (Figure 4.4).

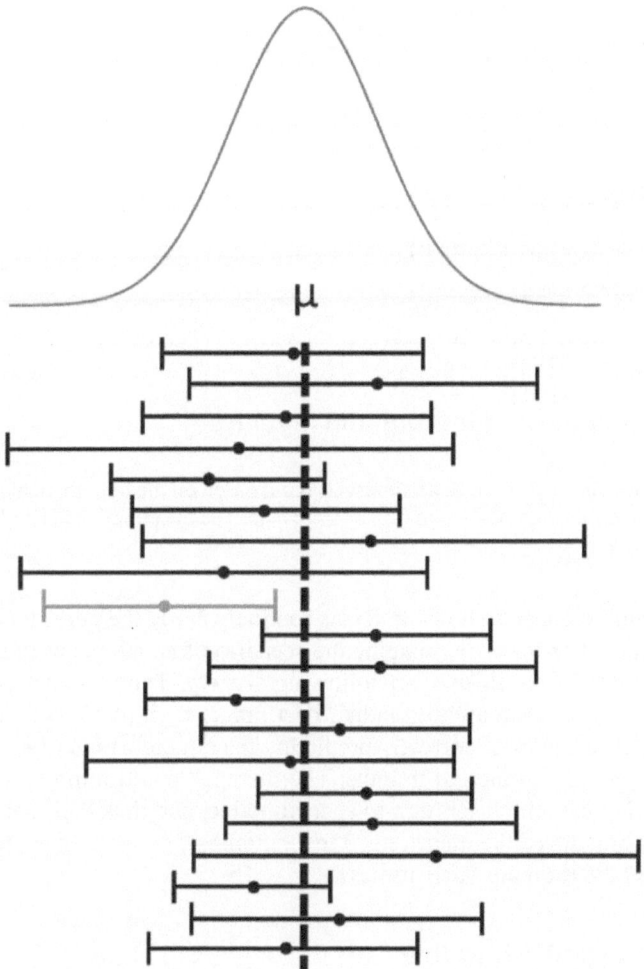

Figure 4.3 Hypothetical confidence intervals based on 20 random samples of size *n*. The brackets represent the lower and upper boundaries of the confidence interval, while the center dot represents the sample mean. The vertical line represents the location of the population mean (μ). Notice that 19 of the 20 (95%) of the intervals include the population mean, while one interval (gray) doesn't include the population mean. In practice, we never really know for sure if the interval we generate includes the population parameter of interest, since we only generate a single confidence interval. However, we have an impression of how likely it is, or how confident we can be, that the confidence interval includes the parameter of interest.

Note: when the sample size is relatively small ($n < {\sim}30$), it's probably more appropriate to generate confidence intervals based on the *t* distribution instead of the standard normal (*z*) distribution. The *t* distribution will be introduced in Chapter 5.

Final thoughts on confidence intervals

Confidence intervals are certainly worth reporting, even if just to highlight the fact that sampling error is built into every parameter we estimate. Expressing some degree of uncertainty is always a good idea when dealing with sample data.

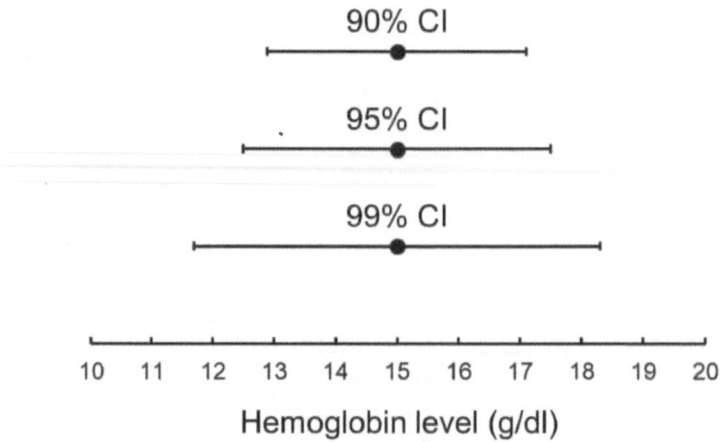

Figure 4.4 90%, 95%, and 99% confidence intervals (CIs) based on the hypothetical hemoglobin data. Notice that the intervals widen (i.e. less precision) as the confidence level increases.

I think it's helpful to consider how clinicians routinely apply the general concept of intervals in daily practice. For instance, imagine the scenario of an athlete asking their therapist when they can expect to return to sport following surgery. The therapist could give them a specific point estimate, such as '9 months', or a range, such as '6 to 12 months'. Obviously, the therapist's chances of correctly predicting the athlete's time of return to sport are better when they provide a range of months. The therapist could improve their chances of accurately predicting the athlete's return to sport timeline, and thus their confidence in their prediction, if they broadened the range (e.g. 3 to 24 months); however, at some point the lack of precision makes the estimate fairly useless.

Introduction to hypothesis testing

In addition to estimating population parameters, such as the population mean, inferential statistics are also used to test hypotheses. For example, we may want to know if a new treatment option is effective, if there is a relationship between variables, or whether groups of individuals differ with respect to a certain characteristic. Addressing any of these types of questions involves sampling from the relevant populations of interest, examining data from these samples, and then making a decision based on the available evidence. To reiterate, the objective of this chapter is simply to introduce the conceptual basis for hypothesis testing. For now, just focus on understanding the general idea. Additional detail will come later in the book.

Two competing hypotheses

A *scientific hypothesis* is essentially a proposed explanation for some observation. Hypothesis testing involves two competing hypotheses: the *null hypothesis*, which is typically denoted H_0 ('H-naught'), and the *alternative hypothesis*, which is typically denoted H_1.

The null hypothesis

The null hypothesis is the hypothesis that's tested statistically. Essentially, we examine evidence from our sample data to determine if it's sufficient to 'reject' (or '*null*ify') the null hypothesis. The null hypothesis will differ based on the specific type of statistical test; however, it generally states that there's no treatment effect, no relationship between variables, no difference between groups, and so on. In other words, the null hypothesis states that any observed effects are simply due to sampling error or 'chance'. When comparing two population means (population A, population B), the null hypothesis can be stated as:

$$H_0: \mu_A = \mu_B \quad \text{or} \quad H_0: \mu_A - \mu_B = 0$$

We can never really prove that the null hypothesis is true, since we aren't testing everyone in the population. Therefore, the terminology 'fail to reject' the null hypothesis is typically used when the evidence isn't sufficient to conclude that the findings are beyond what's likely to occur by chance. This terminology highlights the fact that concluding that there isn't enough evidence to reject the null hypothesis isn't equivalent to proving that the null hypothesis is true. The null hypothesis may still be false; however, the available evidence may have simply been too weak to convince us.

In hypothesis testing, we presume that the null hypothesis is true and then examine the available evidence based on the sample data to determine if it's strong enough for us to reject the null hypothesis. This is analogous to the legal principle that an accused individual is considered 'innocent until proven guilty'. At the beginning of a trial, the defendant is presumed to be innocent. During the trial, the prosecution must present evidence to reject this presumption and convince the jury that the defendant is guilty beyond a reasonable doubt (i.e. reject the presumption of innocence). If the prosecution presents weak evidence, the jury may decide that there's still reasonable doubt and acquit (i.e. fail to reject the presumption of innocence). This doesn't mean that the accused individual is innocent. Instead, the prosecutors simply failed to provide strong enough evidence to reject the presumption of innocence.

The alternative hypothesis

The *alternative hypothesis* contrasts with the null hypothesis and generally states that there is a treatment effect, relationship between variables, difference between groups, and so on. Again, the specifics will vary depending on the type of statistical test. While the null hypothesis is tested statistically, investigators are typically motivated to conduct a study by their belief in the alternative hypothesis, since they typically expect (or at least hope) to observe some type of effect, relationship, difference, and so on. Since the null hypothesis and alternative hypothesis are competing hypotheses, rejecting the null hypothesis results in accepting the alternative hypothesis.

The alternative hypothesis can either be *nondirectional* or *directional*. A nondirectional alternative hypothesis doesn't provide an anticipated direction of the effect, while a directional alternative hypothesis does. When comparing two population means (population A, population B), a nondirectional alternative hypothesis can be stated as:

$$H_1: \mu_A \neq \mu_B \quad \text{or} \quad H_1: \mu_A - \mu_B \neq 0$$

Whereas a directional alternative hypothesis can be stated as:

$$H_1: \mu_A > \mu_B \quad \text{or} \quad H_1: \mu_A - \mu_B > 0$$

or

$$H_1: \mu_A < \mu_B \quad \text{or} \quad H_1: \mu_A - \mu_B < 0$$

Notice that both the null and alternative hypotheses are expressed in terms of population parameters, not sample statistics, since our objective is to make inferences about the populations of interest.

Hypothesis testing outcomes

The results of a hypothesis test come down to one of two decisions: 1) reject the null hypothesis or 2) fail to reject the null hypothesis. It's essentially a 'black-or-white' conclusion that doesn't really allow for shades of gray (which many consider a critical shortcoming). We'll discuss how these decisions are made in the next section; however, let's start by discussing the outcomes in terms of their accuracy.

Type I and Type II errors

The conclusions made based on a hypothesis test can either be correct or incorrect. We are correct when we reject the null hypothesis when it's actually false or fail to reject the null hypothesis when it's actually true. In contrast, we can also be wrong in two different ways. A *Type I error* occurs when we reject the null hypothesis when it's actually true, and a *Type II error* occurs when we fail to reject the null hypothesis when it's actually false (Figure 4.5). While we never really know if we've committed an error, we can consider the potential for error in terms of their probabilities. We pay specific attention to the probability of a Type I error.

Hypothesis testing example

As we move forward in this chapter, let's apply the basic concepts of hypothesis testing to address a hypothetical research question. Imagine that we conduct a study to determine if individuals with low back pain exhibit poorer trunk muscle endurance than individuals

		Reality	
		Null hypothesis is true	Null hypothesis is false
Decision	Reject null hypothesis	**Type I error**	**Correct**
	Fail to reject null hypothesis	**Correct**	**Type II error**

Figure 4.5 Table highlighting each of the four potential scenarios whenever a hypothesis test is conducted. The columns under the 'Reality' heading represent what's actually true, while the rows next to the 'Decision' heading represent the conclusions made based on a hypothesis test.

without low back pain. Our hypothetical study includes a sample of individuals with low back pain (LBP group) and a sample of individuals without low back pain (control group). We assess the endurance of each subject's trunk extensor musculature using the Biering-Sorensen test (Biering-Sorensen, 1984). For the Biering-Sorensen test, the individual lies prone with their lower body secured to an exam table and their trunk extended off the edge of the table. A stopwatch is used to record how long the individual can isometrically maintain their trunk in a horizontal position, with a longer hold time reflecting better trunk muscle endurance.

Based on prior research and anecdotal evidence, we expect individuals with low back pain to exhibit poorer trunk muscle endurance (i.e. shorter hold times). In this case, we've proposed a directional alternative hypothesis (H_1: $\mu_{LBP} < \mu_{Control}$). However, we would test the null hypothesis, which is that there's no difference in hold times between individuals with low back pain and individuals without low back pain (H_0: $\mu_{LBP} = \mu_{Control}$).

Now imagine that the average hold time for the LBP group ($\bar{X}_{LBP}$) was 160 seconds, while the average hold time for the control group ($\bar{X}_{Control}$) was 175 seconds. This observed 15-second difference in sample means has two potential explanations:

1) the observed difference in sample means may be due to sampling error ('chance'). In other words, there's actually no difference in the average hold times for the populations of individuals with low back pain and individuals without low back pain. We just happened to sample individuals for the LBP group with atypically poor trunk muscle endurance and/or individuals for the control group with atypically good trunk muscle endurance. This explanation is consistent with the null hypothesis (H_0: $\mu_{LBP} = \mu_{Control}$).

2) the observed difference in sample means reflects a true difference in the average hold times for the populations of individuals with low back pain and individuals without low back pain. In other words, we observed a difference in sample means because there's actually a difference in the populations. This explanation is consistent with the alternative hypothesis (H_1: $\mu_{LBP} < \mu_{Control}$).

The evidence from our sample data will help us determine if it's reasonable to reject the null hypothesis and conclude that the observed difference in sample means isn't simply due to chance (explanation #2). Essentially, what we're trying to determine is whether the observed 15-second difference in the sample means provides strong enough evidence to convince us that there's a difference in the population means. Obviously, the greater the difference in sample means, the stronger the evidence that the population means differ. For instance, a 30-second difference in sample means (e.g. 145 seconds vs. 175 seconds) would provide more convincing evidence to reject the null hypothesis than a 15-second difference in sample means.

Sampling distribution – trunk endurance example

We've already discussed one type of sampling distribution in this chapter: the distribution of sample means. However, a hypothesis test that involves a comparison of two means is based on a slightly different type of sampling distribution, referred to as the *distribution of the differences in sample means*. The distribution of the differences in sample means is the result of repeatedly sampling from two populations, finding the difference between the sample means ($\bar{X}_{LBP} - \bar{X}_{Control}$), and organizing these differences into a distribution. Notice that it's conceptually the same as the distribution of sample means, except now we're working with the difference between two sample means instead of a single mean.

Now, remember that the null hypothesis states that there's no difference in the mean hold times for the populations (H_0: $\mu_A - \mu_B = 0$). Assuming this were true, we would expect the distribution of the differences in sample means to be normally distributed around a mean of

0, since $\mu_{LBP} - \mu_{Control}$ would equal 0. Some sample mean differences would overestimate the true difference in the population means, while others would underestimate the true difference in the population means because of sampling error; however, relatively large sample mean differences would be rare if the null hypothesis were true. Figure 4.6 includes a theoretical distribution of the differences in sample means based on the null hypothesis. The standard error of this distribution represents the expected sample-to-sample variability in sample mean differences. Notice that this distribution essentially maps out the probability associated with observing any sample mean difference, assuming the null hypothesis is true.

The *p*-value

A hypothesis test involves determining the probability of observing an effect at least as large as what would be observed if the null hypothesis were true. This probability is referred to as a *p-value*. *p*-values are reported in almost every research article you'll read. Therefore, it's important to appreciate what a *p*-value represents and what it doesn't.

Let's revisit the low back pain example. Remember that we observed a sample mean difference of 15 seconds ($\overline{X}_{LBP} - \overline{X}_{Control} = -15$ seconds). In this case, the *p*-value would reflect the probability of observing a 15-second sample mean difference if there were actually no difference in the populations' hold times ($\mu_{LBP} = \mu_{Control}$). Finding the *p*-value would involve determining where our observed sample mean difference ($\overline{X}_{LBP} - \overline{X}_{Control} = -15$ seconds) falls

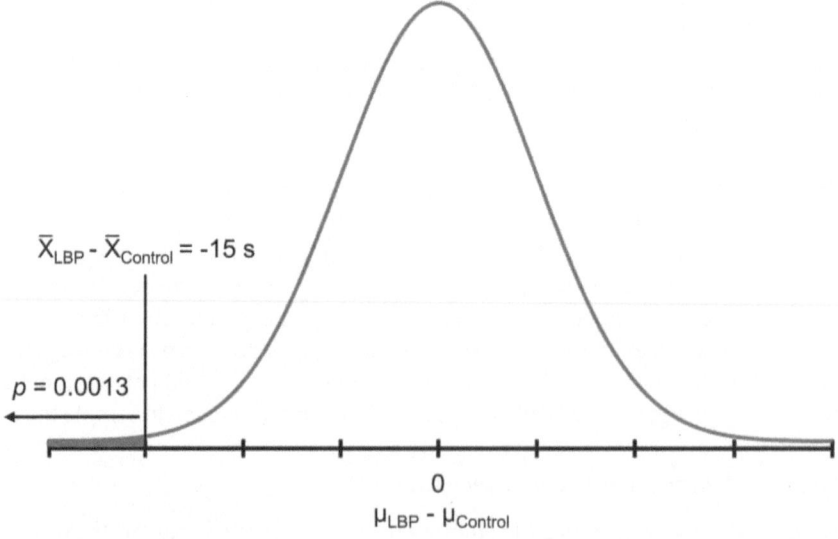

Figure 4.6 Theoretical distribution of the differences in sample means based on the assumption that the null hypothesis is true ($\mu_{LBP} - \mu_{Control} = 0$). Notice that the distribution is normally distributed around a population mean difference of 0, since the null hypothesis states that the population means are equal. The vertical line represents where our observed sample mean difference (-15 seconds, $z = -3.0$) is located within the distribution. The shaded area represents the proportion of sample mean differences that would be expected to be at least this far below the population mean difference of 0. In this case, the probability (*p*-value) of observing a sample mean difference of 15 seconds, if the null hypothesis were true, is 0.0013 (or 0.0026 if both tails are considered).

within a theoretical distribution of differences in sample means based on the assumption that the null hypothesis is true. Let's say that the sampling distribution has a standard error of 5 seconds. If we calculated a z-score, we would find that our observed difference in sample means is located 3.0 standard errors below the center of our theoretical sampling distribution ($z = \dfrac{\bar{X}_{LBP} - \bar{X}_{Control}}{\text{standard error}} = -3.0$).* Notice that this is well into the lower tail of the distribution (Figure 4.6). Using the standard normal distribution table (Appendix C), we could find the proportion of scores that are at least this far into the lower tail of the distribution (Figure 4.6 – shaded region). In this case, only 0.13% of sample mean differences would be expected to be at least this far into the lower tail of the distribution, assuming the null hypothesis were true. In other words, the probability of observing a sample mean difference this extreme, or more extreme, assuming the null hypothesis is true, is 0.0013 ($p = 0.0013$). This probability in the tail of the sampling distribution is the p-value.** In general, it appears that it would be quite unlikely to observe a sample mean difference of 15 seconds if the null hypothesis were true.

* **Note:** z served as our 'test statistic' in this example. We'll discuss other types of test statistics (t statistics, F statistics) in upcoming chapters.

** **Note:** the probabilities in both tails of the distribution are typically combined ('two-tailed test'). In this case, the p-value would be 0.0026 (0.0013 + 0.0013). Two-tailed vs. one-tailed tests will be discussed in Chapter 5.

Hypothesis testing logic

The logic behind a hypothesis test is as follows: if the observed effect is unlikely under the assumption that the null hypothesis is true (i.e. low p-value), then the null hypothesis is likely false, and we should reject the null hypothesis. In contrast, if the observed effect is likely to occur under the assumption that the null hypothesis is true, then the null hypothesis is likely true, and we shouldn't reject the null hypothesis. In essence, the closer the p-value gets to 0, the stronger the evidence against the null hypothesis.* However, the question becomes: when is the evidence strong enough to convince us to reject the null hypothesis?

* **Note:** a p-value can never reach 0, regardless of how extreme an observed result may be. There's always some chance that the observed effect was due to sampling error. Therefore, you should never report a p-value as 0. That said, some statistical analysis software packages, including SPSS, report the p-value as 0 when it's below a certain threshold. For example, when the p-value is less than 0.001, SPSS reports the p-value (or *Sig.* in SPSS terminology) as .000.

Alpha levels

As we've discussed, a hypothesis test comes down to a decision to either reject the null hypothesis or fail to reject the null hypothesis. Prior to conducting an analysis, we establish an *alpha (α) level* (or *significance level*) that essentially serves as the 'line in the sand' for determining whether to reject the null hypothesis. If our observed p-value is below our predefined alpha level ($p < α$), we reject the null hypothesis; if not ($p \geq α$), we don't. The alpha level is conventionally set at a value of 0.05. In this case, we reject the null hypothesis if the p-value is less than 0.05.

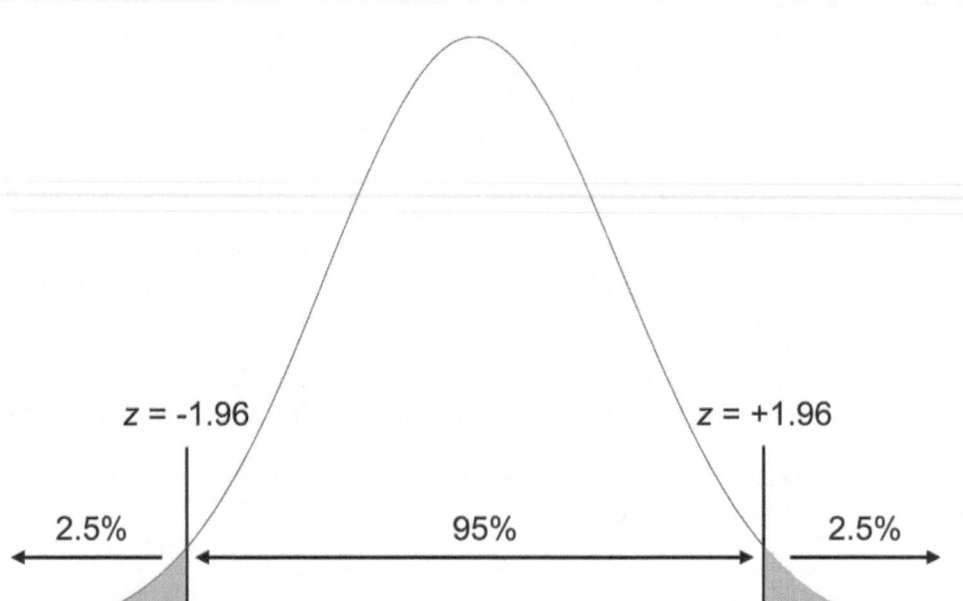

Figure 4.7 Sampling distribution based on the assumption that the null hypothesis is true. When the sampling distribution takes on the shape of the standard normal (*z*) distribution, such as in this example, the critical values are ±1.96 when alpha is 0.05. Notice that when the alpha level is set at 0.05, only 5% of all samples would be expected to produce a test statistic beyond the critical values if the null hypothesis were true. Therefore, observing a test statistic beyond these critical values provides strong evidence to reject the null hypothesis, since it would be unlikely to observe these values by chance. When the test statistic lies beyond the critical values (shaded regions of the distribution), the *p*-value will be less than alpha.

Remember that the *p*-value in our fictitious low back pain example was 0.0013 ($p = 0.0013$). Therefore, based on an alpha level of 0.05, we would reject the null hypothesis and conclude that the difference in hold times is statistically significant. In other words, the observed difference in sample means is probably not due to chance alone, and the population means likely differ.

Note: the alpha level establishes critical values in the sampling distribution that separate observations that are unlikely to occur if the null hypothesis were true (tails of the distribution) from those that would commonly occur by chance alone (body of the distribution) (Figure 4.7). When the test statistic falls beyond these critical values, the *p*-value will be less than α, and we reject the null hypothesis.

The alpha level and Type I error

The alpha level provides us with a degree of control over the risk of committing a Type I error. When the alpha level is set at 0.05, we are accepting a 5% risk of committing a Type I error (i.e. falsely rejecting the null hypothesis when it's actually true). When we conclude that a finding is 'statistically significant', we're essentially signifying that the evidence from our sample data is strong enough to outweigh the potential risk of Type I error that we deemed acceptable prior to the analysis.

Choosing an alpha level

As we've discussed, the alpha level is conventionally set at 0.05. But why 0.05? That's a great question, without a good answer. Surprisingly, the conventional alpha level of 0.05 is an arbitrary standard. The origins of this conventional alpha level of 0.05 are highlighted nicely in a paper by Kennedy-Shaffer (2019). Despite the arbitrary nature, an alpha level of 0.05 has become a well-accepted standard.

While 0.05 tends to be the 'default', there are instances where investigators will use a different alpha level, such as 0.10 or 0.01. Using a higher alpha level, such as 0.10, creates a less stringent cutoff, where the evidence doesn't need to be quite as strong in order to reject the null hypothesis. For instance, let's say we conduct a test to compare two means, and the *p*-value is 0.06. Based on the conventional alpha level of 0.05, this difference wouldn't be statistically significant, since 0.06 isn't less than 0.05. However, if we had chosen to set our alpha level at 0.10, this difference would be statistically significant, since 0.06 is less than 0.10. The benefit of using a higher alpha level is that it reduces the risk of Type II error (failing to reject the null hypothesis when it's false); however, the tradeoff is an increased risk of Type I error (falsely rejecting the null hypothesis). Investigators will sometimes choose to use a higher alpha level, such as 0.10, when they're conducting preliminary analyses to identify factors to consider in subsequent rounds of analyses. Their logic is that they don't want to falsely dismiss certain factors in their preliminary analysis that could prove to be important in future analyses.

Conversely, investigators may choose to use a lower alpha level, such as 0.01, if they want to create a more stringent threshold for statistical significance. When the alpha level is 0.01, the evidence needs to be stronger in order to reject the null hypothesis. Investigators may choose to use a lower alpha level if they want to be more confident that any results deemed 'statistically significant' aren't simply a byproduct of sampling error. For example, imagine that we're studying an intervention with potentially positive effects but also significant risks, side effects, or costs. In this case, we may decide to set our alpha level at 0.01 in order to reduce the risk of committing a Type I error and falsely concluding that the intervention is effective when it actually isn't. Of course, there's a tradeoff in this situation as well. While the lower alpha level reduces the risk of Type I error, it increases the risk of Type II error (i.e. concluding that the intervention isn't effective when it actually is).

Regardless of what alpha level we decide to set, this decision should be made before the analysis is conducted ('*a priori*'). You can imagine the issues that could arise if the alpha level were established after looking at the results of an analysis. For instance, observing a *p*-value of 0.06 could sway us to select an alpha level of 0.10, even if there isn't strong justification for doing so. It's best to avoid this temptation and clearly define what will be considered statistically significant before conducting an analysis. I like to think of it as establishing the 'rules of the game' before play begins.

Criticisms of null hypothesis significance testing

If the logic behind 'null hypothesis significance testing' seems somewhat absurd to you, take solace in the fact that you're certainly not alone. Null hypothesis significance testing has many critics. In fact, some have proposed completely abandoning this approach (e.g.

McShane et al., 2019). One of the main criticisms of conventional null hypothesis significance testing is that it encourages 'black-or-white' thinking, where findings are either statistically significant ($p < \alpha$) or they aren't ($p \geq \alpha$). The notion does seem rather silly if you think about it. There isn't much of a difference between a p-value of 0.049 and a p-value of 0.051, and yet these results lead to completely different conclusions. Opponents of null hypothesis significance testing argue that we should consider effects on more of a continuum (e.g. trivial, small, moderate, large), instead of simply relying on a strict, and arbitrary, threshold. This concept is explored in greater depth in Chapter 13 ('Effect Sizes and Confidence Intervals').

Another criticism of null hypothesis significance testing is that p-values are heavily influenced by sample size. Even if the magnitude of the effect is the same, larger samples will produce lower p-values compared to smaller samples. For example, imagine that we conducted two studies comparing hold times of individuals with and without low back pain. One study included 100 subjects per group, and the other study included 20 subjects per group. Even if both studies showed a sample mean difference of 15 seconds, the p-value for the study with samples of 100 would be much lower than that of the study with samples of 20. As a result, studies with relatively large sample sizes may report statistically significant results even when the effects are relatively small. In contrast, the findings of studies with relatively small sample sizes may not be statistically significant, even when the observed effects are large.

Finally, it's important to realize that there's nothing inherently 'significant' about statistical significance. What I mean is that results that are statistically significant may be of little clinical importance or have minimal 'real-world' value. For example, imagine that we conduct a study to examine the effects of a new, 'accelerated', post-operative rehabilitation protocol on shoulder motion in individuals undergoing rotator cuff repair. As part of the study, we compare shoulder flexion range of motion for a group of patients who completed a conventional protocol and a group of patients who completed the accelerated protocol. Let's say that, on average, the subjects who completed the accelerated protocol exhibited an additional 3° of shoulder flexion motion at the time of discharge, compared to those who completed the conventional protocol. While this 3° difference may be statistically significant, clinicians would probably argue (and rightly so) that this difference in shoulder motion is only meaningful if it results in better shoulder function. When we say that an effect is 'statistically significant', we mean that it's probably not due to chance alone. It's certainly possible for findings to be statistically significant but not important.

So why should I learn this stuff?

While null hypothesis significance testing certainly has its limitations and harsh critics, the scientific community has adopted this approach as the norm to some extent (for better or worse). As a result, it's important to understand the basic concepts so you can critically evaluate primary medical literature. That said, it's also important to appreciate that null hypothesis significance testing is far from an exact science.

Statistical power

So far, we've primarily focused on Type I errors; however, we also need to be conscious of the potential for Type II errors. The probability of committing a Type II error is typically denoted as β ('beta'). *Statistical power* is the probability of rejecting the null hypothesis when it's actually false ($1 - \beta$). In other words, statistical power is the probability of not committing a Type II error.

The concept of statistical power is expanded upon in Chapter 14 ('Sample Size Estimation'). However, at this point, it's good to consider factors that influence the statistical power of a hypothesis test. Some important factors to consider are:

1) The alpha level – as we've discussed, the alpha level will influence the risk of committing a Type II error and thus statistical power. A higher alpha level (e.g. $\alpha = 0.10$), will reduce the risk of committing a Type II error and therefore increase statistical power. In contrast, a lower alpha level (e.g. $\alpha = 0.01$) will reduce statistical power. Essentially, the 'stricter' our cutoff for determining statistical significance, the lower our statistical power.

2) The sample size – as sample size increases, so does statistical power. As a result, studies with larger samples are more likely to produce statistically significant findings. You may hear investigators speak of a study being 'underpowered'. In this case, they're likely referring to the study not having a sufficient number of subjects.

3) The effect size in the population – the larger the effect in the population, the greater the statistical power. For example, if there were a 30-second difference in hold times between the populations of individuals with and without low back pain, it would be much easier to identify a statistically significant difference compared to if there were only a 15-second difference. Of the three factors noted here, the effect size is the only factor that investigators really have no control over.

Final comments

As I mentioned earlier in the introduction, the objective of this chapter wasn't to examine all of the nuances of inferential statistics. In fact, many subtle details were left out of this chapter in an attempt to promote clarity. My goal was simply to introduce some of the core concepts and general logic behind inferential statistics. Subsequent chapters will continue to build on these concepts.

5 *t*-tests

Chapter Objectives

The objectives of this chapter are to . . .

1) describe the general purpose of a *t*-test
2) provide examples of the types of clinical research questions that *t*-tests can be used to address
3) differentiate between independent *t*-tests and paired *t*-tests
4) explain the conceptual basis for independent *t*-tests and paired *t*-tests
5) introduce the *t* distribution and the *t* statistic
6) describe how confidence intervals can be generated to estimate the difference in population means or the mean of the differences in the population
7) differentiate between one-tailed and two-tailed *t*-tests
8) point out key assumptions that should be met in order to conduct a *t*-test
9) demonstrate how to conduct independent *t*-tests and paired *t*-tests using SPSS and Excel software

Introduction

Many clinical research questions involve comparison of the average performance of two independent groups of individuals. For example, we may be interested in comparing the outcomes of patients who underwent two different types of surgical procedures or the characteristics of individuals with and without a certain disorder (i.e. case-control study design). In other instances, we may want to compare the average performance of a single group of individuals in two different conditions or at two time points (e.g. pre- vs. post-intervention). Each of these scenarios involves comparison of two means (e.g. group 1 vs. group 2, condition 1 vs. condition 2, pre vs. post). A *t*-test is a type of hypothesis test that's often used in these circumstances.

Two different types of *t*-tests are commonly utilized. An *independent t-test* (also referred to as an *unpaired t-test*) is used when comparing two distinct groups of subjects (i.e. *independent* samples). For example, Ireland et al. (2003) conducted a study to examine whether women with patellofemoral pain tend to have weaker hip musculature than women without patellofemoral pain. In this case, they used an independent *t*-test to compare hip strength, since their study included two separate groups of subjects (women with patellofemoral pain, women without patellofemoral pain). This type of study is often described as a *between-subjects design*, since the comparison is *between* two different groups of subjects.

DOI: 10.4324/9781003179757-5

In contrast, a *paired t-test* (also referred to as a *dependent t-test*) is used when comparing two different conditions or time points in a single group of subjects. For example, Cholewicki et al. (2007) conducted a study to examine the effects of a lumbosacral orthosis on trunk muscle activity. As part of their study, a group of subjects sat both with and without support from the orthosis. Paired *t*-tests were used to compare trunk muscle activity for the two conditions (with orthosis, without orthosis). A paired *t*-test was appropriate in this case, since muscle activity was recorded in both conditions for a single group of subjects. This type of study is often described as a *repeated measures design* or a *within-subjects design* since *repeated measurements* are taken *within* the same group of subjects.

Learning Activity 5.1 includes additional examples to help you differentiate between independent and paired *t*-tests. Box 5.1 shares the story of the origin of the *t*-test. It's actually quite interesting.

Learning Activity 5.1

Following are five examples of studies that included either an independent *t*-test or a paired *t*-test as part of their analysis. Based on the brief description of each study, try to predict which type of *t*-test the investigators used. The answers are provided at the end of the chapter.

Garcia-Pinillos et al. (2020) conducted a study to examine the effects of fatigue on running mechanics. Their study included a group of 22 male endurance runners. Each subject had their running mechanics analyzed before (non-fatigued) and immediately after (fatigued) completion of a 60-minute run. Running mechanics were compared for the non-fatigued and fatigued conditions.

Kobayashi et al. (2014) conducted a study to compare the gait patterns of older adults who had recently experienced a fall vs. those who hadn't recently fallen. Their study included 18 subjects who had experienced a fall in the past 12 months (fallers) and 19 subjects who hadn't fallen in the past 12 months (non-fallers). The investigators analyzed each subject's gait pattern and compared the walking kinematics of the fallers and non-fallers.

Koontz et al. (2002) conducted a study to compare upper extremity mechanics during wheelchair propulsion at two different speeds. Their study included 27 subjects who used a wheelchair as their primary mode of mobility due to a spinal cord injury. Each subject's upper extremity mechanics were analyzed as they propelled themselves at speeds of 0.9 m/s (slower condition) and 1.8 m/s (faster condition). Upper extremity mechanics were compared for the slower and faster conditions.

Cheung et al. (2016) conducted a study to compare intrinsic foot muscle volume in healthy runners and runners with plantar fasciitis. Their study included 10 runners with plantar fasciitis and 10 runners without plantar fasciitis ('healthy' runners). They measured the volume of each runner's intrinsic foot muscles using MRI. The intrinsic foot muscle volume of the runners with plantar fasciitis and the healthy runners were compared.

Yavuz et al. (2015) conducted a study to compare muscle activity during performance of front squats vs. back squats. Their study included 12 male subjects. Each subject performed front squats and back squats while their lower extremity and trunk muscle activity was recorded via electromyography. Muscle activity was compared for various muscles during performance of the front and back squats.

<hr>

Box 5.1 – Origin of the 'Student's' *t*-test

You may see *t*-tests referred to as 'Student's' *t*-tests. The origin of this name is actually pretty interesting. William Sealy Gosset worked for Guinness Brewery in Dublin, Ireland, during the early 1900s. One of his primary responsibilities was to conduct tests to ensure that the beer being produced met quality standards. As part of his job, Gosset worked to develop analysis techniques that could be applied with small samples. These techniques were quite novel, since most statistical procedures used at the time required relatively large samples.

Gosset believed that his techniques could benefit others and hoped to publish his work. At the time, Guinness didn't allow employees to publish their findings, as they were concerned about revealing trade secrets to competitors. However, they agreed to allow Gosset to publish his techniques as long as he used a pseudonym. Gosset agreed and used the pseudonym *Student* in his publications. His paper, 'The Probable Error of a Mean', which was published in the journal *Biometrika* in 1908, provided the basis for the *t* distribution and thus the *t*-test, hence the term 'Student's' *t*-test.

<hr>

Chapter 1 introduced the concept of independent variables and their corresponding levels. This concept will be applied throughout this section of the book, since identifying the number of independent variables and their levels can be helpful in determining which type of test to conduct. Both independent and paired *t*-tests include a single independent variable with two levels. Chapter 6 will discuss tests that are appropriate when there's a single independent variable with more than two levels (e.g. group 1, group 2, group 3), and Chapter 7 will introduce tests that are appropriate where there is more than one independent variable.

Basis for the independent *t*-test

To help conceptualize the basis for the independent *t*-test, let's consider a study conducted by Eitzen et al. (2012). As part of their study, these investigators compared the gait speeds of individuals with hip osteoarthritis (OA group) and individuals without hip osteoarthritis (control group) (note: they also examined several other variables). Their study involved two distinct populations: those with hip osteoarthritis and those without hip osteoarthritis. Optimally, this question would be addressed by recording the gait speeds of everyone from these populations and then comparing the population means. However, this is obviously not feasible. Instead, the investigators drew samples from the respective populations and compared the mean gait speeds from these samples. The sample means for the OA group and the control group were 1.53 m/s and 1.65 m/s, respectively. This 0.12 m/s sample mean difference has two potential explanations:

1) the observed difference in sample means may simply be due to sampling error ('chance'), which is consistent with the null hypothesis (H_0: $\mu_{OA} = \mu_{Control}$).
2) the observed difference in sample means may reflect a true difference in the gait speeds of the two populations, which is consistent with the alternative hypothesis (H_1: $\mu_{OA} \neq \mu_{Control}$).

Let's elaborate on this concept a bit. While the observed difference in sample means suggests that individuals with hip osteoarthritis walk slower than individuals without hip osteoarthritis, it's possible that this observed difference in gait speeds is simply due to chance (explanation #1). In other words, there may actually be no real difference in the average gait speeds of the populations; however, the investigators could have just happened to sample individuals with atypically slow gait speeds for the OA group and/or atypically fast gait speeds for the control group. When conducting an independent t-test, we're essentially examining the evidence from our sample data to determine if it's strong enough to reject the null hypothesis and conclude that the observed difference in sample means isn't simply due to chance alone. Figure 5.1 includes a diagram to help demonstrate how a difference in sample means can arise by chance, even when there's no difference in the population means.

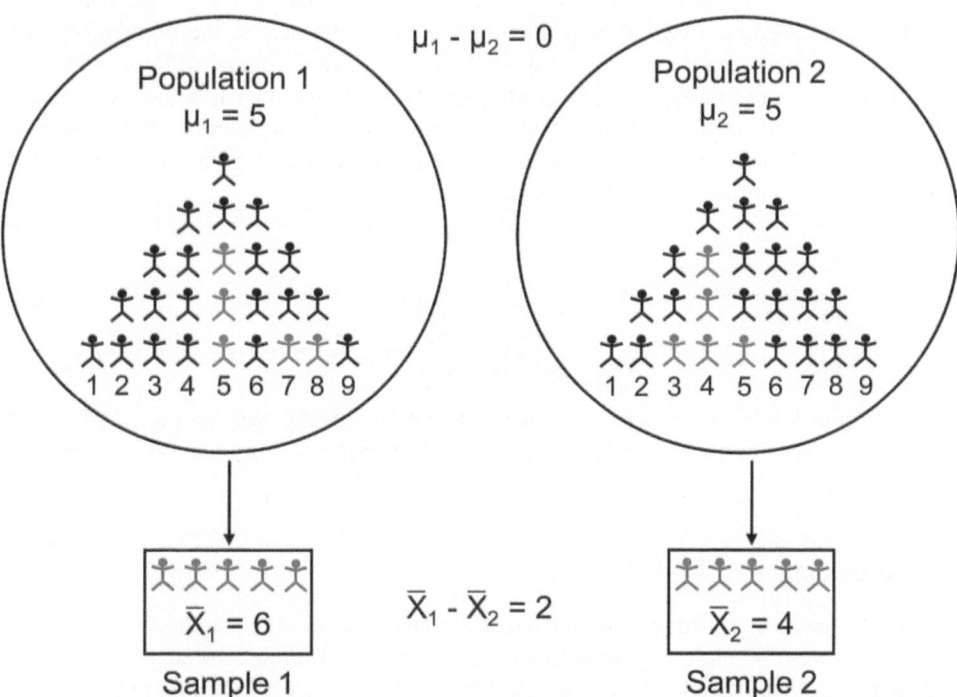

Figure 5.1 Two hypothetical populations, each composed of 25 individuals. The mean (μ) for both populations is equal to 5. As a result, there's no difference in the population means ($\mu_1 - \mu_2 = 0$). A sample of five individuals (gray figures) is selected from each of the populations, and sample means ($\overline{X}$) are calculated. The observed difference in sample means is 2 ($\overline{X}_1 - \overline{X}_2 = 2$), even though the difference in the population means is 0. Notice that in this case, a difference in sample means was observed simply by chance, as there was no real difference in the population means.

Sampling distribution – independent t-test

Chapter 4 introduced the conceptual basis for the *distribution of the differences in sample means*. Remember that the distribution of the differences in sample means is the sampling distribution that would result if we repeatedly sampled from two populations, found the difference in the sample means ($\overline{X}_1 - \overline{X}_2$), and organized these differences into a distribution. While we don't actually go through the process of repeatedly sampling and constructing this distribution, we can contrive a theoretical representation of this distribution using sample data and our knowledge of the typical characteristics of sampling distributions. A *t*-test essentially involves determining where our observed difference in sample means is located within a theoretical distribution of differences in sample means that's based on the assumption that the null hypothesis is true.

Consider that if the null hypothesis were true, the distribution of the differences in sample means would be normally distributed around 0, since $\mu_1 - \mu_2$ would equal 0. Remember that the standard error (often referred to as the *standard error of the differences* in this context) reflects the variability, or spread, of the sampling distribution. In this case, the standard error essentially represents how the differences in sample means are expected to vary about the true difference in the population means. A relatively small standard error indicates that most sample mean differences closely approximate the true difference in the population means, whereas a relatively large standard error indicates that sample mean differences fluctuate more from sample to sample (i.e. greater sampling error). Equation 5.1 includes a form of the equation that can be used to estimate the *standard error of the differences in sample means* ($s_{\overline{X}_1 - \overline{X}_2}$), when the group sizes are equal ($n_1 = n_2$). Essentially, this equation sums the standard errors from each sample.

Equation 5.1

$$s_{\overline{X}_1 - \overline{X}_2} = \sqrt{\frac{s_1^2}{n_1} + \frac{s_2^2}{n_2}}$$

In Equation 5.1, s_1 and s_2 are the standard deviations for the two samples, and n_1 and n_2 are the respective sample sizes. Note that a modified version of this equation is needed when group sizes differ ($n_1 \neq n_2$).

The t distribution

Population standard deviations are needed to directly calculate the standard error; however, these values are rarely known. To work around this, we can estimate the standard error using sample standard deviations. When the standard error is estimated based on sample standard deviations, the *t distribution* is typically used to represent a sampling distribution (hence the terminology '*t*-test') instead of the normal (*z*) distribution. This is done to account for the fact that the estimated standard error will likely underestimate the true standard error.

The *t* distribution is essentially a flatter version of the normal distribution, with more area in the tails and a lower peak. Imagine putting your palm on top of the normal distribution and pushing down so that the distribution bulges out in the tails. That's essentially the shape that the *t* distribution takes on. The *t* distribution is actually a family of distributions, whose exact shapes are dependent on the *degrees of freedom*, which is related to the sample size (see Box 5.2).* The more degrees of freedom, the more the *t* distribution resembles the shape of the normal distribution (Figure 5.2).

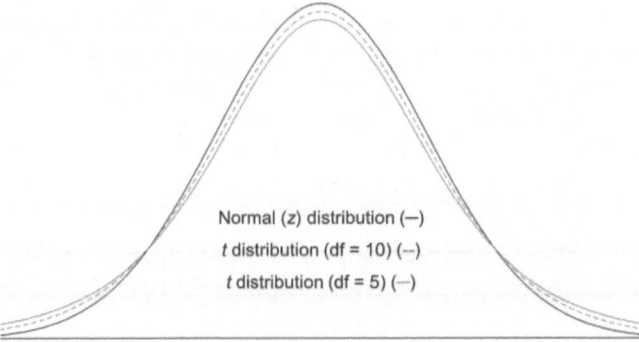

Normal (z) distribution (—)
t distribution (df = 10) (--)
t distribution (df = 5) (--)

Figure 5.2 Plot including the normal (z) distribution, as well as *t* distributions based on 5 degrees of freedom (df = 5) and 10 degrees of freedom (df = 10). Notice that the area in the tails of the *t* distribution is greater when there are fewer degrees of freedom.

Box 5.2 – Degrees of freedom

In statistics, the *degrees of freedom* are the number of values that are free to vary when estimating a parameter. In most cases, the degrees of freedom will be equal to the sample size, minus the number of parameters that need to be estimated. Let's start with a simple example. Imagine that we're estimating a population mean based on data from a sample of five subjects ($n = 5$) and that the sample mean for these five subjects is equal to 10 ($\bar{X} = 10$). The scores for the first four subjects are 8, 14, 12, and 9. In this case, in order for the mean to equal 10, the fifth subject's score would need to be 7 ([8 + 14 + 12 + 9 + 7 = 50; 50/5 = 10). As a result, four of the scores can take on any value (i.e. 'are free to vary'), while the fifth score is constrained (i.e. it can only be 7 if the mean is 10). In this case, the degrees of freedom would be the number of observations (n), minus 1 (5 – 1 = 4 degrees of freedom), since we are trying to estimate a single parameter (μ).

For an independent *t*-test, two parameters need to be estimated (μ_1, μ_2); therefore, the degrees of freedom will be equal to $(n_1 - 1) + (n_2 - 1)$. For instance, a study conducted by Eitzen et al. (2012) included 22 subjects in the control group and 48 subjects in the OA group. Therefore, the degrees of freedom associated with their independent *t*-test was 68 [(22 – 1) + (48 – 1) = 68].

For a paired *t*-test, only one parameter needs to be estimated (μ_D); therefore, the degrees of freedom will be equal to $n - 1$. For instance, a study conducted by Kaji et al. (2010) included 17 subjects. Therefore, the degrees of freedom associated with their paired *t*-test was 16 (17 – 1 = 16).

---

* Note: the degrees of freedom will depend on the specific type of statistical test. The degrees of freedom associated with a test are often reported in the results. Fortunately, most statistical analysis packages, such as SPSS, provide the degrees of freedom for you. The general concept of degrees of freedom is discussed in Box 5.2.

The t *statistic*

The t statistic captures the location of our observed difference in sample means within a t distribution that's based on the assumption that the null hypothesis is true (H_0: $\mu_1 = \mu_2$). Equation 5.2 includes a standard form of the equation for the t statistic for an independent t-test. The numerator is the observed difference in the sample means ($\bar{X}_1 - \bar{X}_2$), while the denominator is the standard error of the differences in sample means ($s_{\bar{X}_1 - \bar{X}_2}$). Remember that the standard error represents the variability of a sampling distribution. Therefore, the t statistic essentially represents how many standard errors the observed difference in sample means is from 0. Note that the order in which the means are subtracted is arbitrary; however, it will influence the sign of the t statistic. The t statistic can be positive or negative.

Equation 5.2

$$t \text{ statistic} = \frac{\bar{X}_1 - \bar{X}_2}{s_{\bar{X}_1 - \bar{X}_2}}$$

Assuming the null hypothesis were true, we would expect most sample mean differences to be located in the center of the t distribution (t statistic close to 0), with fewer sample mean differences in the tails of the distribution. Therefore, if we observe a t statistic that falls into the outer tails of the distribution (either in the upper or lower tail), it provides evidence to suggest that the null hypothesis is false, since it would be unlikely to observe a difference in sample means this extreme if the null hypothesis were true.

Now, let's consider the results of the study conducted by Eitzen et al. (2012). Remember that the average gait speed for their OA group was 1.53 m/s, and the average gait speed for their control group was 1.65 m/s. Their estimated standard error ($s_{\bar{X}_1 - \bar{X}_2}$) was 0.038 m/s. Therefore, the t statistic associated with their observed difference in sample means was −3.16 ($t = \dfrac{1.53 - 1.65}{0.038} = -3.16$). This t statistic is located in the far lower tail of the t distribution (Figure 5.3). As a result, it appears that observing a sample mean difference of 0.12 m/s would be quite rare if the null hypothesis were true.

Another way to conceptualize the t *statistic*

Conceptually, you can also think of the t statistic as a metric that quantifies the degree of separation between the two sample distributions by quantifying the ratio of the difference between the group means relative to variability within the groups. To help visualize this, examine the distributions in Figure 5.4. Both subplot A and subplot B include distributions of scores for two samples of subjects. Notice that in subplot A, the variability among subjects' scores within the groups is small compared to the difference between the groups. In this case, we would be fairly confident that there's actually a difference between the populations from which these subjects were sampled. Now consider subplot B. The difference in the sample means is the same; however, there's much more variability within the groups, resulting in more overlap among the distributions. In this case, we would be less confident that there's a difference in the population means. This ratio of the difference in the group means relative to the variability within the groups is what the t statistic essentially captures. The more the t statistic deviates from 0, the more separation between the sample distributions, and thus, the more likely it is that the population means differ.

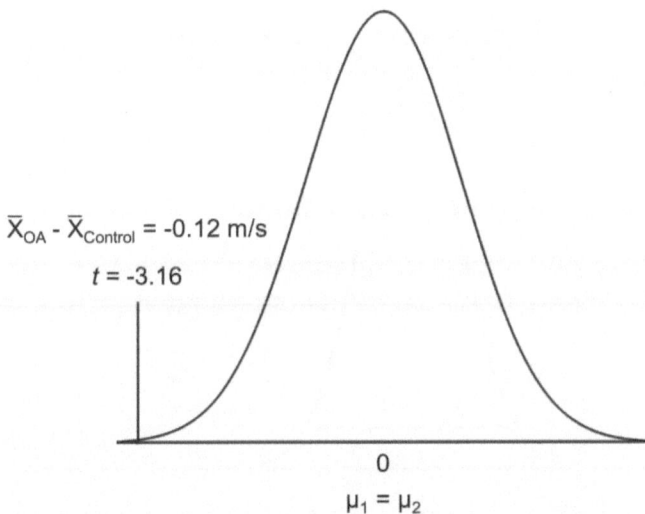

$\overline{X}_{OA} - \overline{X}_{Control} = -0.12$ m/s

$t = -3.16$

0

$\mu_1 = \mu_2$

Figure 5.3 Theoretical distribution of the differences in sample means based on the assumption that the null hypothesis is true ($\mu_1 - \mu_2 = 0$). Notice that the observed difference in sample means of –0.12 m/s is located in the extreme lower tail of the distribution ($t = -3.16$). As a result, it would be quite unlikely to observe a difference in sample means this large by chance alone.

Statistical significance

An independent *t*-test will produce a *p*-value that reflects the probability of observing a difference in sample means as extreme, or more extreme, than what would be observed if the null hypothesis were true (note: the conceptual basis for the *p*-value was discussed in Chapter 4). This *p*-value is the probability that lands in the tails of the distribution, beyond the location of the observed *t* statistic (Figure 5.3).

We compare this *p*-value to a predetermined alpha level (α) in order to determine if the observed difference in sample means provides strong enough evidence to reject the null hypothesis. In this case, the alpha level essentially serves as a cutoff point for determining whether the observed difference in sample means is large enough to conclude that the population means differ. If the *p*-value is less than alpha ($p < \alpha$), we reject the null hypothesis and conclude that the difference in sample means is 'statistically significant'. In other words, the observed difference in sample means likely reflects a true difference in the population means. If the *p*-value is greater than or equal to alpha ($p \geq \alpha$), we conclude that the evidence isn't strong enough to reject the null hypothesis (i.e. the difference in sample means isn't large enough for us to conclude that the population means differ).

Note: the alpha level establishes critical values in the *t* distribution that define when the *t* statistic is extreme enough to reject the null hypothesis. When the *t* statistic falls beyond these critical values, the *p*-value will be less than α, so we reject the null hypothesis. Appendix D includes a table of *t* critical values.

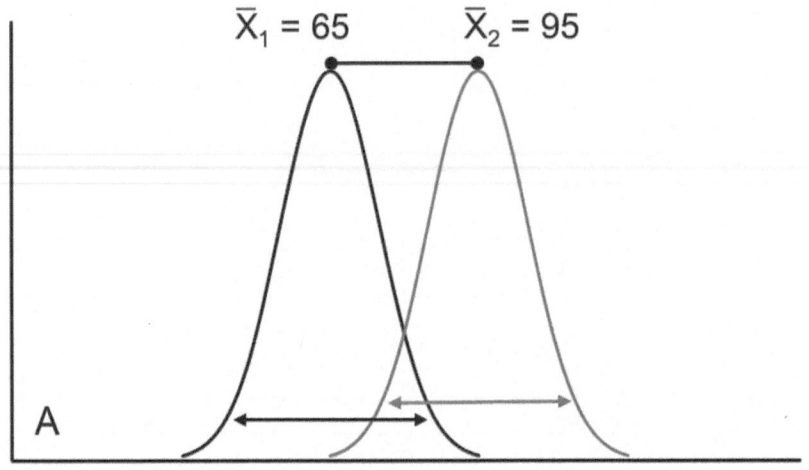

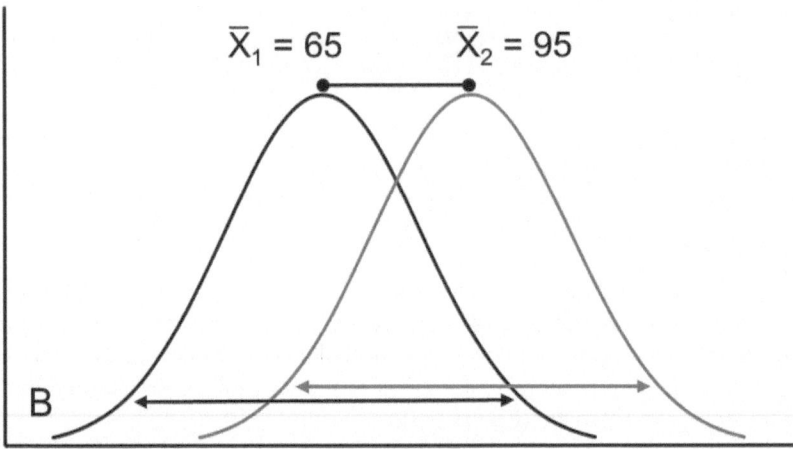

Figure 5.4 Both subplot A (top) and subplot B (bottom) include fictitious distributions of data for two separate samples. In each case, the difference in the sample means ($\overline{X}_1 - \overline{X}_2$) equals 30. However, there is greater separation between the distributions in subplot A, since there's less variance within the groups. Note that the arrows highlight the within-group variance.

The *p*-value based on the *t*-test conducted by Eitzen et al. (2012) was 0.002 ($p = 0.002$), which indicates that if the null hypothesis were true, only 0.2% of all differences in sample means would be expected to be as extreme, or more extreme, than what was observed. Therefore, it appears that it would be quite unlikely to observe a difference in gait speeds of 0.12 m/s by chance alone if the null hypothesis were true. The investigators set their alpha level at 0.05. Since their observed *p*-value ($p = 0.002$) was less than their predefined alpha level ($\alpha = 0.05$), they concluded that the difference in gait speeds was statistically significant. In other words, the observed difference in gait speeds is probably not due to chance alone, and the population means likely differ.

Comparing differences in change scores

In some instances, independent *t*-tests are used to compare the changes exhibited by two different groups of subjects. For example, we may have an experimental group that receives treatment and a control group that doesn't. Or we may have two groups that receive different types of treatment. In these instances, we can calculate *change scores* that reflect the changes exhibited from baseline (pre) to the end of the study period (post) (change score = post – pre). We can then conduct an independent *t*-test to compare these change scores in order to determine if there was a significant difference in how the groups changed over time.

For example, Yavuzer et al. (2008) conducted a study to examine the effects of mirror therapy on upper extremity motor function in individuals with hemiparesis following a stroke. They randomly allocated subjects to either a control group that received conventional rehabilitation or to an experimental group that received conventional rehabilitation, plus mirror therapy training. They used independent *t*-tests to compare the changes in upper extremity motor function (based on the change scores) exhibited by the groups over a 4-week period. In this case, the null hypothesis was that there would be no difference in the changes exhibited by the groups (i.e. the means for the change scores are equal). Their results indicated that the experimental group (conventional rehabilitation + mirror therapy) demonstrated greater improvements in upper extremity function compared to the control group (conventional rehabilitation only) (i.e. they rejected the null hypothesis).

There are other ways to address this type of question (e.g. mixed model ANOVA – Chapter 7; one-way ANCOVA – Chapter 15); however, this approach of using independent *t*-tests to compare change scores is commonly used in clinical research.

Basis for the paired *t*-test

In the case of a paired *t*-test, we typically have a pair of 'scores' for each subject. For instance, if examining the effects of an intervention, we would have values that corresponded with each subject's performance during baseline and post testing, or we may have pairs of scores that correspond with each subject's performance under two different conditions (e.g. single-task vs. dual-task). It's the mean of the differences ($\bar{X}_D$) between these pairs of scores that's analyzed in the case of a paired *t*-test.

To help conceptualize the basis for the paired *t*-test, let's consider a study by Kaji et al. (2010), which examined the immediate effects of 'core stability exercises' on postural sway in a single group of young adult males. The investigators recorded each subject's postural sway in standing before (pre), and shortly after (post), they completed the same set of core stability exercises. Among other variables, the investigators analyzed the amount of sway subjects exhibited in the anterior-posterior direction ('AP sway') (note: higher values correspond with greater sway and may reflect poorer postural control). AP sway was recorded for each subject at both the pre and post time points. On average, the subjects demonstrated a 1.1-mm reduction in AP sway ($\bar{X}_D = -1.1$) from the pre time point to the post time point (post – pre). This –1.1-mm difference in AP sway has two potential explanations:

1) the observed mean of the differences may simply be due to chance. In other words, on average, there's no change in AP sway for the population ($\mu_D = 0$); however, $\bar{X}_D \neq 0$ because of sampling error. This explanation is consistent with the null hypothesis (H$_0$: $\mu_D = 0$).
2) the observed mean of the differences reflects a true effect in the population ($\mu_D \neq 0$). This explanation is consistent with the alternative hypothesis (H$_1$: $\mu_D \neq 0$).

Let's elaborate on this concept before moving forward. When conducting a paired *t*-test, we're examining the evidence from our sample data to determine if it's strong enough to reject the null hypothesis and conclude that, on average, there's a difference between the conditions or time points for the population (i.e. $\mu_D \neq 0$). If we reject the null hypothesis, we're essentially concluding that the evidence suggests that if we administered the intervention (core stabilization exercises in this example) to everyone in the population, the average change in performance would not be 0 ($\mu_D \neq 0$). In other words, there would be a fairly systematic change in performance, either in the positive or negative direction.

Here's another way to conceptualize examining these types of within-subjects changes. Almost every variable we examine will fluctuate a bit from trial to trial, session to session, and day to day. For example, if we examined gait speeds over two time points, we would observe subtle differences in performance across sessions even if we didn't intervene. These fluctuations in performance could be due to any number of factors (e.g. changes in subjects' energy levels or motivation, testing/equipment error). In general, these factors would have a fairly random effect on performance, with some subjects walking faster during the first session and others walking faster during the second session. Therefore, on average, the differences in performance would tend to balance out, and $\bar{X}_D$ would be approximately 0.

Now imagine that we had subjects complete a lower-body strengthening program between the time points. In this case, we may observe more systematic changes in performance, with gait speeds tending to increase from the first testing session to the second testing session for most subjects. You can apply this same logic when considering performance in two conditions. For instance, imagine that we examine gait speeds while subjects walk in both a single-task condition and a dual-task condition. In this case, we would probably find that most subjects walk slower in the dual-task condition. Again, this would be a fairly consistent difference in performance across most, or perhaps all, subjects.

Sampling distribution – paired t-test

For a paired *t*-test, we are interested in the sampling distribution that would result if we repeatedly sampled from a population, found the differences in performance across the two time points or conditions of interest, calculated the mean of these differences ($\bar{X}_D$), and organized these means into a distribution.

Assuming the null hypothesis were true ($\mu_D = 0$), we would expect the sampling distribution to be normally distributed around 0. In this case, the standard error would essentially represent how the means of the differences from the samples are expected to vary about the true mean of the differences in the population. Equation 5.3 includes the equation that can be used to estimate the *standard error* ($s_{\bar{X}_D}$), based on the sample size (n – number of pairs) and the standard deviation of the differences (s_D).

Equation 5.3

$$s_{\bar{X}_D} = \frac{s_D}{\sqrt{n}}$$

Again, the *t* distribution would be used to represent the sampling distribution, since the standard error is estimated based on a sample standard deviation (s_D).

The t *statistic*

In this case, the *t* statistic captures the location of our observed mean of the differences ($\bar{X}_D$) within a *t* distribution that's based on the assumption that the null hypothesis is true ($H_0: \mu_D = 0$). Equation 5.4 includes a standard form of the equation for the *t* statistic for a paired *t*-test. The numerator is the mean of the differences ($\overline{X}_D$), while the denominator is the standard error ($s_{\overline{X}_D}$). Note that the order in which the scores are subtracted is arbitrary; however, it will influence the sign of $\overline{X}_D$ and thus the sign of the t statistic. Again, the t statistic can be positive or negative. Table 5.1 includes an example calculation of the t statistic for a paired t-test.

Equation 5.4

$$t \text{ statistic} = \frac{\overline{X}_D}{s_{\overline{X}_D}}$$

Table 5.1 Hypothetical data set of 6 Minute Walk Test distances.

Subject	Pre	Post	Differences (post – pre)
1	357	450	93
2	477	494	17
3	412	420	8
4	376	378	2
5	540	530	−10
6	339	398	59
7	558	559	1
8	438	450	13
9	312	319	7
10	584	607	23
			$\overline{X}_D = 21$
			$s_D = 31$

6 Minute Walk Test (6MWT) distances (ft) for ten older adults before (pre) and after (post) they completed a lower-body strengthening program. The Differences column includes the difference between the post and pre scores for each subject; positive values reflect a longer 6MWT distance after completing the training program (i.e. greater endurance).
$\overline{X}_D$ is the mean of the differences, and s_D is the standard deviation of the differences. The t statistic for a paired t-test is calculated by dividing the mean of the differences by the estimated standard error of the differences.
$t \text{ statistic} = \dfrac{\overline{X}_D}{s_D/\sqrt{n}} = \dfrac{21}{31/\sqrt{10}} = 2.14$ (upper tail of the distribution)

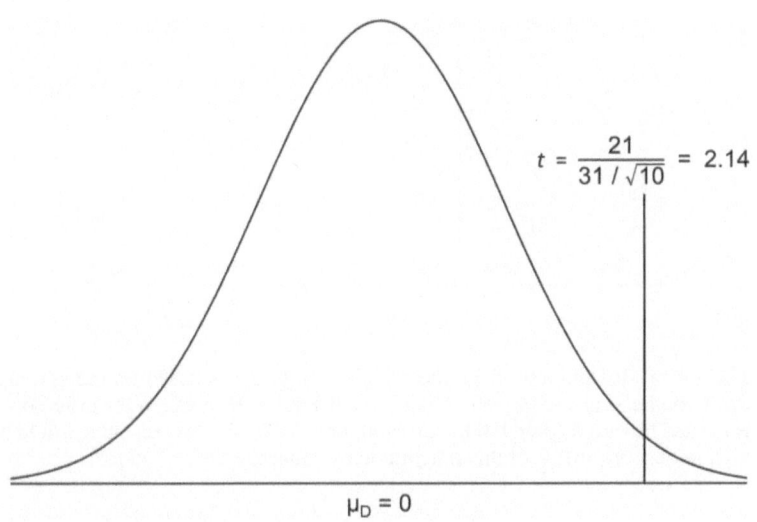

$$t = \frac{21}{31 \,/\, \sqrt{10}} = 2.14$$

$\mu_D = 0$

t statistic within the t distribution, assuming the null hypothesis is true.

Assuming the null hypothesis were true, we would expect most of the means of the differences to be located in the center of the *t* distribution (*t* statistic close to 0). Therefore, if we observe a *t* statistic that falls into the outer tails of the distribution (either in the upper or lower tail), it provides evidence to suggest that the null hypothesis is false, since we would be unlikely to observe a difference this extreme if the null hypothesis were true.

Now, let's consider the results of the study conducted by Kaji et al. (2010). Remember, on average, subjects in their study exhibited a 1.1-mm reduction in AP sway following completion of the core stabilization exercises ($\bar{X}_D = -1.1$ mm). Their estimated standard error $\left(s_{\bar{X}_D} \right)$ was approximately 1.16 mm, and therefore, their *t* statistic was –0.95 ($t = \dfrac{-1.1}{1.16} = -0.95$). Notice that this *t* statistic is located in the lower portion of the *t* distribution; however, it doesn't appear to be that extreme, as it's still within the body of the distribution (Figure 5.5). In other words, it wouldn't be that uncommon to observe an $\bar{X}_D$ of –1.1 mm even if the null hypothesis were true and $\mu_D = 0$.

Statistical significance

A paired *t*-test will produce a *p*-value that reflects the probability of observing a mean of the differences as extreme, or more extreme, than what would be observed if the null hypothesis were true. Again, this *p*-value is the probability that lands in the tails of the distribution, beyond the location of the observed *t* statistic. As with the independent *t*-test, we compare this *p*-value to a predetermined alpha level, which is conventionally 0.05, in order to determine if the observed mean of the differences provides strong enough evidence to reject the null hypothesis.

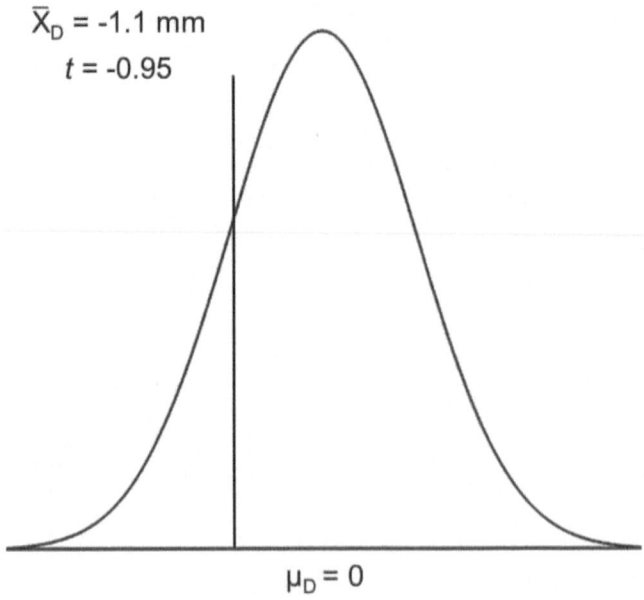

Figure 5.5 Theoretical distribution of the means of the differences based on the assumption that the null hypothesis is true ($\mu_D = 0$). Notice that the observed mean of the differences of –1.1 mm is located toward the body of the distribution ($t = -0.95$). As a result, it would be fairly common to observe an $\bar{X}_D$ of this magnitude by chance alone.

The *p*-value based on the *t*-test conducted by Kaji et al. (2010) was 0.356 (*p* = 0.356), which indicates that if the null hypothesis were true, 35.6% of all $\bar{X}_D$ values would be expected to be as extreme, or more extreme, than what was observed. Therefore, it appears that the observed sample data ($\bar{X}_D = -1.1$ mm) isn't that unlikely to occur if the null hypothesis is true. In other words, the sample data doesn't provide very strong evidence to reject the null hypothesis. The investigators set their alpha level at 0.05. Since their observed *p*-value (*p* = 0.356) was greater than their predefined alpha level ($\alpha = 0.05$), they concluded that the change in AP sway wasn't statistically significant.*

* **Note:** the investigators did observe statistically significant reductions in medial-lateral sway, as well as reductions in sway velocity, following completion of the core stabilization exercises.

Confidence intervals

Chapter 4 introduced the conceptual basis for developing a confidence interval when estimating a population mean. We can also generate confidence intervals when estimating the difference in population means ($\mu_1 - \mu_2$) or the mean of the differences in the population (μ_D). In either case, the boundaries of the confidence interval provide a range of values that's expected to include the true population parameter.

As an example, Eitzen et al. (2012) generated a 95% confidence interval for the mean difference in gait speeds they observed for their samples of subjects with and without hip osteoarthritis ($\bar{X}_{OA} - \bar{X}_{Control} = -0.12$ m/s). The lower and upper boundaries of their 95% confidence interval ($CI_{95\%}$) were -0.196 m/s and -0.045 m/s, respectively ($CI_{95\%} = [-0.196, -0.045]$). Based on this interval, the true difference in population means ($\mu_{OA} - \mu_{Control}$) is expected to fall within a range of -0.196 m/s and -0.045 m/s. Since it was a 95% confidence interval, there's a 95% probability that the true difference in population means falls within this interval. Notice that 0 m/s isn't included within this range of values. Therefore, it's unlikely that the difference in the population means is 0 m/s, which supports the results of their test of statistical significance.

The same logic can be applied to paired data. In this case, the confidence interval will include a range of values that's expected to include the true mean of the differences in the population (μ_D).

Confidence intervals are discussed in greater detail in Chapter 13 ('Effect Sizes and Confidence Intervals').

Two-tailed vs. one-tailed tests

Conventionally, we examine both the upper and lower tails of the *t* distribution when conducting a *t*-test, which is referred to as a *two-tailed test*. With a two-tailed test, we establish critical values that define areas in both tails of the distribution which include outcomes that are unlikely to be observed if the null hypothesis were true (i.e. 'extreme observations'). When the alpha level is set at 0.05, these outer tails make up 5% of the total area of the distribution (2.5% in each tail). If our *t* statistic falls within one of these areas in the upper or lower tail of the distribution, we conclude that the observed difference is statistically significant. For example, imagine that we conducted a study to compare the trunk muscle activity of individuals with and without low back pain during performance of a standardized lifting task. A two-tailed *t*-test would allow us to determine whether the observed mean difference in muscle activity is located in the extremes of either tail of the *t* distribution.

With a *one-tailed test*, we only examine one tail of the distribution (either the upper or lower tail, not both). In the case where the alpha level is set at 0.05, this area in either the upper or lower tail would make up 5% of the total area of the distribution (all 5% in one tail). Figure 5.6 includes a comparison of the boundaries created based on one-tailed and two-tailed tests.

The benefit of a one-tailed test is that it provides greater statistical power since the *t* statistic doesn't need to be as extreme in order to be considered statistically significant. However, a drawback of a one-tailed test is that we must (or at least should) determine which side of the distribution to examine before conducting the analysis. Therefore, there's the potential for differences to go undetected simply because they occurred in the opposite direction of what was expected. For example, if we conducted a one-tailed *t*-test to determine whether individuals with low back pain exhibit less trunk muscle activity than individuals without low back pain, our test would essentially ignore the possibility of the individuals with low back pain exhibiting greater trunk muscle activity, since we only tested for an effect in the other direction.

I don't go into detail about one-tailed tests because I generally don't think they're a good idea, and many agree with me (e.g. Wright & London, 2009). If you want greater statistical power, it's probably better to increase your sample size or potentially adjust your alpha level. That said, I wanted to introduce the concept because you'll come across one-tailed tests when reading the literature. If investigators run a one-tailed test, they should provide strong evidence that the observed effect would only be expected to occur in the direction they tested.

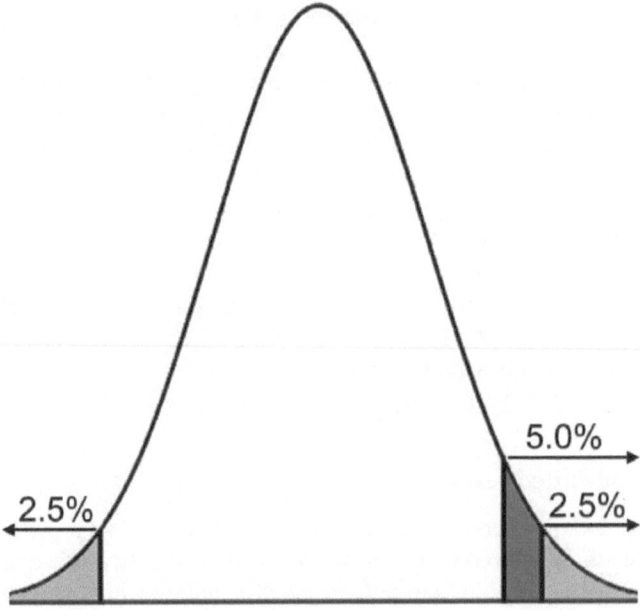

Figure 5.6 *t* distribution with critical regions defined based on an alpha level of 0.05. With a two-tailed test, critical regions are defined in both the upper and lower tails of the distribution (light gray). These regions make up 5% of the total area under the curve (2.5% in each tail). With a one-tailed test, a critical region is only defined for one tail of the distribution (dark gray). Notice that in the case of a one-tailed test, the *t* statistic doesn't need to be as extreme in order to be located in the critical region, and therefore, it's easier to reject the null hypothesis. However, with a one-tailed test, only one side of the distribution is examined.

Many statistical analysis software packages provide you with the option of running either a one-tailed or two-tailed *t*-test. If not, you can simply take the *p*-value that results from a two-tailed test and divide it in half. For example, a *p*-value of 0.06 based on a two-tailed test would be equivalent to a *p*-value of 0.03 for a one-tailed test ($0.06/2 = 0.03$). Notice that if the alpha level were set at 0.05, a one-tailed test would be considered statistically significant in this case (since $0.03 < 0.05$), whereas a two-tailed test wouldn't (since $0.06 > 0.05$), which reflects the fact that one-tailed tests tend to have greater statistical power.

Assumptions

This section highlights key assumptions that should be met in order to conduct a *t*-test (paired and/or independent).

1) The dependent variable is continuous

This isn't an assumption that's tested statistically. Instead, it's related to the nature of the dependent variable of interest.

Options if this assumption isn't met

Other tests can be used with different types of data. For example, the Mann-Whitney U test or the Wilcoxon signed-rank test can be used when comparing ordinal data. These non-parametric tests are introduced in Chapter 12 ('Non-Parametric Tests').

2) No significant outliers

An outlier is essentially a data point that differs significantly from the other observations in the data set (i.e. an extremely high or low value for the dependent variable of interest). When an outlier is present, the first step should be to attempt to determine whether the data point was entered erroneously or if there was some type of equipment malfunction that could explain the outlier. You should also consider whether the atypical value is within a range of what's possible. Outliers due to data entry errors, equipment miscalibration, and so on are relatively easy to address by re-entering the correct data or removing a data point that's obviously erroneous.

Options if this assumption isn't met

When the reason for an outlier is unclear, we must carefully consider how to proceed. In some cases, investigators will remove an outlier from the analysis; however, this is generally discouraged when there's no obvious reason to believe that an error occurred. A better option is to report the results of the analysis both with the outlier included and with the outlier removed. This allows readers to appreciate how the outlier influenced the results of the analysis and make their own decision about how to interpret the study findings. Another option is to perform a non-parametric test, such as the Mann-Whitney U test or Wilcoxon signed-rank test, since these tests tend to be less affected by outliers. Non-parametric tests are discussed in Chapter 12 ('Non-Parametric Tests').

3)   The dependent variable should be normally distributed

For an independent *t*-test, the dependent variable should be normally distributed for both groups. In the case of a paired t-test, it's the difference scores that should be normally distributed. Appendix A describes ways to assess normality. It should be noted that in most cases, minor deviations from normality won't have a major influence on the results of a *t*-test. In other words, *t*-tests are fairly 'robust' to violations of the assumption of normality.

Options if this assumption isn't met

If the assumption of normality isn't met, it may be possible to transform the data so that it's more normally distributed. Data transformation is discussed in Appendix B. Another option is to conduct a non-parametric test, such as the Mann-Whitney U test or the Wilcoxon signed-rank test (Chapter 12), since these tests don't require the data to be normally distributed.

4)   Homogeneity of variance – *independent t-tests only**

For an independent *t*-test, it's assumed that the variance is the same for both populations of interest (i.e. *homogeneity of variance*). Since the variance of the populations are unknown, we compare the sample variances to get an idea of whether this assumption is met. If the sample variances are similar, the data satisfies the assumption of homogeneity of variance; however, if the sample variances differ substantially, the assumption is violated. While independent *t*-tests tend to be robust to violations of the assumption of homogeneity of variance, there can be issues (mainly an inflated risk of Type I error) when there are marked differences in variance, especially when group sizes differ.

Levene's test is commonly used to test the assumption of homogeneity of variance. In fact, SPSS includes the results of Levene's test as part of its standard output. Levene's test tests the null hypothesis that the population variances are equal (H_0: $\sigma_1 = \sigma_2$). If the *p*-value generated from Levene's test is less than alpha (typically 0.05), it suggests that the population variances differ, which reflects a violation of the assumption of homogeneity of variance. This can be counterintuitive, as we are hoping to observe a non-significant result for Levene's test (*p*-value ≥ 0.05), since this indicates that our data satisfies the assumption of homogeneity of variance.

* **Note:** this assumption only pertains to independent *t*-tests, since paired *t*-tests only involve one group of subjects, with the variance of the difference scores incorporated in the analysis.

*Options if this assumption isn't met**

As part of its standard output, SPSS provides two different sets of results whenever an independent *t*-test is performed. One set should be used when the assumption is satisfied (i.e. Levene's test isn't significant, *p*-value ≥ 0.05), and the other set should be used when the assumption isn't satisfied (i.e. Levene's test is significant, *p*-value < 0.05). When the assumption is violated, SPSS includes an adjustment to the degrees of freedom to reduce the inflated risk of Type I error.

* **Note:** there are certainly other ways to test for, and account for, violations of the assumption of homogeneity of variance. I've chosen to highlight this approach simply because it's built into the standard SPSS output.

Application opportunities

Example data set #1

This example is based on a data set published by Mistry et al. (2021) (DOI: 110.7717/ peerj.11252/supp-1), which includes data for 31 women with upper extremity lymphedema resulting from breast cancer ('cases') and 31 age-matched women without lymphedema or a history of breast cancer ('controls'). As part of the study, subjects' maximal grip strength (units – kg) was tested using a hand dynamometer. The objective of this analysis is to determine if there's a statistically significant difference in grip strength between the cases and controls.

Data files

BrCa_grip_data.xlsx – Excel file that includes grip strengths for the cases (involved upper extremity) and controls (non-dominant upper extremity). Grip strength values for the cases and controls are organized in separate columns ('Cases', 'Controls').

   BrCa_grip_data.sav – SPSS file that includes grip strengths for the cases (involved upper extremity) and controls (non-dominant upper extremity). The file includes two columns: column 1 ('Group') designates whether the subject was a member of the cases group (coded – 1) or the control group (coded – 0); column 2 ('GripStrength') includes the grip strength values for each subject.

Video

IndependentTTest.mp4 – video that includes a demonstration of how to conduct an independent *t*-test using SPSS and the Excel Analysis ToolPak.

Sample write-up

A two-tailed, independent *t*-test was conducted to compare the grip strengths of women with upper extremity lymphedema resulting from breast cancer (cases) and an age-matched control group. An alpha level of 0.05 was used for this test of statistical significance.

   The mean ± standard deviation grip strengths for the cases and controls were 24.42 ± 9.87 kg and 29.26 ± 7.09 kg, respectively. The difference in grip strength between the groups was statistically significant ($t(54) = 2.22$; $p = 0.031$), with women in the cases group demonstrating weaker grip strength compared to controls.

Notes: *t* is the *t* statistic, with its corresponding (adjusted) degrees of freedom (54). *p* is the *p*-value associated with the test. It would also be a good idea to report that the degrees of freedom were adjusted, since the data appeared to violate the assumption of homogeneity of variance based on the results of Levene's test.

Example data set #2

This example is based on a data set published by MacLennan et al. (2020) (DOI: 10.7717/ peerj.8224/supp-1), which includes data for 13 subjects who participated in a study designed to examine the effects of knee immobilization on quadriceps muscle size and composition. As part of their study, the investigators measured the cross-sectional area of each subject's vastus lateralis muscle before (pre) and after (post) a 2-week period of knee immobilization. The objective of this analysis is to determine whether there was a statistically significant change in vastus lateralis cross-sectional area following the immobilization period.

Data files

VL_CSA_data.xlsx – Excel file that includes vastus lateralis cross-sectional area (CSA) values for each subject at the pre and post time points. Pre and post values are included in separate columns (Pre, Post).

VL_CSA_data.sav – SPSS file that includes vastus lateralis cross-sectional area values for each subject at the pre and post time points. Pre and post values are included in separate columns (VL_CSA_pre, VL_CSA_post).

Video

PairedTTest.mp4 – video that includes a demonstration of how to conduct a paired *t*-test using SPSS and the Excel Analysis ToolPak.

Sample write-up

A two-tailed, paired *t*-test was conducted to determine if there was a statistically significant change in vastus lateralis cross-sectional area following the 2-week knee immobilization period. An alpha level of 0.05 was used for this test of statistical significance.

The mean ± standard deviation cross-sectional areas for the vastus lateralis at the pre and post time points were 16.71 ± 2.85 cm^2 and 15.60 ± 2.38 cm^2, respectively. This 1.11 cm^2 change in cross-sectional area was not statistically significant ($t(12) = 2.06$; $p = 0.06$).

Notes: *t* is the *t* statistic, with its corresponding degrees of freedom (12). *p* is the *p*-value associated with the test.

Answers to learning activity

Learning Activity 5.1

Answers

Garcia-Pinillos et al. (2020) – used paired *t*-tests to compare running mechanics for the non-fatigued and fatigued conditions.

Kobayashi et al. (2014) – used independent *t*-tests to compare gait kinematics of the fallers and non-fallers.

Koontz et al. (2002) – used paired *t*-tests to compare upper extremity mechanics for the slower and faster speeds.

Cheung et al. (2016) – used independent *t*-tests to compare intrinsic foot muscle volume for the healthy runners and the runners with plantar fasciitis.

Yavuz et al. (2015) – used paired *t*-tests to compare muscle activity for the front and back squats.

6 Introduction to analysis of variance

Chapter Objectives

The objectives of this chapter are to . . .

1) describe the general purpose of one-way and repeated-measures analysis of variance and to provide examples of the types of research questions that these analyses can be used to address
2) explain the general function of an omnibus test
3) describe the theoretical basis for one-way analysis of variance and summarize the computations involved
4) introduce the F distribution and F-tests
5) explain how one-way analysis of variance can be used to compare changes in performance across multiple groups
6) highlight how the results of a one-way analysis of variance can be summarized in an ANOVA table
7) describe the theoretical basis for repeated-measures analysis of variance
8) highlight the key advantage of repeated-measures analysis of variance compared to one-way analysis of variance
9) describe the concept of familywise error and explain how analysis of variance is used to control the risk of Type I error
10) introduce the general concept of post hoc testing
11) point out key assumptions that should be met in order to conduct one-way or repeated-measures analysis of variance
12) demonstrate how to conduct one-way and repeated-measures analysis of variance using SPSS and Excel software

Introduction

Chapter 5 discussed the t-test, which is commonly used to compare two means. This chapter will introduce analyses that can be used to compare more than two means. For instance, we may want to compare the average performance of several groups. Or we may want to compare the average performance of a single group in three or more conditions or at three or more time points. Each of these situations involves comparison of more than two means (e.g. group 1, group 2, group 3 or pre, post, follow-up). Analysis of variance (ANOVA) can be used in these situations to determine if there are any differences across the multiple

DOI: 10.4324/9781003179757-6

groups, conditions, or time points of interest.* In this chapter, we'll discuss two specific types of ANOVA: one-way ANOVA and repeated-measures ANOVA. You can think of these analyses as extensions of the independent and paired *t*-tests discussed in Chapter 5. More advanced types of ANOVA will be introduced in Chapter 7 ('Factorial Analysis of Variance').

* **Note:** technically, ANOVA can also be used to compare two means; however, *t*-tests are typically used in these circumstances, mostly because *t*-tests are easier to implement. In the end, the result will be the same regardless of whether you use a *t*-test or ANOVA to compare two means.

One-way ANOVA is used in instances where there's a single 'between-subjects factor' with three or more levels, such as when comparing three or more different groups of individuals (note: 'factor' = independent variable; 'levels' = subcategories of the independent variable).* For example, Carville et al. (2007) compared quadriceps isometric force output in younger adults, older adults who had recently experienced a fall ('fallers'), and older adults who hadn't recently fallen ('non-fallers'). Since their study consisted of three distinct groups, or samples, of subjects (younger adults, fallers, non-fallers – three levels), they used one-way ANOVA to compare quadriceps force output. Note that each group represented a level of the independent variable. One-way ANOVA is essentially an extension of the independent *t*-test discussed in Chapter 5. Remember that an independent *t*-test is used to compare two distinct groups (i.e. *independent* samples) of individuals. One-way ANOVA is used to address similar questions, except it can accommodate more than two groups.

* **Note:** the terminology 'one-way' reflects the fact that the analysis includes one independent variable or factor. Chapter 7 will introduce analyses that incorporate two factors, which is referred to as 'two-way ANOVA'.

Repeated-measures ANOVA is used when there's one 'within-subjects factor' with three or more levels (note: you'll also see this described as 'one-way ANOVA with repeated measures'). In this case, performance is compared across three or more conditions, or time points, in a single group of subjects. In other words, *repeated measurements* are taken from the same group of subjects. For example, Hannigan and Pollard (2020) compared impact forces while a group of recreational runners ran in three different types of running shoes: a traditional running shoe, a 'minimal' running shoe that provided limited foot support, and a 'maximal' running shoe that provided extra foot support. The investigators used a repeated-measures ANOVA to compare the impact forces across the three types of shoes (traditional shoe, minimal shoe, maximal shoe – three levels). A repeated-measures ANOVA was appropriate in this case since all subjects ran in each of the different types of shoes. In other words, *repeated measurements* were recorded across the three conditions *within* a single group of runners. Repeated-measures ANOVA is essentially an extension of the paired *t*-test discussed in Chapter 5. Remember that a paired *t*-test is used to compare performance of a single group of subjects in two conditions or at two time points (e.g. post vs. pre). Repeated-measures ANOVA can address the same types of questions, except it can accommodate more than two conditions or time points.

Learning Activity 6.1 includes additional examples to help you differentiate between when it's appropriate to use one-way ANOVA vs. repeated-measures ANOVA.

Learning Activity 6.1

Following are five examples of studies that included either a one-way ANOVA or a repeated-measures ANOVA as part of their analysis. Based on the brief description of each study, try to predict which type of analysis the investigators used. The answers are provided at the end of the chapter.

Grenier et al. (2012) conducted a study to examine energy cost as soldiers marched with different body-borne loads. Their study included a single group of former infantrymen. Each subject marched while carrying a light load (≤1 kg), a moderate load (~20 kg), and a heavy load (~38 kg). The investigators compared energy cost for the three different load conditions (light load, moderate load, heavy load).

Khalaj et al. (2014) conducted a study to examine postural stability in individuals with knee osteoarthritis (OA). Their study included 20 subjects without knee OA ('healthy'), 20 subjects with mild knee OA ('mild OA'), and 20 subjects with moderate knee OA ('moderate OA'). Each subject's postural stability was assessed, and the amount of postural sway was compared across the groups (healthy, mild OA, moderate OA).

Zaffagnini et al. (2006) conducted a study to compare knee-related function in individuals who underwent different types of anterior cruciate ligament (ACL) reconstruction surgeries. As part of their study, individuals who had experienced an ACL tear received one of three different ACL reconstruction surgeries. In total, the study included 75 subjects, with 25 subjects undergoing each type of surgery. The investigators conducted a 5-year follow-up and compared knee-related function for the three groups at that time point.

Schucker et al. (2009) conducted a study to examine how attentional focus influences running economy. Their study included 24 trained runners. Each runner completed separate blocks where they were asked to focus on their surroundings, their running pattern, or their breathing while running. Oxygen consumption was compared for the three running conditions (focus on surroundings, focus on running pattern, focus on breathing).

Reinold et al. (2004) conducted a study to compare shoulder muscle activity during performance of seven different common shoulder external rotation exercises. Their study included ten subjects, who all completed each of the exercises. Electromyography was used to record muscle activation, and shoulder muscle activity was compared across the seven exercises.

Omnibus tests

One-way and repeated-measures ANOVA can help us determine if there's a statistically significant difference among all groups, conditions, or time points of interest. However, these tests won't inform us about which specific pair, or pairs, of groups, conditions, or time points differ. For example, when comparing quadriceps isometric force output among younger adults, older fallers, and older non-fallers, one-way ANOVA would help us determine if there are any differences among the groups means; however, the results wouldn't tell us which specific groups differ (e.g. younger adults vs. older fallers, younger adults vs. older non-fallers, or older fallers vs. older non-fallers). Tests of this nature that evaluate the overall differences across multiple levels of an independent variable are referred to as *omnibus tests*.

In most cases we use ANOVA to determine if there are any differences among the levels of an independent variable and then conduct *post hoc tests** to determine where the differences exist (note: post hoc tests are also commonly referred to as *multiple comparisons tests*). Essentially, the ANOVA test will tell us if there are any differences overall, and the post hoc tests will tell where the differences exist. If the ANOVA results aren't significant, there's typically no need to conduct post hoc tests, since we already know that there are no differences among the levels of the independent variable. Post hoc tests function like *t*-tests in that they compare pairs of means; however, in most cases, they include some type of 'adjustment' to reduce the risk of Type I error. The concept of post hoc testing will be revisited later in this chapter ('Post Hoc Tests' section).

* **Note:** *post hoc* is Latin for 'after this', which is appropriate since these tests are performed as a follow-up to a significant omnibus test.

As an example, let's return to the study conducted by Carville et al. (2007), which compared quadriceps isometric force output in younger adults, older fallers, and older non-fallers. The results of the one-way ANOVA indicated that there was a statistically significant difference in quadriceps force steadiness among the groups. The investigators then conducted post hoc tests and found that the older fallers demonstrated less force steadiness than the younger adults and the older non-fallers. They also found that there wasn't a significant difference in force steadiness between the younger adults and the older non-fallers. Notice that the ANOVA results didn't provide information about which groups differed, they simply indicated that the groups differed in some manner. It was the post hoc tests that provided information about which specific groups differed.

Note: so far, each example has included three levels (e.g. younger adults, older fallers, older non-fallers); however, both one-way ANOVA and repeated-measures ANOVA can be extended to include more than three levels.

Focus on conceptual understanding

The next two sections will include an overview of the computational basis for one-way ANOVA and repeated-measures ANOVA. One of the nice things about ANOVA is that, while the computations are somewhat labor intensive, none are overly complex. In addition, they involve metrics that were introduced in earlier chapters, such as means, sums of squares, and variances. That said, I encourage you to focus on developing a conceptual understanding of these analyses instead of focusing too much on the specific details of the computations. In the end, if you understand what we're trying to achieve when using ANOVA, the computational procedures should make sense.

Basis for one-way ANOVA

In general, one-way ANOVA is used in situations where we want to examine data from three or more samples in order to determine if there's strong enough evidence to conclude that there are differences among the respective populations. To help conceptualize the basis for this analysis, let's consider a study by Bologna et al. (2016), which was conducted to examine motor performance in individuals with varying stages of Parkinson's disease. As part of their study, investigators recorded movement speed during a repetitive finger tapping task for three distinct groups, or independent samples, of subjects: 1) individuals without Parkinson's disease ('controls'), 2) individuals with early-stage Parkinson's disease ('early PD'), and 3) individuals with more advanced Parkinson's disease ('advanced PD'). They then conducted a one-way ANOVA test to determine if there was a statistically significant difference in movement speeds among the three groups (controls, early PD, advanced PD).

In the case of the study conducted by Bologna et al. (2016), the null hypothesis was that there was no difference in the average movement speeds of the populations of individuals without Parkinson's disease, individuals with early-stage Parkinson's disease, and individuals with more advanced Parkinson's disease (H_0: $\mu_{\text{Control}} = \mu_{\text{early PD}} = \mu_{\text{advanced PD}}$, where μ represents the population mean). In other words, the null hypothesis states that any observed difference in movement speeds is simply due to chance or sampling error. In contrast, the alternative hypothesis states that there's a difference among the population means (i.e. not all of the population means are equal). Remember that the null hypothesis is what's tested statistically. In this case, the investigators analyzed the results of the one-way ANOVA in order to determine if there was sufficient evidence to reject the null hypothesis and conclude that the populations differed with respect to their average movement speeds. Notice again that the results of this type of omnibus test don't provide information about which groups differ; they just reflect whether there are any differences among the groups overall.

The F statistic

In the case of ANOVA, the *F* statistic (or *F* ratio) serves as our test statistic. In fact, ANOVA is part of a group of statistical tests generally referred to as '*F*-tests' (note: other applications of *F*-tests will be discussed in subsequent chapters). In the case of one-way ANOVA, the *F* statistic captures the amount of variance among the group means ('between-groups variance') relative to the amount of variance within the groups ('within-groups variance' or 'error variance') (Equation 6.1).

Equation 6.1

$$F \text{ statistic} = \frac{\text{between-groups variance}}{\text{within-groups variance}}$$

Note: the concept of variance was first introduced in Chapter 2. Remember that, in general, variance reflects how a set of values tend to deviate, or vary, about a mean.

Between-groups variance

The between-groups variance represents the extent to which the different sample means vary in relation to one another. The first step in finding the between-groups variance involves calculating the *between-groups sum of squares* (SS_{Between}), which is the sum (Σ) of the squared deviations of the sample means ($\overline{X}_{1-k}$, where *k* represents the number of groups) about the *grand mean* ($\overline{X}_G$). The grand mean ($\overline{X}_G$) is simply the average of all the scores, regardless of their group (note: imagine taking the entire collection of scores from across all groups and finding the average; this is the grand mean). Equation 6.2 includes a general form of the equation for calculating SS_{Between}.

Equation 6.2

$$SS_{\text{Between}} = \sum n_k \left(\overline{X}_k - \overline{X}_G \right)^2$$

In Equation 6.2, n_k is the number of subjects in each group, with *k* representing the group number (1, 2, 3 . . . *k*).

The between-groups variance is then calculated by dividing SS_{Between} by the corresponding between-groups degrees of freedom (df_{Between}), which is the number of groups (k), minus 1 ($df_{\text{Between}} = k - 1$). It's important to note that in the context of ANOVA, we typically refer to variance using the terminology 'mean square' (MS). Don't let this confuse you; the term 'mean square' is simply referring to some form of variance. Equation 6.3 includes a general form of the equation for calculating the between-groups mean square (MS_{Between}) – in other words, the between-groups variance. This between-groups variance (MS_{Between}) makes up the numerator of the F statistic (Equation 6.1).

Equation 6.3

$$MS_{\text{Between}} = \frac{SS_{\text{Between}}}{k-1}$$

Before moving on to discuss the within-groups variance, let's revisit the study conducted by Bologna et al. (2016). In this case, the between-groups variance represents how the sample means ($\bar{X}_{\text{Control}}$, $\bar{X}_{\text{EarlyPD}}$, $\bar{X}_{\text{AdvancedPD}}$) differed among the three groups: in other words, how the group means varied about the grand mean. Note that in the case of the study by Bologna et al. (2016), the grand mean reflected the average movement speed for all subjects in the study, regardless of which group they were in. The more the group means differ from one another, the greater the between-groups variance.

Within-groups variance

Within-groups variance represents how the individual values tend to deviate about their respective sample means within the separate groups (note: within-groups variance is also commonly referred to as 'error variance' in the case of one-way ANOVA). The first step in finding the within-groups variance involves calculating the *within-groups sum of squares* (SS_{Within}). SS_{Within} is simply the total of the sums of squares [$SS = \Sigma(X - \bar{X})^2$] from each of the groups ($SS_{\text{Within}} = SS_1 + \ldots SS_k$, where k represents the number of groups). The within-groups variance, which is referred to as the within-groups mean square (MS_{Within}), is then calculated by dividing SS_{Within} by the corresponding within-groups degrees of freedom (df_{Within}), which is the total number of subjects across all groups (N) minus the number of groups (k) ($df_{\text{Within}} = N - k$). Equation 6.4 includes a general form of the equation for the within-groups mean square (MS_{Within}) (i.e. the within-groups variance). This within-groups variance (MS_{Within}) makes up the denominator of the F statistic (Equation 6.1).

Equation 6.4

$$MS_{\text{Within}} = \frac{SS_{\text{Within}}}{N-k}$$

For the study conducted by Bologna et al. (2016), the within-groups variance represents the cumulative amount of subject-to-subject variability in movement speed within the groups (control, early PD, advanced PD). While the between-groups variance reflects the variance between the groups, the within-groups variance reflects the variance within the control, early PD, and advanced PD groups. It's important to consider that performance (movement speed in this case) will vary, even within a comparable group of individuals (e.g. all members of the control group will move at different speeds).

Note: in the case of one-way ANOVA, the between-groups variance and the within-groups variance make up the total variance in the data set (total variance = between-groups variance + within-groups variance). The terminology 'analysis of variance' reflects the fact that we're partitioning out the variance associated with the independent variable (between-groups variance) and the rest of the variance that isn't associated with the independent variable (within-groups variance). As you can see, the terminology *analysis of variance* is quite appropriate, since ANOVA involves analyzing the different types of variance.

F *statistic*

Finally, the F statistic is calculated by dividing $MS_{Between}$ (between-groups variance) by MS_{Within} (within-groups variance) (Equation 6.5). It's important to note that since we're working with squared values (sums of squares), the F statistic will always be non-negative (F statistic ≥ 0).

Equation 6.5

$$F \text{ statistic} = \frac{\text{between-groups variance}}{\text{within-groups variance}} = \frac{MS_{Between}}{MS_{Within}} = \frac{SS_{Between}/df_{Between}}{SS_{Within}/df_{Within}}$$

In the case of one-way ANOVA, the F statistic essentially captures the amount of separation among the distributions for the various groups. If the F statistic is relatively large, it indicates that the differences between the group means are much greater than the variation within the groups, which provides strong evidence to suggest that the population means differ, since there's a lot of separation among the groups (Figure 6.1). In contrast, if the F statistic is relatively small ($F = \sim 1$), it indicates that the differences between the group means are small in relation to the variation within the groups (i.e. minimal separation), which doesn't provide strong evidence to suggest that the population means differ. Therefore, the larger the F statistic, the more likely we are to reject the null hypothesis.

The F distribution

Chapter 5 described how a *t*-test involves determining where an observed t statistic lies within a t distribution based on the assumption that the null hypothesis is true. ANOVA relies on the same concept, except we use a different sampling distribution, the F distribution (hence the terminology F-test). The F distribution is a theoretical distribution that represents what would likely happen if we repeatedly sampled, calculated an F statistic, and then organized these F statistics into a distribution. Since F statistics can only be non-negative, the F distribution starts at 0 and is positively skewed, with a single tail that extends indefinitely in the positive direction (Figure 6.2).

An F-test involves determining where the observed F statistic is located within an F distribution that's based on the assumption that the null hypothesis is true. Assuming the null hypothesis were true, we would expect most F statistics to lie within the body of the F distribution. Therefore, if we observe an F statistic that falls into the extreme tail of the

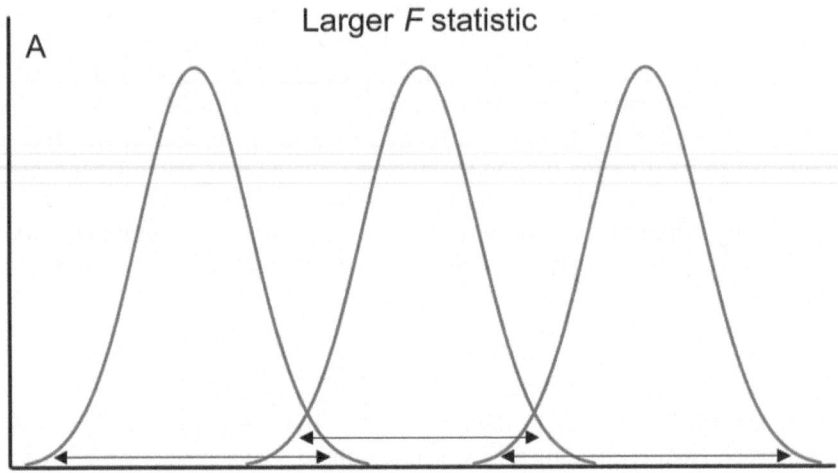

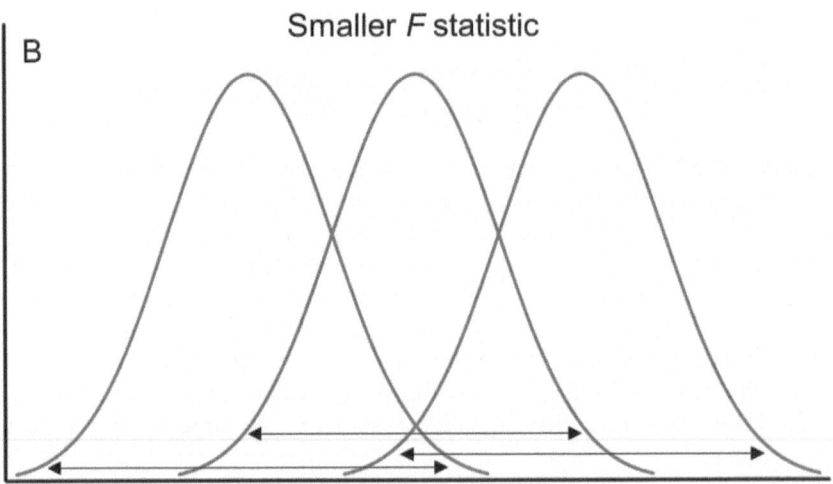

Figure 6.1 Both subplot A (top) and subplot B (bottom) include fictitious distributions of scores for three separate groups (note: the arrows highlight the within-groups variance). Notice that there's greater separation (i.e. less overlap) between the distributions in subplot A vs. subplot B, since there's less within-group variance in the case of subplot A. As a result, the *F* statistic would be larger for the data depicted in subplot A, since the *F* statistic captures the amount of between-groups variance relative to the amount of within-groups variance.

F distribution, it provides strong evidence to suggest that the null hypothesis is false (i.e. there's some difference in the population means).

For example, Bologna et al. (2016) reported an *F* statistic of 16.7 (*F* = 16.7) based on their comparison of the movement speeds of their control, early PD, and advanced PD groups. This indicates that the between-groups variance was over 16 times greater than the within-groups variance. If you look at where this observed *F* statistic would fall within the

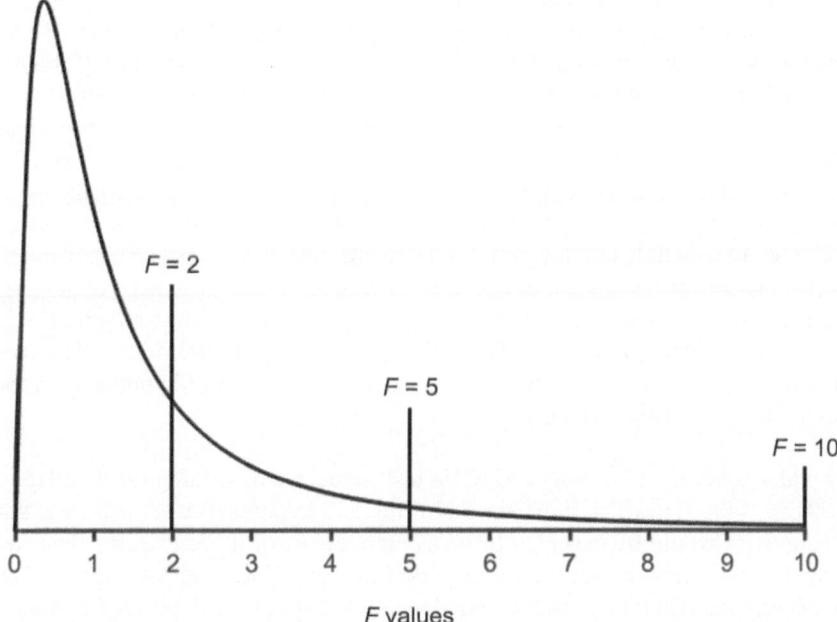

Figure 6.2 Example of an F distribution. The locations of different F statistics ($F = 2$, $F = 5$, $F = 10$)
are highlighted within the F distribution. Notice that the larger the F statistic, the farther it
lies into the tail of the distribution. Note: the exact shape of the F distribution depends on
the degrees of freedom.

theoretical F distribution included in Figure 6.2, you'll see that observing an F statistic this
extreme would be very unlikely if the null hypothesis were true.

Note: like the t distribution, the F distribution is actually a family of distributions, whose
exact shape is dependent on the number of degrees of freedom in both the numerator and the
denominator of the F statistic.

Statistical significance

An ANOVA test will produce a p-value that reflects the probability of observing an F statistic
as extreme or more extreme than what would be observed if the null hypothesis were true.
This p-value is the probability that lands in the tail of the distribution beyond the location of
the observed F statistic.* The lower the p-value, the more 'extreme' the observed F statistic
is considered. In other words, the lower the p-value, the less likely it is that the null hypothesis is true.

* **Note:** the F distribution is asymmetrical, with only one tail. Therefore, unlike a t-test,
it isn't necessary to differentiate between one- and two-tailed tests in the case of an
F-test.

In order to determine if the observed F statistic provides strong enough evidence to reject the null hypothesis, we compare the observed p-value to a predetermined alpha level (α). The alpha level essentially serves as a cutoff point for determining if the observed F statistic is large enough to conclude that the population means differ in some manner. If the p-value is less than alpha ($p < \alpha$), we reject the null hypothesis and conclude that there's a 'statistically significant' difference among the population means. In other words, the sample means differ more than what would be expected by chance. If the p-value is greater than or equal to alpha ($p \geq \alpha$), we don't reject the null hypothesis (i.e. we 'fail to reject the null hypothesis'). Failing to reject the null hypothesis essentially indicates that the evidence from our sample data isn't strong enough to conclude that the population means differ.

Note: the alpha level establishes a critical value in the F distribution that defines when the F statistic is extreme enough to reject the null hypothesis. When the F statistic exceeds this critical value, the p-value will be less than α, so we reject the null hypothesis. Appendix E includes a table of F critical values.

The p-value based on the one-way ANOVA test conducted by Bologna et al. (2016) was less than 0.001 ($p < 0.001$), which indicates that if the null hypothesis were true, less than 0.1% of all F statistics would be expected to be as extreme as, or more extreme than, what was observed. The investigators set their alpha level at 0.05. Since their observed p-value ($p < 0.001$) was less than their predefined alpha level ($\alpha = 0.05$), they concluded that there was a statistically significant difference in movement speeds among the groups (control, early PD, advanced PD).

As a follow-up to their significant omnibus test, the investigators conducted post hoc tests to compare the movement speeds of each of the groups. Their results indicated that the advanced PD group exhibited slower movement speeds compared to both the control group and the early PD group, while the early PD group exhibited slower movement speeds than the control group. In other words, all groups differed with respect to their movement speed.

Comparing differences in change scores

Chapter 5 discussed how independent t-tests can be used to compare the changes exhibited by two different groups of subjects by comparing the groups' change scores. One-way ANOVA can be used in the same manner, with the added potential for comparing the changes exhibited by more than two groups. For example, Parker et al. (1988) conducted a study to examine the effects of cognitive-behavioral training in patients with rheumatoid arthritis. Patients were randomly allocated to one of three groups: a cognitive-behavioral training group, a placebo group, or a control group. The cognitive-behavioral training group completed a program where they learned ways to manage and cope with their pain. The placebo group completed a program that provided general education about rheumatoid arthritis; the program was designed so that the placebo group had a similar amount of contact with investigators but didn't receive any type of cognitive-behavioral training. The control group didn't participate in any type of program. The investigators used one-way ANOVA to compare the changes (based on change scores, post–pre) exhibited by the three groups (cognitive-behavioral training group, placebo group, control group) for several pain-related variables over a 12-month period. Interestingly, patients who participated in the cognitive-behavioral training program reported feeling that they had gained more control over their pain compared to patients in the placebo and control groups.

As you can see, one-way ANOVA can be used to compare the changes exhibited by different groups of subjects. As was the case in the study conducted by Parker et al. (1988), this approach is commonly used to compare the changes exhibited by groups of patients who receive different types of treatment, such as in the case of a randomized controlled trial.

ANOVA table

The results of a one-way ANOVA are often summarized within a table, which is commonly referred to as an 'ANOVA table' (note: you may also see this described as a 'source table'). This ANOVA table typically includes the sums of squares, degrees of freedom, mean squares, and F statistic. It may also include the p-value and/or the F critical value. Table 6.1 provides an example of the general layout of an ANOVA table.

Table 6.1 General layout of an ANOVA table.

	Sum of squares (SS)	Degrees of freedom (df)	Mean squares (MS)	F statistic
Between groups	$SS_{Between}$	$df_{Between}$	$MS_{Between} = $ $SS_{Between}/df_{Between}$	$F = $ $MS_{Between}/MS_{Within}$
Within groups (error)	SS_{Within}	df_{Within}	$MS_{Within} = $ SS_{Within}/df_{Within}	
Total	$SS_{Total} = $ $SS_{Between} + SS_{Within}$	$df_{Total} = $ $df_{Between} + df_{Within}$		

Between-groups ($SS_{Between}$), within-groups (SS_{Within}), and total (SS_{Total}) sums of squares.
Between-groups ($df_{Between}$), within-groups (df_{Within}), and total (df_{Total}) degrees of freedom.
Between-groups ($MS_{Between}$) and within-groups (MS_{Within}) mean squares.
F statistic (F).

In the past, it was common to report the complete ANOVA table in the results section of a research article; however, this isn't as common anymore. Most investigators simply report the F statistic and degrees of freedom, along with a p-value, when reporting ANOVA results. Regardless, an ANOVA table tends to be standard output for most statistical analysis software packages, so it's good to be familiar with the general layout.

Basis for repeated-measures ANOVA

In general, repeated-measures ANOVA is used in situations when we want to compare performance in a single group of subjects across three or more different conditions or time points. I won't go into the same level of computational detail for repeated-measures ANOVA as I did for one-way ANOVA, since repeated-measures ANOVA is a bit more involved. Instead, I'll focus almost exclusively on the general principles of the analysis.

To help conceptualize the basis for repeated-measures ANOVA, let's consider a study by Reinold et al. (2008), which was conducted to examine the acute effects of pitching on shoulder motion. The study included a single group of professional baseball pitchers. The investigators measured the pitchers' shoulder range of motion using a goniometer before pitching (pre), immediately after a pitching session (post), and 24 hours after the pitching session had ended (follow-up). They then used repeated-measures ANOVA to determine if there was a statistically significant difference in shoulder motion among the time points (pre, post, follow-up). In this case, the null hypothesis was that there are no differences in shoulder motion among the time points: in other words, any observed differences in shoulder motion are simply due to random variation, not the pitching session. In contrast, the alternative hypothesis stated that there would be a difference in shoulder motion among the time points. Again, the null hypothesis is what's tested statistically.

The F statistic

As was the case with one-way ANOVA, the *F* statistic serves as our test statistic for repeated-measures ANOVA. With repeated-measures ANOVA, it's the within-subjects variance that we're particularly interested in analyzing, since our goal isn't to compare the different individuals but rather to determine how each individual's performance tends to vary across the different conditions. Some of this within-subjects variance is simply due to random variation in performance ('error variance'); however, some can be explained by the different experimental conditions ('between-conditions variance' or 'treatment variance'). If the different experimental conditions influence performance, the between-conditions variance should greatly exceed the error variance. In other words, there should be a fairly systematic pattern to how performance varies across the conditions.

The *F* statistic captures the ratio of the between-conditions variance relative to the error variance. A conceptual form of the *F* statistic for repeated-measures ANOVA is included in Equation 6.6.

Equation 6.6

$$F \text{ statistic} = \frac{\text{between-conditions variance}}{\text{error variance}}$$

Between-conditions variance

Notice that the between-conditions variance makes up the numerator of Equation 6.6. This between-conditions variance represents how the means for the different conditions vary about the grand mean ($\overline{X}_G$). In this case, the grand mean is the overall mean based on all scores, regardless of condition. Notice that this is conceptually the same as the between-groups variance described for one-way ANOVA, except now we're discussing the variance among the means for different conditions instead of means for different groups (remember, repeated-measures ANOVA only includes a single group, so we don't have between-groups variance).

Error variance

The error variance makes up the denominator of the *F* statistic. This error variance represents random variation in performance among the conditions or time points. It's important to note that this error variance doesn't include the variation among subjects (i.e. individual differences in performance). A key benefit of repeated-measures ANOVA is that we can partition out, and essentially remove, the variation among subjects from the analysis. This isn't possible in one-way ANOVA (note: I'll revisit this later in the chapter – 'Advantage of Repeated-Measures ANOVA').

F statistic

The F statistic will be relatively large when performance differs in a consistent pattern across conditions, such as when performance tends to get better for most subjects after treatment or over time. A small F statistic ($F = {\sim}1$) indicates that differences in performance across conditions tend to vary among subjects, such as when some subjects show improved performance, some show worse performance, and others show minimal change after treatment or over time (i.e. differences in performance tend to be unsystematic or random).

Degrees of freedom

In the case of repeated-measures ANOVA, the degrees of freedom for the between-conditions term will be the number of conditions (k), minus 1 ($df_{\text{Between}} = k - 1$). The degrees of freedom for the error term (df_{Error}) will be equal to ($k - 1$) × ($n - 1$), where n is the number of subjects. For example, the study conducted by Reinold et al. (2008) included three time points (pre, post, follow-up) and 67 subjects. Therefore, df_{Between} was 2 ($df_{\text{Between}} = 3 - 1 = 2$) and df_{Error} was 132 ($df_{\text{Error}} = [3 - 1] \times [67 - 1] = 132$).

Statistical significance

As was the case with one-way ANOVA, with repeated-measures ANOVA, we determine where our observed F statistic falls within an F distribution that's based on the assumption that the null hypothesis is true. If the F statistic falls into the outer tail of the distribution, it provides strong evidence that the differences in performance across the conditions aren't simply due to random variation. In other words, the different experimental conditions likely contributed to the observed differences in performance. We can compare the p-value associated with this F statistic to a predefined alpha level (typically 0.05) in order to determine if the differences among the conditions or time points are statistically significant. As you can see, the general process involved in repeated-measures ANOVA is essentially the same as one-way ANOVA, except for some differences in the way the F statistic is derived.

Now, let's return to the example introduced at the beginning of this section. Remember that Reinold et al. (2008) compared shoulder motion in pitchers immediately before (pre), immediately after (post), and 24 hours after a pitching session (follow-up). Prior to the pitching session, the pitchers exhibited an average of 54.1° (±11.4°) of shoulder internal rotation; immediately after (post), they exhibited an average of 44.6° (±11.9°) of shoulder internal rotation; and 24 hours later (follow-up), they exhibited an average of 46.5° (±10.0°) of shoulder internal rotation. The p-value associated with the repeated-measures ANOVA test comparing shoulder internal rotation motion across the three time points (pre, post, follow-up) was less than 0.001 ($p < 0.001$), which was well below the investigators' predefined alpha level. As a result, they concluded that there was a statistically significant difference in shoulder internal rotation motion among the time points.

Again, the results of this type of omnibus test don't inform us about which specific conditions or time points differ; they only tell us whether there are any differences overall. Therefore, the investigators conducted post-hoc tests to compare shoulder internal rotation motion for each pair of time points (post vs. pre, follow-up vs. pre, follow-up vs. post). Their results indicated that shoulder internal rotation motion was significantly less for the post and follow-up time points compared to the pre time point but that there wasn't a statistically significant difference between the post and follow-up time points. In general, these results appear to suggest that the pitching session resulted in an immediate reduction in shoulder internal rotation motion and that this reduction in shoulder motion persisted 24 hours after the session ended.

Advantage of repeated-measures ANOVA

As we've discussed already, one of the key advantages of repeated-measures ANOVA (vs. one-way ANOVA) is that individual differences in performance (i.e. 'between-subjects variance') can be isolated and accounted for in the analysis. This isn't possible with one-way ANOVA, where individual differences contribute to observed differences between the groups. The ability to partition out inter-subject variance from the analysis with repeated-measures ANOVA helps to accentuate the variance among the conditions, resulting in a larger F statistic. This tends to result in greater statistical power for repeated-measures ANOVA compared to one-way ANOVA, which allows us to detect smaller differences in performance with fewer subjects. In general, you can think of repeated-measures ANOVA as a more 'efficient' analysis.

Obviously, there are times when repeated-measures designs aren't appropriate or even possible. For example, think of the study conducted by Bologna et al. (2016), where movement speed was compared for individuals without Parkinson's disease, individuals with early-stage Parkinson's disease, and individuals with more advanced Parkinson's disease (control, early PD, advanced PD). Obviously, it isn't possible to conduct this study using a repeated-measures design, since these are mutually exclusive groups (i.e. subjects can't be in the control group and then be in the PD groups). This necessitates the use of a between-groups design, with one-way ANOVA for analysis. However, when possible, there's a tremendous advantage to the repeated-measures study design and repeated-measures ANOVA.

Why ANOVA?

At some point in this chapter, you've probably asked yourself, 'Why not just forget about the omnibus test and use t-tests to compare the pairs of means?' That's a great question, since in most cases, we want to know if there are differences between the pairs of groups, conditions, or time points. The most common reason for using an omnibus test is to attempt to control the risk of Type I error, which occurs when we falsely reject the null hypothesis.

Remember, that the alpha level allows us to establish the level of risk of a Type I error we're willing to accept. In most cases, the alpha level is set at 0.05. When the alpha level is set at 0.05, we're essentially accepting a 5% chance of committing a Type I error. However, it's important to note that this 5% chance of committing a Type I error applies to each statistical test conducted. Therefore, when we conduct multiple comparisons, the overall risk of committing a Type I error accumulates and exceeds 5%. The cumulative probability of committing a Type I error across multiple tests is typically referred to as the 'familywise error rate' (note: you'll also see this referred to as the 'experiment-wise error rate'*). The term 'familywise' reflects that this is the combined risk of error that results when a series, or 'family', of statistical tests are conducted.

* Note: there's a subtle difference between the concepts of familywise and experiment-wise error rates. The familywise error rate is the risk of Type I error that accumulates across a group ('family') of tests, such as when comparisons are made between the levels of an independent variable. The experiment-wise error rate is the risk of Type I error that accumulates across all of the tests conducted as part of an experiment. That said, the terms are often used interchangeably, since they reflect the same concept.

For example, imagine we're interested in comparing the performance of three different groups (group 1, group 2, group 3). Instead of conducting a one-way ANOVA, we simply use independent *t*-tests to compare each of the pairs of groups (groups 1 vs. 2, groups 1 vs. 3, and groups 2 vs. 3). If we used an alpha of 0.05 for each test, our chances of committing at least one Type I error would no longer be 5%. Instead, the familywise error rate would be around 14% once all three tests were conducted (Equation 6.7 is an equation for calculating the familywise error rate). In other words, the cumulative probability of committing a Type I error would be around 0.14, not the originally intended 0.05 (familywise error rate = $1 - [1 - 0.05]^3 = \sim 0.14$). This familywise error rate would become even greater if more comparisons were made, such as if there were more than three groups (Figure 6.3). Learning Activity 6.2 provides an opportunity for you to calculate a familywise error rate using Equation 6.7.

Equation 6.7

$$\text{familywise error rate} = 1 - (1 - \alpha)^c$$

In Equation 6.7, α is the alpha level associated with each test, and c is the number of comparisons.

Learning Activity 6.2

Imagine we're conducting a study to compare the time spent participating in physical activity among individuals without hypertension ('normal blood pressure'), individuals with pre-hypertension, individuals with stage I hypertension, and individuals with stage II hypertension. In this case, our study would include four distinct groups: normal blood pressure, pre-hypertension, stage I hypertension, and stage II hypertension. What would the familywise error rate be if we conducted independent *t*-tests (alpha level = 0.05) to compare the time spent participating in physical activity for each pair of groups?
The answer is provided at the end of the chapter.

Now, imagine that instead of comparing the group means using *t*-tests, we use one-way ANOVA. In this case, the familywise error rate would be equal to our designated alpha level of 0.05, since we would be comparing the group means with a single statistical test. Again, the general idea of conducting a preliminary ANOVA test is to avoid the inflation of the risk of Type I error that occurs when multiple comparisons are made.

Post hoc tests

As we've discussed throughout this chapter, post hoc tests are often conducted as a follow-up to a significant ANOVA test in order to determine which groups, conditions, or time points differ. There are a number of different options available for post hoc testing. Some of the more commonly used post hoc tests are the Bonferroni test, Tukey's test, and Scheffe's test. However, these are just a few of the many post hoc tests available.

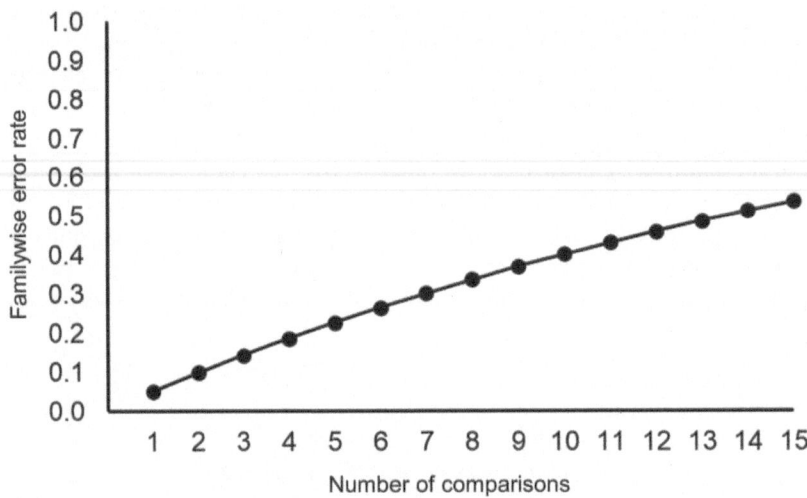

Figure 6.3 Plot of the familywise error rate (*y*-axis) based on the number of comparisons made (*x*-axis) when the alpha level is 0.05. Notice that the probability of committing a Type I error increases as the number of comparisons increases.

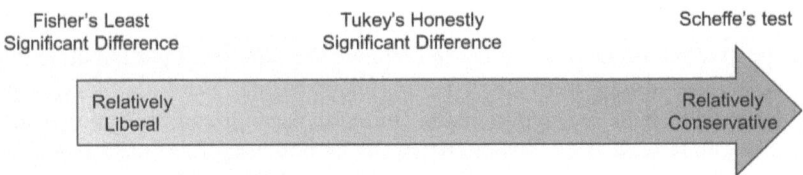

Figure 6.4 Three different post hoc tests that vary with respect to their degree of Type I error protection and statistical power. Fisher's least significant difference test offers no protection against Type I error but maximizes statistical power ('relatively liberal'). In contrast, Scheffe's test offers strong protection against Type I error but at the expense of statistical power ('relatively conservative'). Tukey's honestly significant difference test is generally considered more neutral on the liberal-conservative continuum. Note: these are just three examples of many different options for post hoc testing.

Almost all post hoc tests incorporate some adjustment to control the risk of Type I error that accumulates when multiple comparisons are made (i.e. the familywise error rate). The difference among the various post hoc tests lies in how much protection they provide against Type I error. Some tests are more 'liberal', with minimal protection against Type I error, while others are more 'conservative', offering greater protection against Type I error. Although conservative tests provide more protection against Type I error, the tradeoff is a loss of statistical power and therefore an increase in the risk of committing a Type II error (i.e. failing to detect differences that actually exist). While there's no consensus regarding which post hoc test to use, it's important to consider the tradeoff between the risk of Type I and Type II errors when selecting from the various options for post hoc testing (Figure 6.4).

I won't discuss the nuances of each of the different post hoc tests in this book (there really are a lot, and they differ quite a bit in their approaches to limiting the risk of Type I error). However, Box 6.1 includes a description of one common procedure used in post hoc testing.

Box 6.1 Post hoc test example

Bonferroni post hoc tests are commonly used to compare pairs of levels of an independent variable. Bonferroni post hoc tests involve adjusting the alpha level ('Bonferroni correction') based on the number of comparisons made in order to limit familywise error.* The adjustment is fairly simple, which is why I selected this as an example to highlight. Other types of post hoc tests involve different procedures, but their overall objective is the same (i.e. to control the risk of Type I error).

For Bonferroni post hoc tests, a series of t-tests are performed for the pairs of levels of the independent variable, with an adjustment to the alpha level. The adjustment simply involves dividing the original alpha level by the number of comparisons. For instance, if we conducted a study with three groups and we wanted to compare each pair of groups (group 1 vs. group 2, group 1 vs. group 3, group 2 vs. group 3), we would divide our original alpha level (let's say $\alpha = 0.05$) by the number of comparisons (3). In this case, our adjusted alpha level would be 0.0167 ($\alpha_{Adjusted} = 0.05/3 = 0.0167$). We would then compare our observed p-values based on the pairwise comparisons of the group means (independent t-tests) to this adjusted alpha level of 0.0167. Notice that this adjustment essentially functions to preserve the familywise error rate at the originally defined alpha level of 0.05. As an example, imagine that the p-value associated with the comparison of group 1 vs. group 2 was 0.03 ($p = 0.03$). In this case, we would conclude that there isn't a statistically significant difference between the groups, since the observed p-value is greater than the adjusted alpha level (0.03 > 0.0167).

Bonferroni post hoc tests are fairly conservative. In fact, they're often criticized for being overly conservative, especially when a lot of comparisons are made (e.g. Streiner & Norman, 2011). Again, I'm not necessarily recommending Bonferroni post hoc tests or suggesting they're the best, or even a good, option. This section is simply meant to highlight an example of what post hoc tests involve.

* **Note:** for Bonferroni post hoc tests, SPSS adjusts the p-values instead of the alpha level so that the observed (adjusted) p-values can still be compared to our predefined alpha level (typically 0.05). This adjustment involves multiplying the observed (unadjusted) p-values by the number of comparisons. This adjustment to the p-values is equivalent to adjusting the alpha level. Therefore, the results (significant vs. not significant) will be the same regardless of whether the Bonferroni correction is applied to the alpha level or the p-values.

Assumptions

This section highlights some of the key assumptions that should be met in order to conduct a one-way ANOVA or a repeated-measures ANOVA. Most of the assumptions are the same as those discussed for t-tests (Chapter 5). Therefore, I'll just briefly highlight the assumptions that were already discussed in Chapter 5.

1) The dependent variable is continuous

This isn't an assumption that's tested statistically. Instead, it's related to the nature of the dependent variable of interest.

2)   No significant outliers

An outlier is essentially a data point that differs significantly from the other observations in the data set (i.e. an extremely high or low value for the dependent variable of interest).

3)   The dependent variable should be normally distributed

The dependent variable should be normally distributed for each level of the independent variable, whether it's a between-subjects (one-way ANOVA) or a within-subjects (repeated-measures ANOVA) factor.

4)   Homogeneity of variance – *one-way ANOVA only*

For one-way ANOVA, it's assumed that the variance is the same for each of the populations of interest (i.e. *homogeneity of variance*). Since the variances of the populations are unknown, we compare the sample variances to get an idea of whether this assumption is met. If the sample variances are similar, the data satisfies the assumption of homogeneity of variance; however, if the sample variances differ substantially, the assumption is violated.

SPSS includes the option to run Levene's test for homogeneity of variance (described in Chapter 5) as part of its one-way ANOVA package, as well as an alternative option for one-way ANOVA if the assumption of homogeneity of variance isn't met (Welch's ANOVA). It's worth exploring these options if you suspect that your data may fail to satisfy the assumption of homogeneity of variance, especially if you're working with groups of different sizes.

5)   Sphericity – *repeated-measures ANOVA only*

For repeated-measures ANOVA, it's assumed that the variances of the differences between each pair of conditions or time points are equal (i.e. *sphericity*). For example, a study with three conditions (e.g. pre, post, follow-up) would have three sets of difference scores (pre vs. post, pre vs. follow-up, and post vs. follow-up). Repeated-measures ANOVA assumes that each of these differences exhibits similar variance. The assumption of sphericity is similar to the assumption of homogeneity of variance for one-way ANOVA, except we're examining the variance of the differences between conditions or time points instead of group variances (note: the assumption of sphericity is essentially the repeated-measures equivalent of homogeneity of variance). We didn't need to worry about this assumption in the case of a paired *t*-test, since there was only one set of differences between the two levels of the independent variable.

Mauchly's test is commonly used to test the assumption of sphericity. In fact, SPSS includes the results of Mauchly's test as part of its standard output. Mauchly's test tests the null hypothesis that the variances of the differences are equal. If the *p*-value generated from Mauchly's test is less than alpha (typically 0.05), it suggests that the assumption of sphericity has been violated. This can be counterintuitive, as we're hoping to observe a non-significant result for Mauchly's test (*p*-value ≥ 0.05), since this indicates that our data satisfies the assumption of sphericity.

Options if this assumption isn't met

When the assumption of sphericity is violated, it's common to adjust the degrees of freedom associated with the repeated-measures ANOVA test in order to control the increased risk of Type I error that occurs when the variances differ. Two common adjustments used when the assumption of sphericity is violated are the Greenhouse-Geisser correction and the Huynh-Feldt correction. Fortunately, SPSS automatically generates results with these adjustments as part of its standard output.

Application opportunities

Example data set #1

This example is based on a data set published by Jerez-Mayorga et al. (2019) (DOI: 10.7717/peerj.7471/supp-1), which includes data for 14 older adults with hip osteoarthritis ('OA group'), 14 older adults without hip osteoarthritis ('older group'), and 14 younger adults without hip osteoarthritis ('younger group') (note: the original data set included additional subjects in the older and younger groups; however, I modified the data set so the groups sizes are equivalent). As part of the study, subjects completed the Sit-to-Stand test, which involves standing and sitting as fast as possible for 10 repetitions. The investigators recorded the time required to complete the Sit-to-Stand test using a stopwatch (units – seconds). The objective of this analysis is to determine if there's a statistically significant difference in Sit-to-Stand test time among the groups (OA group, older group, younger group).

Data files

HipOA_STStest_data.xlsx – Excel file that includes Sit-to-Stand test times for the younger group, older group, and OA group. Sit-to-Stand test times are organized in separate columns ('Younger', 'Older', 'OA').

   HipOA_STStest_data.sav – SPSS file that includes Sit-to-Stand test times for the younger group, older group, and OA group. The file includes two columns. Column 1 ('Group') designates whether the subject was a member of the younger group (coded – 1), the older group (coded – 2), or the OA group (coded – 3). Column 2 ('STStest_time') includes the Sit-to-Stand test times for each subject.

Video

OneWayANOVA.mp4 – video that includes a demonstration of how to conduct a one-way ANOVA using SPSS and the Excel Analysis ToolPak.

Sample write-up

One-way analysis of variance was conducted to compare the Sit-to-Stand test times of younger adults (younger group), older adults without hip osteoarthritis (older group), and older adults with hip osteoarthritis (OA group). In the case of a significant omnibus test, Bonferroni post hoc tests were conducted to compare each of the groups. An alpha level of 0.05 was used for all tests of statistical significance.

   The mean (± standard deviation) Sit-to-Stand test times for the younger group, older group, and OA group were 8.2 ± 1.4 s, 10.7 ± 1.6 s, and 12.9 ± 2.5 s, respectively. There was a statistically significant difference in Sit-to-Stand test times among the groups [$F_{(2, 39)} = 21.49$; $p < 0.001$]. Post hoc tests indicated that Sit-to-Stand test times were shorter for the younger group, compared to both the older group ($p = 0.004$) and the OA group ($p < 0.001$). Sit-to-Stand test times were also shorter for the older group compared to the OA group ($p = 0.011$).

Notes: *F* is the *F* statistic, with its corresponding between-groups (2) and within-groups (39) degrees of freedom. *p* are the *p*-values associated with the one-way ANOVA and the post hoc tests.

Example data set #2

This example is based on a study I conducted with some of my former students (Almonroeder et al., 2020). The purpose of the study was to examine the influence of different types of verbal instructions on leg stiffness during landing in female athletes. The data set includes leg stiffness values during a drop landing task for 16 female athletes in three conditions: 1) baseline condition, 2) internal focus condition, and 3) external focus condition. The data for the baseline condition was recorded before the athletes received any type of instructions. The data for the internal focus condition was recorded after the athletes received instructions that encouraged them to attend to a specific aspect of their body's movement during the landing (i.e. adopt an 'internal focus'). The data for the external focus condition was recorded after the athletes received instructions that encouraged them to attend to the effects of their movement (i.e. adopt an 'external focus'). For the internal focus condition, athletes were instructed to 'focus on bending your knees when you land', whereas for the external focus condition, they were instructed to 'focus on landing softly'. All athletes completed trials in the baseline, internal focus, and external focus conditions. The objective of this analysis is to determine if there's a statistically significant difference in leg stiffness among the three conditions (baseline, internal focus, external focus).

Note: higher values for the leg stiffness variable reflect a 'stiffer' landing; units are Nkg^{-1}/m.

Data files

FoA_land_data.xlsx – Excel file that includes leg stiffness values for each subject in the baseline ('Base'), internal focus ('IF'), and external focus ('EF') conditions. Leg stiffness values are included in separate columns for each condition (Base, IF, EF).

FoA_land_data.sav – SPSS file that includes leg stiffness values for each subject in the baseline ('stiffness_base'), internal focus ('stiffness_IF'), and external focus ('stiffness_EF') conditions. Leg stiffness values are included in separate columns for each condition (stiffness_base, stiffness_IF, stiffness_EF).

Video

RM_ANOVA.mp4 – video that includes a demonstration of how to conduct a repeated measures ANOVA using SPSS and the Excel Analysis ToolPak.

Sample write-up

Repeated-measures analysis of variance was conducted to compare leg stiffness across the baseline, internal focus, and external focus conditions. In the case of a significant omnibus test, Fisher's least significant difference post hoc tests were conducted to compare the means for each of the conditions. An alpha level of 0.05 was used for all tests of statistical significance.

The mean (± standard deviation) leg stiffness values for the baseline, internal focus, and external focus conditions were 110.4 ± 38.8 Nkg^{-1}/m, 84.0 ± 38.1 Nkg^{-1}/m, and 69.5 ± 17.9 Nkg^{-1}/m, respectively. There was a statistically significant difference in leg stiffness among the conditions [F (2, 30) = 19.92; $p < 0.001$]. Post hoc tests indicated that leg stiffness was lower for both the internal focus ($p < 0.001$) and external focus ($p < 0.001$) conditions compared to the baseline condition, as well for the external focus condition compared to the internal focus condition ($p = 0.047$).

Notes: F is the F statistic, with its corresponding degrees of freedom (2, 30). p are the p-values associated with the repeated-measures ANOVA and the post hoc tests.

Answers to learning activities

Learning Activity 6.1

Answers

  Grenier et al. (2012) – used repeated-measures ANOVA to compare energy cost for the three load conditions (light load, moderate load, heavy load).

  Khalaj et al. (2014) – used one-way ANOVA to compare postural sway for the three groups (healthy, mild OA, moderate OA).

  Zaffagnini et al. (2006) – used one-way ANOVA to compare knee-related function for the three groups.

  Schucker et al. (2009) – used repeated-measures ANOVA to compare oxygen consumption for the three running conditions (focus on surroundings, focus on running pattern, focus on breathing).

  Reinold et al. (2004) – used repeated-measures ANOVA to compare shoulder muscle activity for the seven shoulder external rotation exercises.

Learning Activity 6.2

Answer

  The study would involve six total comparisons:

1) Normal blood pressure vs. pre-hypertension
2) Normal blood pressure vs. stage I hypertension
3) Normal blood pressure vs. stage II hypertension
4) Pre-hypertension vs. stage I hypertension
5) Pre-hypertension vs. stage II hypertension
6) Stage I hypertension vs. stage II hypertension

  Familywise error rate $= 1 - (1 - 0.05)^6 = 0.26$ or 26%

In this instance, there's a 26% chance of committing a Type I error for at least one of the six comparisons.

7 Factorial analysis of variance

Chapter Objectives

The objectives of this chapter are to . . .

1) describe the general purpose of factorial analysis of variance
2) provide examples of the types of research questions that factorial analysis of variance can be used to address
3) differentiate between between-subjects and within-subjects factors and provide examples of how these different types of factors can be combined within a statistical model
4) provide an overview of the conceptual basis for two-way analysis of variance
5) distinguish between interaction effects and main effects and describe the basis for statistically testing these effects
6) define and provide examples of marginal means
7) introduce the general structure of an interaction plot and describe how these plots can be used to help interpret the results of a two-way analysis of variance
8) describe the typical order of interpretation for factorial analysis of variance
9) highlight how additional statistical tests are often conducted as a follow-up to factorial analysis of variance
10) provide examples of studies that have used different types of factorial designs
11) demonstrate how to conduct a mixed-model analysis of variance using SPSS software

Introduction

Chapters 5 and 6 described tests that are used when dealing with a single independent variable (e.g. *t*-tests, one-way analysis of variance). In this chapter, we'll discuss factorial analysis of variance (ANOVA), which can be used to examine the effects of multiple categorical independent variables, or 'factors', within a single statistical model.* A key benefit of factorial ANOVA is that we can look at how the different factors in the model interact with one another or, in other words, how the effects of one factor are influenced by the other. This allows us to address more complex questions than what's possible when only analyzing a single factor in isolation. Considering the multifaceted nature of health and medicine, you can probably already appreciate the importance of being able to consider how different factors (e.g. disease severity, treatment type) interact with one another.

* **Note:** in the context of ANOVA, independent variables are typically referred to as 'factors'. Each factor includes two or more subcategories, which are referred to as 'levels'.

DOI: 10.4324/9781003179757-7

This chapter will primarily focus on instances where two factors are being analyzed ('two-way ANOVA'), since this is what you'll come across most often in the medical literature. While factorial ANOVA can include more than two factors, interpretation becomes more challenging as additional factors are added to the model. At this point, it's probably best to focus on two-way ANOVA and then progress to more advanced forms of factorial ANOVA once you're comfortable with the general concepts.

Although very useful, factorial ANOVA is one of the more conceptually challenging types of analyses covered in this book. Therefore, I'll focus on the general concepts instead of diving into the details of the computations involved, especially since the computational details will depend on the specifics of the statistical model, such as the number and type(s) of factors included.

Types of factors

A factorial ANOVA model can incorporate multiple between-subjects factors, multiple within-subjects factors, or a combination of between- and within-subjects factors ('mixed-model ANOVA'). As a reminder, a 'between-subjects factor' is one in which the levels of the independent variable are composed of different groups of individuals (e.g. injured, uninjured). In contrast, a 'within-subjects factor' is one where a single group of subjects is tested under multiple conditions or at multiple time points (e.g. pre, post, follow-up). In other words, repeated measurements are taken *within* a single group of subjects in the case of a within-subjects factor.

Conceptual basis of factorial ANOVA

Factorial ANOVA allows us to examine the effects of the individual factors ('main effects'), as well as how the factors interact with one another ('interaction effects'). While we may be interested in the main effects, we're often specifically interested in the interaction effect(s), since the ability to examine how the different factors interact with, or influence, one another is a key element of factorial ANOVA. In the case of a two-way ANOVA, we'll have two main effects and an interaction effect to examine.

Let's start by considering a hypothetical case where our analysis would include two factors (i.e. 'two-way ANOVA'). Imagine that we're interested in examining whether sex differences in anterior cruciate ligament thickness are dependent on age.* To address this question, we conduct a cross-sectional study where we record ACL thickness in male and female adolescents ranging from 10 to 18 years of age. We categorize the adolescents into three different age groups: 10–12 years of age, 13–15 years of age, and 16–18 years of age. These groups make up the three levels of our factor 'age'. We also have a factor 'sex', which has two levels (male, female). Therefore, our factorial ANOVA model includes two between-subjects factors: 'age' and 'sex'.

* **Note:** this example is based on a study conducted by Hosseinzadeh and Kiapour (2021), which serves as a nice example of a factorial ANOVA with two between-subjects factors.

In this case, the results of a two-way factorial ANOVA would allow us to address the following three questions:

1) does sex have an effect on ACL thickness?
2) does age have an effect on ACL thickness?

3)   do the factors age and sex interact with one another? In other words, are sex differences in ACL thickness dependent on age? Or another way to think of it is: are age differences in ACL thickness dependent on sex?

Questions 1 and 2 are related to the main effects, while question 3 is related to the interaction effect. For each of these questions, we have a null hypothesis that can be tested. The statistical significance of the main effects and the interaction effect are determined based on the results of three different F-tests, two associated with the main effects and one associated with the interaction effect (note: the basis for the F-test was introduced in Chapter 6).

Figure 7.1 (subplot A) includes a table to help you conceptualize the different factors included in our analysis. Within this table, the levels of the factor 'sex' (Factor A) are denoted A1 and A2, while the levels of the factor 'age' are denoted B1, B2, and B3. The individual cells in the table represent sample means for each of the 6 unique samples of subjects across the two factors ($\bar{X}_{A1B1}$, $\bar{X}_{A1B2}$, $\bar{X}_{A1B3}$, $\bar{X}_{A2B1}$, $\bar{X}_{A2B2}$, $\bar{X}_{A2B3}$). For instance, the cell denoted $\bar{X}_{A1B2}$ includes the sample mean for the 13–15-year-old males, while the cell denoted $\bar{X}_{A2B1}$ includes the sample mean for the 10–12-year-old females. The table also includes *marginal means*. A marginal mean is the average for one level of a factor across all levels of the other factor. For instance, $\bar{X}_{A1}$ is the mean for all male subjects, regardless of their age (i.e. the average ACL thickness for all males, across the age groups), while $\bar{X}_{B1}$ is the mean for all 10–12-year-olds, regardless of their sex (i.e. the average ACL thickness for all 10–12-year-olds, regardless of whether they are male or female). Notice that in this case we have two

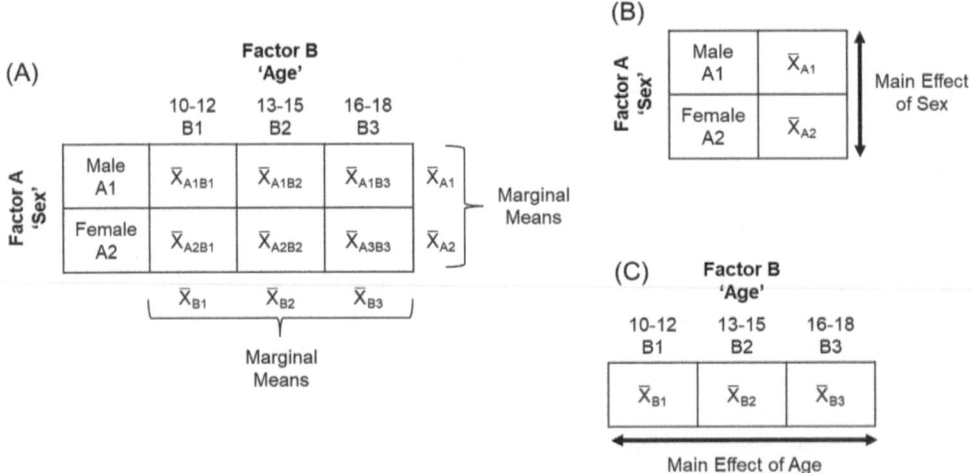

Figure 7.1 Subplot A (left) includes a table to help you conceptualize the factors involved in our hypothetical study examining how sex (Factor A) and age (Factor B) influence ACL thickness. The rows of the table represent the levels for the factor 'sex' (Male – A1, Female – A2), while the columns represent the levels for the factor 'age' (10–12 – B1, 13–15 – B2, 16–18 – B3). Each cell includes a sample mean for one of the six different subgroups. The table also includes the marginal means associated with each factor. Subplot B (top-right) includes a table that represents the main effect of sex, while subplot C (bottom-right) includes a table that represents the main effect of age. Notice that examining the main effects essentially involves analyzing the data as if the other factor didn't exist. You can think of analyzing the main effects as conducting two separate single-factor analyses.

marginal means associated with the factor 'sex' ($\bar{X}_{A1}$, $\bar{X}_{A2}$) and three marginal means associated with the factor 'age' ($\bar{X}_{B1}$, $\bar{X}_{B2}$, $\bar{X}_{B3}$). The main effects will be based on the differences among these marginal means.

Main effect – sex

The main effect of 'sex' is based on the difference between the marginal means, $\bar{X}_{A1}$ and $\bar{X}_{A2}$ (Figure 7.1, subplot B). In this case, the null hypothesis states that there's no difference in ACL thickness between the populations of males and females (H_0: $\mu_{Males} = \mu_{Females}$). Since we're working with samples, we need to consider the fact that we'll likely observe some difference in ACL thickness between males and females simply by chance alone, even if there's no difference in the populations. Remember, we always need to be mindful of sampling error.

The results of the *F*-test for the main effect of sex would allow us to determine whether the observed difference in ACL thickness between males and females is greater than what's expected by chance alone (i.e. 'statistically significant'). If the *p*-value associated with this *F*-test was less than our predefined alpha level (typically 0.05), we would reject the null hypothesis and conclude that the main effect of sex is statistically significant. In this case, a significant main effect of sex would indicate that our observed difference in ACL thickness is unlikely to be due to chance alone. In other words, the evidence from our sample data is strong enough to conclude that the populations of males and females differ with respect to their ACL thickness.

Main effect – age

The main effect of 'age' is based on the variance among the marginal means, $\bar{X}_{B1}$, $\bar{X}_{B2}$, and $\bar{X}_{B3}$ (Figure 7.1, subplot C). In this case, the null hypothesis states that there's no difference in ACL thickness among the age groups (H_0: $\mu_{10-12} = \mu_{13-15} = \mu_{16-18}$). The results of the *F*-test for the main effect of age would indicate whether there's a statistically significant difference in ACL thickness among the age groups (10–12 years, 13–15 years, 16–18 years).

If the *p*-value associated with the *F*-test of the main effect of age was less than our predefined alpha level (typically 0.05), we would reject the null hypothesis and conclude that the main effect of age is statistically significant. In other words, the observed difference in ACL thickness among the age groups is unlikely to be due to chance alone (i.e. the populations of 10–12-, 13–15-, and 16–18-year-olds likely differ with respect to their ACL thickness).

Main effects

Notice that examining the main effects basically involves conducting separate one-way analyses that neglect the potential influence of the other factor. For instance, examining the main effect of age involves comparing ACL thickness across all age groups, regardless of the subjects' sex, since males and females are grouped together. You can think of this as ignoring the potential influence of sex and simply comparing the different age groups. The opposite is true when the main effect of sex is analyzed, since this comparison of the males and females doesn't account for the different age groups. The interaction effect goes beyond these main effects and would allow us to determine the extent to which the factors sex and age influence, or interact with, one another.

Interaction effect

When examining the interaction between two factors, we're essentially trying to determine if the effect of one factor is dependent on the level of the other factor. For example, imagine we observe that the difference in ACL thickness between males and females is negligible for the 10–12 age group but that males tend to have much thicker ACLs compared to females for the 13–15 and 16–18 age groups (note: this finding is depicted in Figure 7.2). This is an example of what could be described as a 'sex-by-age' interaction effect, as the effect of sex is dependent on age. You can also consider this from the opposite perspective, in that the differences among the age groups depends on sex.

As with the main effects, an F-test is conducted to determine if the interaction effect is statistically significant. If the p-value associated with the F-test of the interaction effect is less than our predefined alpha level (typically 0.05), we conclude that the interaction effect is statistically significant. In other words, we reject the null hypothesis that there isn't an interaction between the factors in the population.

Now imagine that you're trying to explain the findings of our hypothetical study to a colleague who asks whether there's a sex difference in ACL thickness. In the case of our observed sex-by-age interaction effect, the best answer would probably be, 'it depends on age'. When you start needing to include caveats such as 'it depends' when explaining results, it probably means that you're dealing with some type of interaction effect.

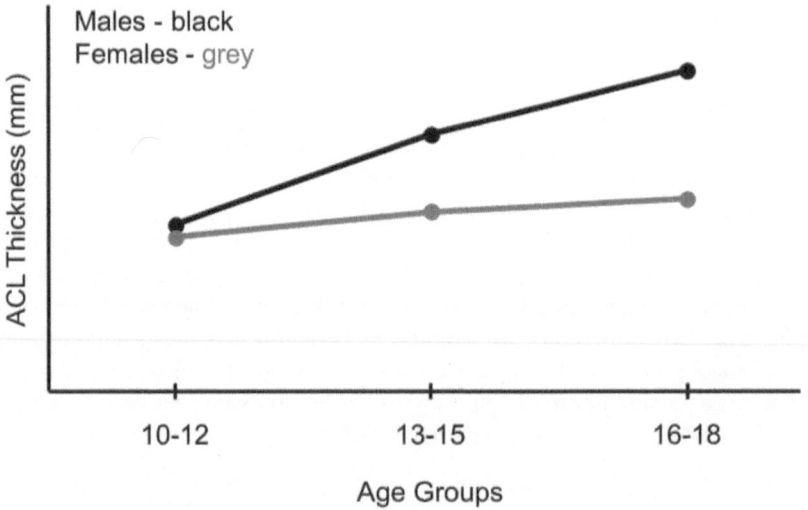

Figure 7.2 Interaction plot of the average ACL thickness for males and females (separate lines) across the different age groups (x-axis). Notice that the difference between males and females is dependent on age ('sex-by-age' interaction effect). Note: these results were contrived for this example; they aren't based on actual data.

Degrees of freedom

As discussed in previous chapters, we typically report the degrees of freedom associated with any statistical test we conduct, including an F-test. In the case of a two-way ANOVA, we need to report the degrees of freedom associated with the F-tests of the main effects and the interaction effect. The degrees of freedom (df) for the main effects are equal to the number of levels associated with each factor (k), minus 1 ($df_{FactorA} = k - 1$; $df_{FactorB} = k - 1$). The degrees of freedom for the interaction effect (df_{AxB}) is equal to the product of the degrees of freedom associated with the main effects ($df_{AxB} = df_A \times df_B$).

For instance, in the case of our hypothetical study examining the effects of sex and age on ACL thickness, the degrees of freedom associated with the main effect of 'sex' would be 1, since there are two levels for this factor ($df_{sex} = 2 - 1$). The degrees of freedom associated with the main effect of 'age' would be 2, since there are three levels for this factor ($df_{age} = 3 - 1$). The degrees of freedom associated with the interaction effect would be 2 ($df_{sex \times age} = df_{sex} \times df_{age} = 2 \times 1 = 2$).

We report these degrees of freedom, along with the 'error' degrees of freedom (df_{error}), with each of the corresponding F statistics. An example is included at the end of this chapter ('Application opportunity').

Interaction plots

A specific type of plot, often referred to as an *interaction plot*, is commonly used to help interpret the results of a two-way ANOVA. These plots are also often included as figures in research articles where some type of two-way ANOVA was performed. In an interaction plot, separate lines differentiate the levels of one factor, while the levels of the second factor are displayed on the x-axis. The y-axis includes the dependent variable of interest. Figure 7.2 includes an example of an interaction plot based on the results of our hypothetical study examining the effects of sex and age on ACL thickness. In this case, separate lines were used to differentiate between the males and females, while the different age groups were displayed along the x-axis.

An interaction effect may be present if the lines on the interaction plot don't run parallel to each other, such as what's depicted in Figure 7.2. If the lines run parallel to one another, then there isn't an interaction effect. Main effects may be present if there's a notable difference in performance across the levels of one factor, independent of the other factor included in the analysis. Figure 7.3 includes examples of interaction plots depicting different main and interaction effects.

It's important to note that simply examining an interaction plot doesn't allow us to determine if there are statistically significant interaction or main effects. For example, there may appear to be an interaction effect based on the plot, but it may not be statistically significant once we consider what's likely to occur by chance. Investigators will typically use interaction plots as a first look at their data before moving forward with significance testing or to help them understand the results of their significance tests.

Order of interpretation

With two-way ANOVA, we should start by examining the interaction effect. If the interaction effect isn't statistically significant, we can then move on to examine the main effects. If the interaction effect is significant, we typically explain this interaction effect and don't move on to consider the main effects. This may seem counterintuitive at first, but think of it this way: if we know that the factors are dependent on one another (i.e. a significant interaction effect exists), it probably doesn't make sense to consider the factors independently. Again, the ability to examine how multiple factors interact with one another is an important feature of factorial ANOVA.

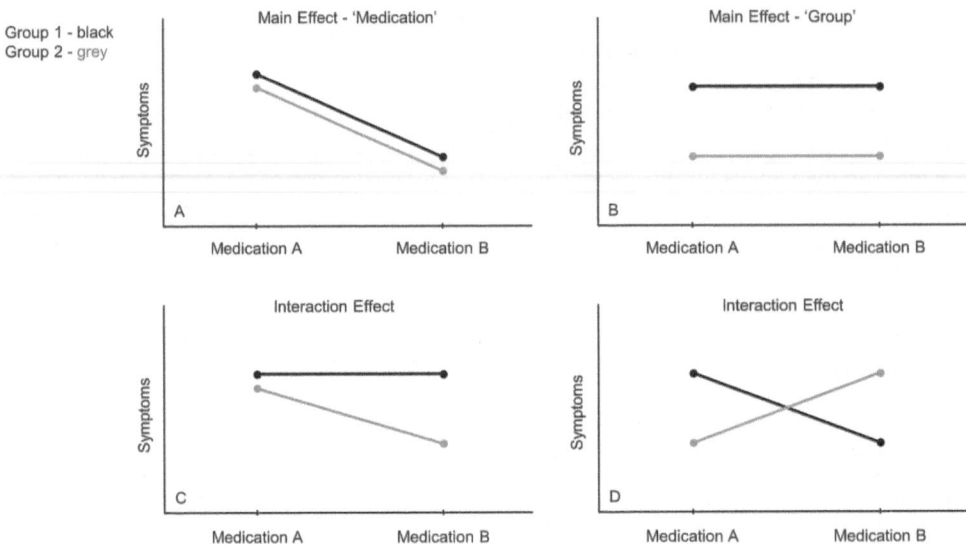

Figure 7.3 Interaction plots (A–D) based on four different outcomes for a hypothetical study comparing the effects of two medications (Medication A, Medication B) on 'symptoms' in two
groups of patients (Group 1 – black lines, Group 2 – gray lines). Subplot A represents
an example where there's a main effect of 'medication', as both groups experience fewer
symptoms with Medication B. Subplot B represents an example where there's a main effect
of 'group', as Group 1 experiences greater symptoms regardless of the medication they
use. Subplots C and D represent examples where there's a 'group-by-medication' interaction effect. In the case of subplot C, Group 1 experiences no difference in symptoms
with Medication A vs. Medication B; however, Group 2 experiences fewer symptoms with
Medication B. In the case of subplot D, Medication B is more effective (fewer symptoms)
than Medication A for Group 1, while the opposite is true for Group 2. Note: you may see
interaction effects described as 'disordinal' or 'ordinal'; when the lines on the plot cross
(e.g. subplot D), the interaction is considered disordinal, and when they don't (e.g. subplot
C), the interaction is considered ordinal.

That said, there are some instances where it makes sense to examine the main effects even
if there's a significant interaction effect. In the end, if the main effects provide additional
insight, they should probably be reported, even if it's a bit unconventional.

Follow-up tests

In many cases, additional statistical tests are conducted to further explore the factorial
ANOVA results, especially when there's a significant interaction effect. For example, let's
revisit our hypothetical study examining the effects of sex and age on ACL thickness. Again,
imagine that we observed the 'sex-by-age' interaction effect described earlier, where the difference between males and females differed across the age groups (depicted in Figure 7.2). In
this case, we may decide to conduct pairwise comparisons of the males and females for each
age group. In other words, we could compare the ACL thickness of the males and females
in the 10–12 age group, the 13–15 age group, and then the 16–18 age group. We could also

examine ACL thickness across the age groups separately for the males and females (often referred to as examining the 'simple effects' or 'simple main effects'). You can think of this as conducting a one-way ANOVA comparing the 10–12, 13–15, and 16–18 age groups for the males and then doing the same for the females in a separate analysis.

These are just examples. The type of tests used as a follow-up to a preliminary factorial ANOVA will depend on the specifics of the analysis, and in some instances, it's not necessary to conduct any follow-up tests.

Additional examples

In this section, I'll provide additional examples to highlight different types of factorial ANOVA models. The examples will include a two-way ANOVA with one between-subjects factor and one within-subjects factor ('mixed-model ANOVA') (Example #1) and a two-way ANOVA with two within-subjects factors (Example #2).

Example #1: Two-way mixed-model ANOVA

A 'mixed-model' ANOVA includes a combination, or *mix*, of between-subjects and within-subjects factors. As an example, let's consider a study conducted by Llamas-Ramos et al. (2014) to compare the effects of dry needling and manual therapy on neck pain. As part of the study, patients with chronic neck pain were randomly allocated to receive either dry needling ('dry needling group') or manual therapy ('manual therapy group') to address trigger points in their upper trapezius.* Both groups were treated for two sessions per week over a 2-week period (four total sessions). Patients were asked to rate their neck pain intensity on a 0–10 scale (0 = no pain; 10 = maximum pain) prior to treatment (baseline), immediately after the last treatment session (post), 1 week later (1-week follow-up), and 2 weeks later (2-week follow-up). The investigators conducted a two-way mixed-model ANOVA (alpha level = 0.05) with a between-subjects factor of 'group' (dry needling, manual therapy) and a within-subjects factor of 'time' (baseline, post, 1-week follow-up, 2-week follow-up).

* **Note:** a 'trigger point' is a hypersensitive area in a muscle that can contribute to pain in another region (i.e. 'refer' pain). Trigger points in the upper trapezius often refer pain to the neck.

The results of their analysis indicated that there wasn't a statistically significant 'group-by-time' interaction effect ($p = 0.516$); however, the main effect of 'time' was statistically significant ($p < 0.001$), as both groups reported similar reductions in pain intensity over the course of the study period. In other words, there was a significant change in pain intensity over time, but the change in pain intensity didn't differ between the groups.

Figure 7.4 includes an interaction plot based on the results reported by Llamas-Ramos et al. (2014). Notice that both groups (dry needling, manual therapy) exhibited a similar decrease in pain from baseline to post and then more subtle reductions in pain over the follow-up time points. As you can see, the lines tend to run parallel to one another, which is consistent with the lack of a significant interaction effect.

The mixed-model ANOVA design is very commonly utilized in medical research, especially in studies examining intervention effectiveness. For instance, consider the structure of a typical randomized controlled trial, where patients are randomly allocated to either a control group or a treatment group (or perhaps to two different treatment groups) and then

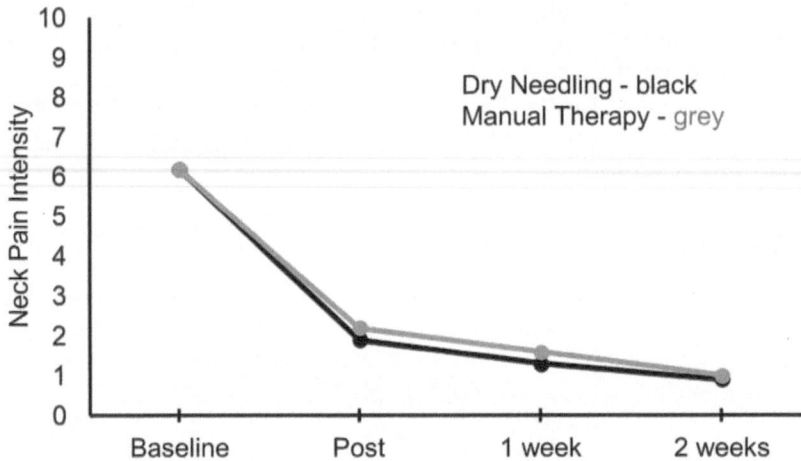

Figure 7.4 Interaction plot based on the results reported by Llamas-Ramos et al. (2014). The two groups (dry needling, manual therapy) are represented by separate lines, while the different time points (baseline, post, 1-week follow-up – '1 week', 2-week follow-up – '2 weeks') are included on the *x*-axis. Pain intensity (0–10 scale) is the dependent variable and is included on the *y*-axis. Notice that both groups experienced similar changes in pain over time (main effect of 'time').

monitored over time. This type of study design involves a *mix* of a between-subjects factor ('group') and a within-subjects factor of ('time'), and therefore, mixed-model ANOVA is often included as part of the analysis.

Note: the 'Application opportunity' at the end of the chapter provides another example of a mixed-model ANOVA.

Example #2: Two-way ANOVA with two within-subjects factors

A factorial ANOVA model can also incorporate multiple within-subjects factors. For example, Roberts et al. (2014) conducted a study to examine the effects of cold-water immersion on muscle recovery following a session of resistance training. As part of the study, subjects completed two rounds of high-intensity resistance training separated by 2 weeks. After one of the sessions, subjects immersed their bodies in a pool of cold water for 10 minutes ('cold-water immersion' condition). After the other session, they biked for 10 minutes ('active recovery' condition). The order of the conditions (cold-water immersion, active recovery) was randomized. Subjects were asked to report their perceived level of leg muscle soreness during squatting on a 0–100 visual analog scale (0 = no soreness; 100 = maximal soreness) before (baseline) and immediately after training (post), as well as 2 hours, 4 hours, and 6 hours after each of the recovery conditions.* The investigators conducted a two-way ANOVA (alpha level = 0.05) with within-subjects factors of 'condition' (cold-water immersion, active recovery) and 'time' (baseline, post, 2 hours, 4 hours, 6 hours).** Notice that the factor 'condition' is a within-subjects factor in this instance since subjects completed both the cold-water immersion and active recovery protocols (often referred to as a 'cross-over study design').

* Note: the investigators also examined several other variables, including muscle force output, muscle temperature, inflammatory markers, and jump performance.

** Note: this type of analysis may also be referred to as a 'two-way ANOVA with repeated measures' or a 'repeated-measures two-way ANOVA'.

The results of their analysis indicated that there was a significant 'condition-by-time' interaction effect ($p < 0.001$). The significant interaction effect was a result of the subjects experiencing greater recovery in the cold-water immersion condition compared to the active recovery condition.

Figure 7.5 includes an interaction plot based on the results reported by Roberts et al. (2014). Notice that for both conditions (cold-water immersion, active recovery), subjects experienced an increase in leg muscle soreness after training (post vs. baseline) and then a reduction in soreness over the 6-hour recovery period. However, the reduction in soreness was greater in the cold-water immersion condition vs. the active recovery condition. In other words, the change in muscle scores over time was dependent on the recovery condition, hence the significant interaction effect.

Learning Activity 7.1 provides additional opportunities for you to identify the number and types of factors included in a factorial ANOVA model.

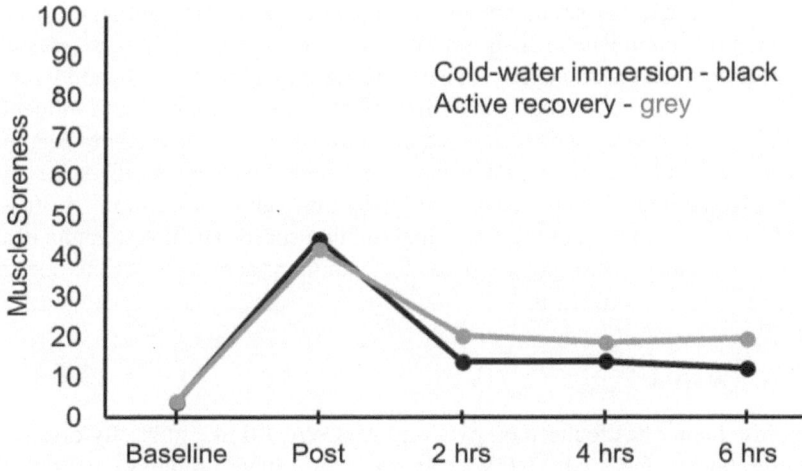

Figure 7.5 Interaction plot based on the results reported by Roberts et al. (2014). The two conditions (cold-water immersion, active recovery) are represented by separate lines, while the different time points (baseline, post, 2 hours – '2 hrs', 4 hours – '4 hrs', 6 hours – '6 hrs') are included on the *x*-axis. Leg muscle soreness (0–100; 0 = no soreness, 100 = maximal soreness) is the dependent variable and is included on the *y*-axis. Notice that subjects tended to experience less leg muscle soreness during the recovery period (2 hrs, 4 hrs, 6 hrs) for the cold-water immersion condition vs. the active recovery condition ('condition-by-time' interaction effect).

Learning Activity 7.1

Following are four examples of studies that included some type of factorial ANOVA design. Based on the following brief descriptions, try to predict the number of factors included in the analysis, the number of levels associated with each factor, and whether the factors were between-subjects or within-subjects factors. The answers are included at the end of the chapter.

Hollman et al. (2007) conducted a study to examine the effects of a secondary cognitive task on gait speed in individuals of varying ages. Their study included groups of older adults (>70 years of age), middle-aged adults (40–55 years of age), and younger adults (20–35 years of age). All subjects completed walking trials without performing a secondary cognitive task (normal condition) and while performing a secondary cognitive task (dual-task condition), which involved spelling a random word backwards. Walking speed was recorded during both the normal and dual-task walking conditions.

Lariviere et al. (2015) conducted a study to determine if sex and low back pain status influence postural control while sitting on an unstable surface. Their study included a group of subjects with chronic low back pain, as well as a control group without low back pain. Both groups were composed of male and female subjects. Postural sway was recorded as subjects sat on an unstable surface.

Magadle et al. (2007) conducted a study to examine the effectiveness of inspiratory muscle training for patients with chronic obstructive pulmonary disease (COPD). As part of their study, patients with COPD were randomly allocated to an experimental group that completed inspiratory muscle training or to a control group that completed a sham training program. The investigators assessed lung function upon enrollment in the study (baseline), and after 3, 6, and 9 months.

Hobara et al. (2019) conducted a study to explore how running speed influences leg stiffness in sprinters who had undergone a transfemoral ('above-knee') amputation and ran with a prosthetic limb. Running mechanics were recorded for the sprinters' unaffected limb and prosthetic limb while they ran on a treadmill at 30%, 40%, 50%, 60%, and 70% of their maximal running speed. The investigators examined leg stiffness during the stance phase for both limbs across the various speeds.

Three-way ANOVA

Although this chapter has focused on two-way ANOVA, I'd like to briefly discuss the more complex 'three-way' factorial ANOVA. As you could have probably guessed, three-way ANOVA incorporates three factors. In the case of three-way ANOVA, we can consider the interaction among the three factors, the interaction between each pair of factors, and the main effects for each factor. We typically start by examining the highest-order interaction effect (i.e. the interaction among all factors), then move to the lower-order interaction effects (i.e. the interaction among the pairs of factors) and finally to the main effects.

To help you conceptualize what a three-way ANOVA would involve, let's consider a study conducted by Paterno et al. (2011). The investigators were interested in determining whether differences in the degree of side-to-side asymmetry in limb loading, between athletes with and without a history of ACL reconstruction, is dependent on sex. They recorded the forces acting on the lower limbs during a double-leg landing task in a group of male and female athletes who had undergone ACL reconstruction (ACLR group) and a group of uninjured male and female athletes (control). Their three-way ANOVA model included the between-subjects factors of 'group' (ACLR, control) and 'sex' (male, female) and the within-subjects factor of 'limb' (uninvolved, involved for the ACLR group; dominant, non-dominant for the control group).

The investigators started by examining the 'group-by-sex-by-limb' interaction effect in order to determine if the degree of side-to-side asymmetry in limb loading between the ACLR and control groups differed for males and females. The results of an *F*-test of this three-way interaction effect indicated that there wasn't a statistically significant 'group-by-sex-by-limb' interaction effect ($p = 0.622$). Therefore, the investigators moved on to examine the lower-order interaction effects. Interestingly, they observed a significant 'group-by-limb' interaction effect ($p = 0.002$), as the ACLR group tended to exhibit more side-to-side asymmetry in limb loading compared to the control group, regardless of sex. In other words, individuals who had undergone ACL reconstruction tended to exhibit more side-to-side differences in limb loading compared to controls, and this effect was consistent across males and females.

As you can see, additional factors allow us to address more nuanced questions; however, interpretation becomes more challenging. In fact, interpretation becomes almost impossible when four factors are included in an ANOVA model, which is why you probably won't come across many four-way ANOVAs in your readings. Additional factors also tend to increase the total sample size needed, which is another drawback.

If you're considering conducting a four-way ANOVA for your own research, I'd consider simplifying your study, collapsing a variable across levels, or getting a statistician involved.

Different terminology

Factorial ANOVA models can also be described based on the number of levels associated with the factors they include. As an example, let's return to our hypothetical study examining the effects of sex and age on ACL thickness. Remember that the factor 'sex' had two levels (male, female), while the factor 'age' had three levels (10–12 years, 13–15 years, 16–18 years). In this case, our analysis could be described as a 2 × 3 (read '2-by-3') factorial ANOVA, with '2 × 3' referring to the fact that one factor had two levels, while the other factor had three levels. If we expanded our study to include an additional age group of 7–9-year-olds, our analysis would then be described as a 2 × 4 factorial ANOVA, since the factor 'age' would now have four levels (7–9 years, 10–12 years, 13–15 years, 16–18 years).

As another example, let's consider the three-way ANOVA conducted by Paterno et al. (2011), which included three factors ('group', 'sex', 'limb'), each with two levels. In this case, the analysis could be described as a 2 × 2 × 2 factorial ANOVA.

Again, this is just a different way of describing a factorial ANOVA design. You'll often see this convention when reading research articles since it allows the authors to express both the number of factors and the number of levels associated with these factors simultaneously.

Assumptions

The assumptions associated with factorial ANOVA will depend on the specifics of the factors included in the model. For example, if we have a within-subjects factor with more than two levels, we should determine whether the assumption of sphericity is met. As another example, if our model is composed of between-subjects factors, we should consider whether our data satisfies the assumption of homogeneity of variance. Again, the specifics will depend on the nature of the factors included in the analysis. You can look back at Chapters 5 and 6 as a starting point for determining which specific assumptions you may need to consider.

Application opportunity

Example data set

This example is based on a data set published by Lehecka et al. (2019) (DOI: 10.7717/peerj.7287/supp-1). The data set is from a study conducted to compare the effects of two different hip-strengthening exercises on gluteal strength, power, endurance, and girth. The two exercises examined were 1) gluteal squeezes and 2) supine bilateral bridges. As part of the study, subjects were assigned to either a group that completed gluteal squeezes ('squeeze group') or to a group that completed supine bilateral bridges ('bridge group') over the course of 8 weeks. The dependent variables of interest were recorded before (pre) and after (post) the 8-week period.

The data set provided includes hip extension force measurements (units – kg) for the right limb at the pre and post time points for both groups (squeeze, bridge). The objective of this analysis is to examine the changes in hip strength for the two groups. More specifically, we want to determine if there's a statistically significant 'group-by-time' interaction effect, indicating that the changes in hip strength over time differed between the groups.

Data files

Bridge_vs_Squeeze_data.sav – SPSS file that includes hip extension force ('strength') values for the subjects in the 'bridge group' ($n = 14$) and the 'squeeze group' ($n = 16$) at the pre and post time points. The file includes three columns. Column 1 ('Group') designates whether the subject was a member of the bridge group (coded – 1) or the squeeze group (coded – 2). Columns 2 and 3 include the hip extension force values for each subject at the pre ('HipExtStr_Pre') and post ('HipExtStr_Post') time points, respectively.

Video

MixedANOVA.mp4 – video that includes a demonstration of how to conduct a mixed-model ANOVA using SPSS.

Sample write-up

A mixed-model analysis of variance, with a between-subjects factor of 'group' (squeeze, bridge) and a within-subjects factor of 'time' (pre, post), was conducted to compare the changes in hip extension strength over the course of the 8-week training period. The alpha level was set at 0.05.

There was not a significant group-by-time interaction effect [$F (1, 28) = 0.838$; $p = 0.368$] or a significant main effect of group [$F (1, 28) = 0.372$; $p = 0.547$]. However, there was a significant main effect of time [$F (1, 28) = 28.190$; $p < 0.001$], as both groups demonstrated comparable improvement in hip extension strength over the 8-week period (16.7% increase for the squeeze group, 11.0% increase for the bridge group) (Figure 7.6).

Notes: *F* is the *F* statistic, along with its corresponding degrees of freedom (effect, error). *p* represents the *p*-values associated with the *F*-tests of the interaction effect and main effects.

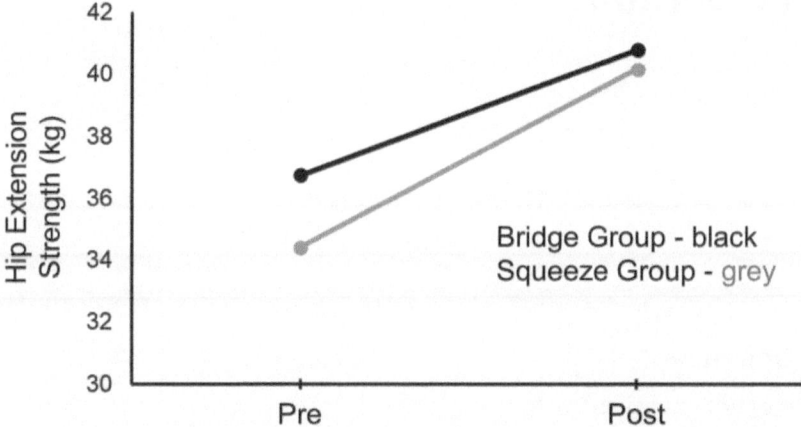

Figure 7.6 Interaction plot based on the results of the mixed-model ANOVA conducted as part of the Application Opportunity. The two groups (bridge, squeeze) are represented by separate lines, while the time points (pre, post) are included on the *x*-axis. Hip extension strength (kg) is the dependent variable and is included on the *y*-axis. Notice that both groups demonstrated a similar increase in hip extension strength over the course of the training period (main effect of 'time'). Note: this figure is based on data reported by Lehecka et al. (2019).

Answers to learning activity

Learning activity 7.1

Hollman et al. (2007)

- Two factors: 'group' (three levels – older adults, middle-aged adults, younger adults); 'condition' (two levels – normal, dual-task)
- Group is a between-subjects factor, while condition is a within-subjects factor (mixed-model ANOVA)

Lariviere et al. (2015)

- Two factors: 'sex' (two levels – male, female); 'low back pain status' (two levels – low back pain, control)
- Both factors are between-subjects factors

Magadle et al. (2007)

- Two factors: 'group' (two levels – experimental, control); 'time' (four levels – baseline, 3 months, 6 months, 9 months)
- Group is a between-subjects factor, while time is a within-subjects factor (mixed-model ANOVA)

Hobara et al. (2019)

- Two factors: 'limb' (two levels – prosthetic, uninvolved); 'speed' (five levels – 30%, 40%, 50%, 60%, 70%)
- Both factors are within-subjects factors

8 Correlation

Chapter Objectives

The objectives of this chapter are to . . .
1) describe the general purpose of bivariate correlation
2) provide examples of the types of clinical research questions that bivariate correlation can be used to address
3) summarize the key features of a scatter plot
4) explain how to interpret a Pearson product-moment correlation coefficient
5) describe the concept of covariance in the context of correlation
6) define the coefficient of determination and explain what it represents
7) explain the basis for examining the statistical significance of a correlation coefficient
8) highlight how sample size can influence the results of a test of the statistical significance of a correlation coefficient
9) explain what confidence intervals represent in the context of correlation coefficients
10) provide examples of correlation analyses that incorporate change scores
11) distinguish between correlation and causation
12) point out key assumptions that should be met in order to conduct a Pearson product-moment correlation analysis
13) demonstrate how to conduct a Pearson product-moment correlation analysis using SPSS and Excel software

Introduction

In general, correlation involves examining the relationship between variables. There are many different types of correlation analyses, which can be used to address different research questions and to examine various types of data. However, the focus of this chapter will be on bivariate correlation for continuous variables (i.e. variables measured on an interval or ratio scale).

The purpose of bivariate correlation is to examine the relationship between two variables, often denoted X and Y. It's important to note that, unlike the analyses discussed in Chapters 5–7 (i.e. t-tests, analysis of variance), the goal of correlation isn't to determine if there's a difference between the X and Y variables. Instead, the intent is to examine the extent to which the two variables are related or 'go together'. It's also important to note that in the case of correlation, we typically don't attempt to manipulate the variables, as our goal is generally to observe how the variables naturally coexist.

With bivariate correlation, we'll have an X and Y pair for each subject. For example, if we wanted to examine the relationship between age and walking speed, we would need to record age and measure walking speed for everyone in our sample.

DOI: 10.4324/9781003179757-8

Scatter plots

A scatter plot is often used to visualize the relationship between the X and Y variables. With a scatter plot, the variable denoted X is plotted along the x-axis (horizontal axis), while the variable denoted Y is plotted along the y-axis (vertical axis). Each point on the plot represents an X/Y pair for an individual subject. You can also think of these X/Y pairs as coordinates that describe the position of the point in a plane.

Note: the variable denoted X vs. Y is often arbitrary in correlation; however, this will not be the case with regression, where the intent is typically to use the X variable to predict the Y variable. Regression will be introduced in Chapter 9.

Now let's look at an example of a scatter plot. Figure 8.1 includes a scatter plot based on the results of a study conducted by Wisloff et al. (2004). The purpose of the study was to examine the relationship between lower body strength and vertical jump height in elite soccer players. Lower body strength was assessed by determining the maximum amount of weight each player could squat for a single repetition (one repetition maximum). The scatter plot in Figure 8.1 includes the one repetition maximum squat weights (x-axis) and the vertical jump heights (y-axis) for 16 athletes who participated in the study. Each point on the scatter plot represents an X/Y pair for an individual athlete. As an example, the athlete whose data point is circled was able to squat 170 kilograms of weight and jump 64 centimeters high. The scatter plot also includes a *line of best fit* (or trend line) that travels through the center of the distribution of data points. This line of best fit represents the single line that gets as close as possible to each X/Y pair (i.e. this line 'best fits' the data points). Chapter 9 includes additional information about deriving a line of best fit, since this is a critical aspect of simple linear regression.

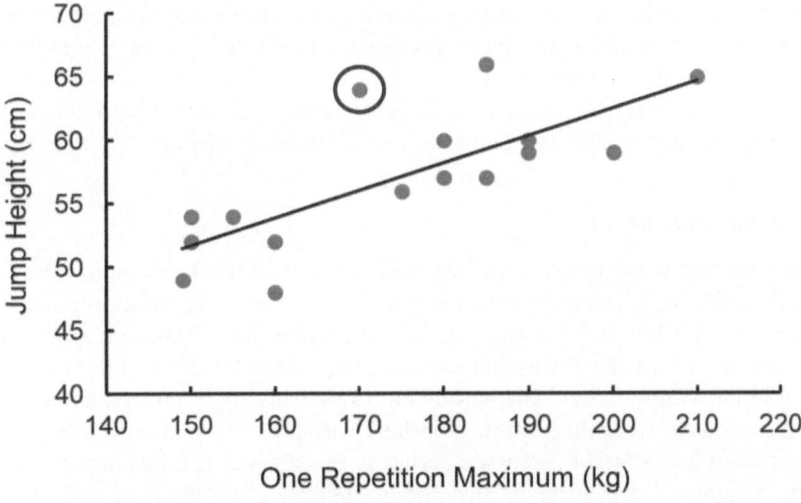

Figure 8.1 Scatter plot based on one repetition maximum squat weights (x-axis) and vertical jump heights (y-axis) for 16 athletes who participated in a study conducted by Wisloff et al. (2004). The line of best fit is represented by the solid black line running diagonally through the data points.

As you progress through this chapter, you'll learn more about how to both qualitatively and quantitatively examine the relationship between variables, as well as other key information that can be gleaned from a scatter plot. However, as a primer, let's start by simply describing some general things that can be observed from the scatter plot in Figure 8.1. First, you'll notice that there appears to be a general pattern to the data points, as they tend to start in the bottom-left corner and move toward the top-right corner of the scatter plot. This indicates that athletes with stronger lower bodies (i.e. greater one repetition maximum weights) tended to be able to jump higher. You'll also notice that most data points appear to be located fairly closely to the line of best fit but that very few data points lie directly on the line. Finally, you'll see that some of the data points are located farther from the line of best fit than others. For example, the athlete whose data point is circled didn't appear to fit the general pattern observed for the sample, as his lower body strength was slightly below average, but he was able to jump higher than almost all of the other athletes in the study.

As you can already see, scatter plots provide a tremendous amount of information. Examining a scatter plot is often done as a preliminary step to qualitatively visualize the nature of the relationship (or lack thereof) between variables before performing a more quantitative analysis. Scatter plots can also help us determine whether our data meets some of the key assumptions associated with bivariate correlation (discussed at the end of this chapter). Fortunately, scatter plots are fairly easy to generate and are often standard output when conducting a bivariate correlation analysis using most statistical analysis software packages. Scatter plots are also commonly included as figures in research articles that report the results of a bivariate correlation analysis.

An introduction to correlation coefficients

While examining a scatter plot allows us to qualitatively assess the relationship between two variables, correlation coefficients help to quantitatively characterize the nature of the relationship. The Pearson product-moment correlation coefficient, which is typically represented by a lowercase, italicized *r* and often referred to as the '*r* value', is commonly used to quantitatively describe the relationship between two continuous variables. Throughout this chapter, any reference to a correlation coefficient, or *r* value, is referring to the Pearson product-moment correlation coefficient.

Correlation coefficients describe two key aspects of the relationship between variables: 1) the direction of the relationship and 2) the strength of the relationship.

Direction of the relationship

Correlation coefficients can range from values of -1.00 to $+1.00$. The sign of the correlation coefficient describes the direction of the relationship. A positive correlation coefficient ($r > 0.00$) represents a positive relationship (or 'direct relationship') between variables, meaning that as the values for the X variable increase, the values for the Y variable also tend to increase. In other words, individuals who exhibit relatively high values for the X variable also tend to exhibit relatively high values for the Y variable. The relationship between lower body strength and jump height discussed earlier in this chapter is an example of a positive relationship, as athletes with stronger lower bodies tended to be able to jump higher.

A negative correlation coefficient ($r < 0.00$) represents a negative relationship (or 'inverse relationship') between variables, meaning that as the values for the X variable increase, the values for the *Y* variable tend to decrease. In other words, individuals who exhibit relatively high values for the *X* variable tend to exhibit relatively low values for the *Y* variable, and vice versa. Consider the relationship between age and walking speed in adults. This is an example of a negative relationship, since walking speed tends to become slower with age (i.e. walking speed decreases as age increases).

Strength of the relationship

In addition to the direction of the relationship, correlation coefficients also describe the strength of the relationship between the variables. A correlation coefficient of +1.00 represents a perfect positive relationship between the variables, whereas a correlation coefficient of −1.00 represents a perfect negative relationship between the variables. Essentially, the closer the correlation coefficient is to the ±1.00 limits, the stronger the relationship. Another way to think about it is that the closer the correlation coefficient is to 0.00, the weaker the relationship. It's important to clarify what's meant by a 'perfect' relationship. With a perfect relationship, all data points lie directly on the line of best fit. This is true for both perfect positive and perfect negative relationships.

Of course, very few relationships are perfect. In fact, many are quite poor. The more the data points deviate from the line of best fit, the weaker the relationship between the variables and the closer the correlation coefficient gets to 0.00. For example, consider the relationship between lower body strength and jump height. While there does appear to be a positive relationship between lower body strength and jump height, it's apparent when viewing the scatter plot in Figure 8.1 that most data points don't lie directly on the line of best fit. This is an example of an imperfect relationship. The correlation coefficient associated with the lower body strength and jump height data is +0.76, which isn't perfect, but also isn't close to 0.00.

Figure 8.2 includes scatter plots and their associated correlation coefficients for relationships of varying directions and strengths. Learning Activity 8.1 also provides you with an opportunity to match different correlation coefficients with their corresponding scatter plots.

Interpreting correlation coefficients

There are many guidelines available to assist with interpreting the strength of a relationship based on the magnitude of a correlation coefficient. For example, Table 8.1 includes a set of guidelines proposed by Portney (2020). These types of general guidelines serve as a good starting point; however, it's important to note that these are just guidelines, not strict rules. You still need to use your judgment. Even a relatively 'weak' relationship is potentially meaningful if it provides useful insight that could improve clinical practice, help to establish a new theory, or expand upon our understanding of a phenomenon. Conversely, a relatively 'strong' relationship may have little relevance or could be unimpressive in some circumstances. It's also important to note that guidelines for interpreting the strength of a correlation coefficient vary considerably across disciplines.

When conducting your own research, it's generally a good idea to make a prediction about the direction and strength of the relationship you expect before beginning to look at your data. Otherwise, it can be easy to convince yourself that the correlation coefficient you observe is exactly what you expected. The reality is that many (perhaps most) analyses won't turn out as anticipated, which is okay. In fact, these unexpected findings are part of what makes research exciting!

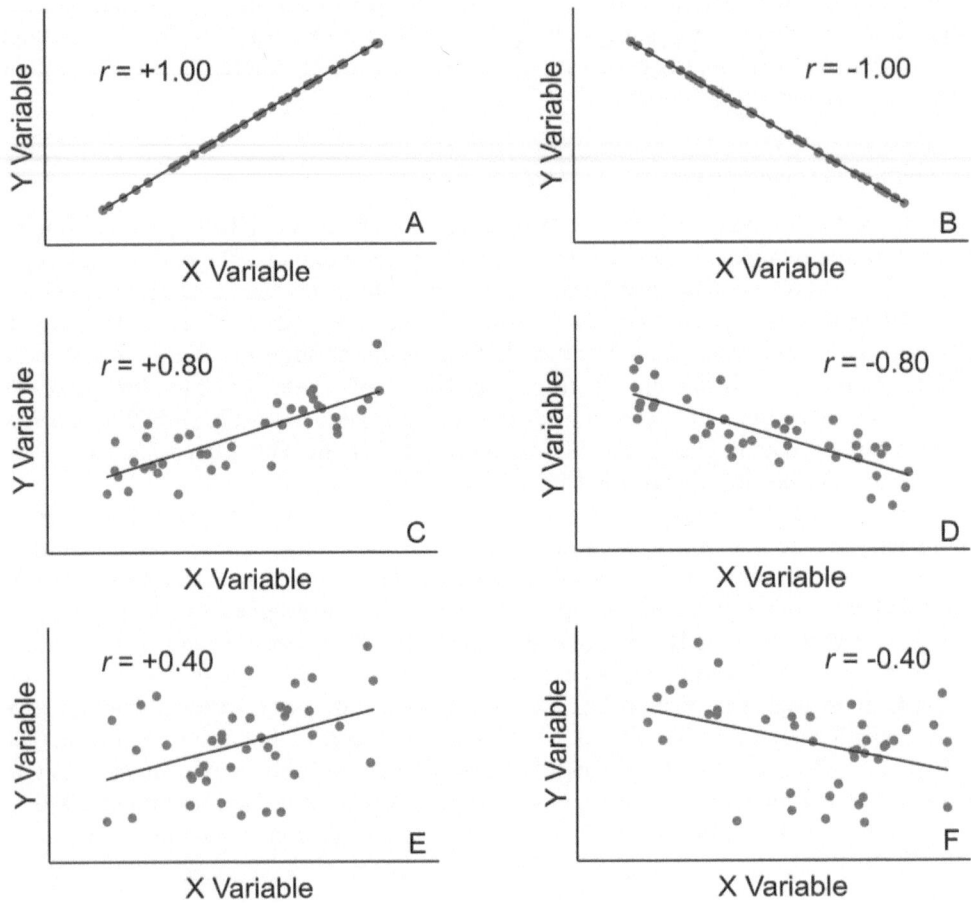

Figure 8.2 Example scatter plots (A–F) for relationships of varying directions and strengths. Each scatter plot includes the correlation coefficient (*r*) associated with the data points. Subplots A, C, and E include examples of positive relationships, while subplots B, D, and F include examples of negative relationships.

Table 8.1 Proposed guidelines for interpreting correlation coefficients.

Positive r value	Interpretation	Negative r value	Interpretation
0 to 0.25	Little or no relationship	0 to –0.25	Little or no relationship
0.25 to 0.50	Weak, positive relationship	–0.25 to –0.50	Weak, negative relationship
0.50 to 0.75	Moderate, positive relationship	–0.50 to –0.75	Moderate, negative relationship
≥0.75	Strong, positive relationship	≤–0.75	Strong, negative relationship

Note the overlap between categories; this is meant to highlight that these are general guidelines, not strict cutoff points.
Guidelines proposed by Portney (2020).

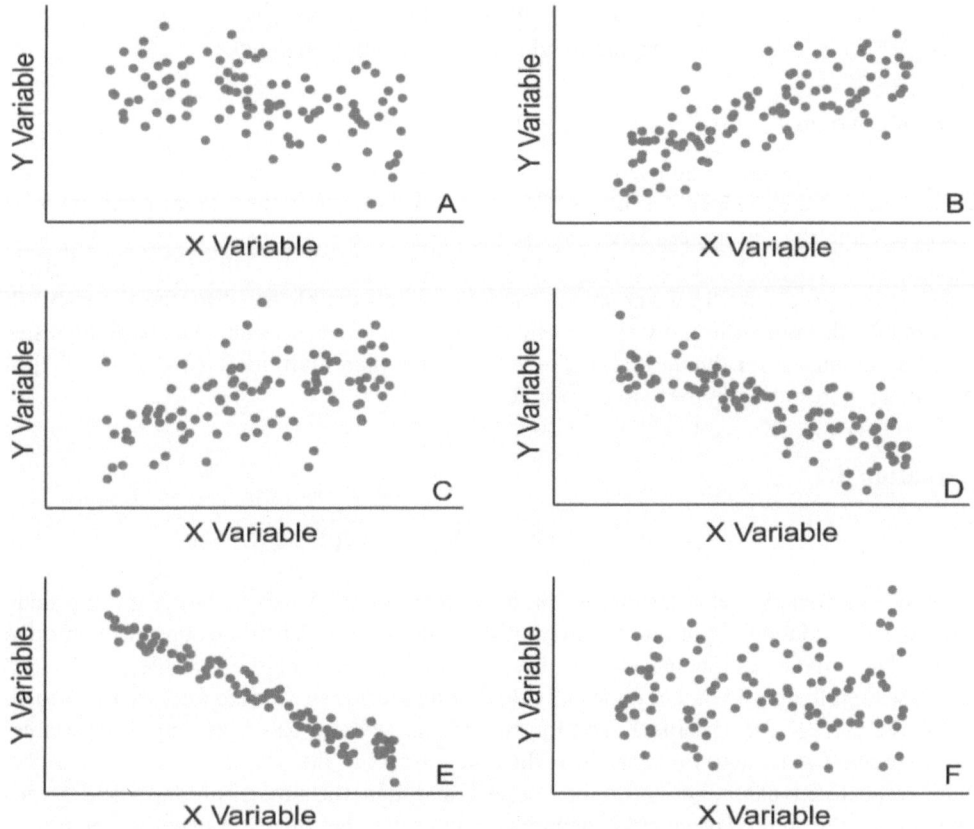

Learning Activity 8.1 The scatter plots included in panels A–F depict relationships of varying directions and strengths. Attempt to match the following correlation coefficients with their corresponding scatter plots: $r = -0.97$; $r = -0.81$; $r = -0.46$; $r = +0.07$; $r = +0.52$; $r = +0.94$. The answers are included at the end of the chapter.

Basis for the correlation coefficient

At this point, you should have a general understanding of what a correlation coefficient represents and how it's interpreted. Now let's take a more in-depth look at how a correlation coefficient is derived.

The concept of *covariance* is critical to understanding bivariate correlation and the correlation coefficient. Covariance represents the extent to which the X and Y variables vary together and is based on the *sum of products* (discussed in the next subsection). Before considering how a correlation coefficient is calculated, it's good to think about correlation coefficients more conceptually. Equation 8.1 presents the conceptual basis for the correlation coefficient (r). As you can see, the correlation coefficient captures how the variables vary together (i.e. the covariance) relative to how they vary individually.

Equation 8.1

$$r = \frac{\text{degree to which } X \text{ and } Y \text{ vary together}}{\text{degree to which } X \text{ and } Y \text{ vary separately}}$$

Sum of products

The sum of products can be used to capture the extent to which the X and Y variables vary together about their respective means. Equation 8.2 shows how the sum of products is calculated. First, the differences between each subject's score for the X variable (X) and the overall sample mean for the X variable ($\bar{X}$) are calculated, as well as the differences between each subject's score for the Y variable (Y) and the overall sample mean for the Y variable ($\bar{Y}$). Essentially, this quantifies how much each subject's X and Y scores deviate about the respective sample means for the variables. These values are then multiplied [$(X - \bar{X}) (Y - \bar{Y})$] and summed ($\Sigma$), resulting in the sum of products.

Equation 8.2

$$\text{Sum of products} = \sum \left(X - \bar{X} \right)\left(Y - \bar{Y} \right)$$

Now let's consider what the sum of products represents. The sign of the sum of products provides information about the direction of the relationship. When the sum of the products is positive, it indicates that there's a positive relationship between the variables. Think about it this way: if there's a tendency for individuals who are above average for variable X to also be above average for variable Y, and for individuals who are below average for variable X to also be below average for variable Y, then the product of the deviations for X and Y about their respective means will tend to be positive, and thus, the sum of products will be positive. When the sum of products is negative, it indicates that there's a negative relationship between the variables. In this case, there's a tendency for individuals who are above average for variable X to be below average for variable Y, and vice versa. As a result, the product of the deviations for X and Y about their respective means will tend to be negative, and thus, the sum of products will be negative.

The consistency of this pattern across all subjects, and therefore the strength of the relationship, is related to the magnitude of the sum of products. If the sum of products is 0 (or close to 0), it indicates that there's no real relationship between the variables. In this case, some individuals will be above or below average for both variables, while others will be above average for one variable but below average for the other. Essentially, these positive and negative values cancel each other out and result in a sum of products of approximately 0. This is a situation where there's clearly no pattern to how X and Y vary.

Standardizing the sum of products

As you can see, the magnitude of the sum of products is related to the strength of the relationship between the variables; however, simply examining the raw magnitude of the sum of products can be misleading, since the size of the deviation scores will depend on the measurement scales of the variables. For example, think about what would happen to the sum of products for the relationship between lower body strength and jump height if vertical jump height were recorded in meters instead of centimeters. In this case, recording vertical jump height in meters (vs. centimeters) would reduce the deviation scores for the jump height variable, resulting in a smaller sum of products. Because of this dependence on the measurement scales of the variables, it's not possible to develop generic guidelines for interpreting the sum of products or to compare the sum of products across different studies. To create a metric that can be more easily interpreted and compared across studies, we need to 'standardize' the sum of products.

Calculating a correlation coefficient essentially involves standardizing the sum of products by accounting for the inherent variance associated with the individual variables. To standardize the sum of products, we first quantify the degree to which the X and Y variables vary separately. One way to do this is to calculate the sum of squares associated with each variable. The sum of squares captures how the X and Y scores for each subject deviate (or vary) from the respective sample means associated with the variables ($\bar{X}$ and $\bar{Y}$) (note: the sum of squares was first introduced in Chapter 2). Equations 8.3 and 8.4 show how the sum of squares can be calculated for the X (SS_x) and Y (SS_y) variables.

Equation 8.3

$$SS_X = \sum \left(X - \bar{X} \right)^2$$

Equation 8.4

$$SS_Y = \sum \left(Y - \bar{Y} \right)^2$$

Once we have the sum of squares, the correlation coefficient (r) can be calculated by dividing the sum of products by the square root of the product of the sum of squares (Equation 8.5). This final step standardizes the sum of products so that the resulting correlation coefficient can potentially range from -1.00 to $+1.00$, regardless of the measurement scales of the variables. Having this type of standardized metric, which is independent of the measurement scales of the variables, allows for more uniform interpretation and easier comparison across studies.

Equation 8.5

$$r = \frac{\text{Sum of products}}{\sqrt{SS_X SS_Y}}$$

or

$$r = \frac{\sum \left(X - \bar{X} \right) \left(Y - \bar{Y} \right)}{\sqrt{SS_X SS_Y}}$$

Note: the equation (or equations) for calculating a correlation coefficient can be presented in several different ways. Don't be alarmed if you see this equation in a different convention. The general concept and interpretation will be the same.

Working through the calculations

While working through calculations may not always be the best way to learn concepts, in this instance, I think a lot can be gained from performing the calculations involved in deriving a correlation coefficient. Table 8.2 shows the steps involved in calculating a correlation coefficient. The X and Y values in Table 8.2 are heights (inches) and reaction times (milliseconds) for a group of ten college-aged females who were in a study I conducted a few years ago. The reaction

Table 8.2 Heights and reaction times for ten college-aged females.

	X/Y variables		Deviations		Squared deviations		Products
Subject	Height (in)	Reaction time (ms)	$(X - \bar{X})$	$(Y - \bar{Y})$	$(X - \bar{X})^2$	$(Y - \bar{Y})^2$	$(X - \bar{X}) * (Y - \bar{Y})$
1	66	289	0	+9	0	81	0
2	67	342	+1	+62	1	3844	62
3	63	253	−3	−27	9	729	81
4	64	269	−2	−11	4	121	22
5	69	268	+3	−12	9	144	−36
6	63	309	−3	+29	9	841	−87
7	66	272	0	−8	0	64	0
8	68	291	+2	+11	4	121	22
9	65	258	−1	−22	1	484	22
10	70	249	+3	−31	9	961	−93
	$\bar{X} = 66$	$\bar{Y} = 280$			$SS_x = 46$	$SS_Y = 7390$	$SoP = -7$

$\bar{X}$ = sample mean for height; $\bar{Y}$ = sample mean for reaction time.
SS_x = sum of squares for height; SS_Y = sum of squares for reaction time.
SoP = sum of products.

$$r = \frac{\sum(X - \bar{X})(Y - \bar{Y})}{\sqrt{SS_x SS_Y}} = \frac{-7}{\sqrt{46 * 7390}} = -0.01$$

As you can see based on the r value and the scatter plot, there's really no relationship between height and reaction time ($r \sim 0$). This shouldn't be surprising based on the sum of products, as there's no clear pattern to how the variables vary in relation to one another. Some subjects were above average height but exhibited below-average reaction times, others were below average height but exhibited above-average reaction times, and others were above/below average for both variables. Essentially, most of the positive and negative values ended up cancelling each other out, resulting in a sum of products close to zero.

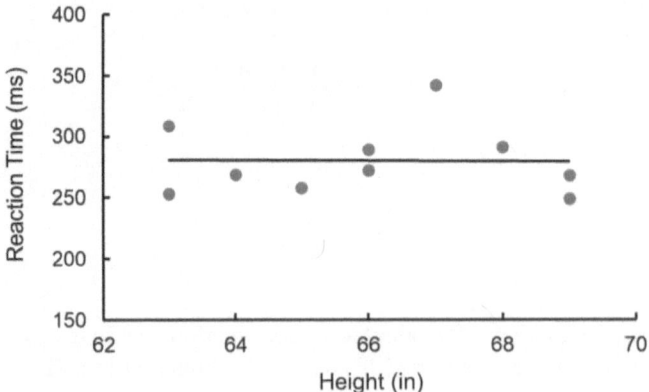

Scatter plot of the heights (*x*-axis) and reaction times (*y*-axis) for the ten subjects.

time values in this example represent the time required for the individual to press a button on a keyboard in response to a visual stimulus that appeared on a screen in front of them. Obviously, this is a fairly silly example, as there's no logical reason to believe that height would be related to reaction time (at least in my mind). That said, this is a good example to work through to get an appreciation for a situation where there's no consistent pattern to the covariance and thus no relationship ($r \sim 0.00$). I encourage you to work through these calculations by hand. When doing so, focus on the concepts instead of just 'plugging and chugging'.

Another way to think about scatter plots

Now that the concepts of covariance and the sum of products have been discussed, it may be helpful to examine a few more scatter plots. Figure 8.3 includes four scatter plots (A, B, C, D). Scatter plot A (top-left) represents a strong positive relationship ($r = +0.80$), scatter plot B (top-right) represents a strong negative relationship ($r = -0.80$), scatter plot C (bottom-left) represents no relationship ($r = 0.00$), and scatter plot D (bottom-right) represents a perfect positive relationship ($r = +1.00$). The dashed vertical lines on the scatter plots are positioned at the location of the mean for the X variable, and the dashed horizontal lines are positioned at the location of the mean for the Y variable. These dashed lines divide the scatter plots into four quadrants. The top-right quadrant includes data points that are above average for both the X and Y variables, the bottom-left quadrant includes data points that are below average for both the X and Y variables, the top-left quadrant includes data points that are below average for the

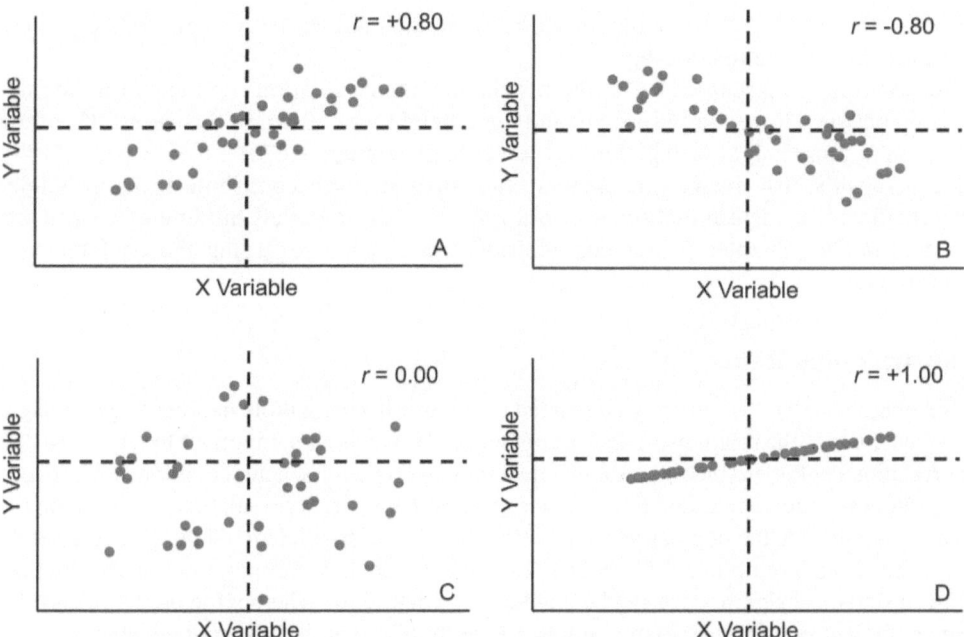

Figure 8.3 Example scatter plots (A–D) for relationships of varying directions and strengths. Each scatter plot includes the correlation coefficient (*r*) associated with the data points. The dashed vertical lines on the scatter plots are positioned at the location of the mean for the *X* variable, and the dashed horizontal lines are positioned at the location of the mean for the *Y* variable.

X variable but above average for the *Y* variable, and the bottom-right quadrant includes data points that are above average for the *X* variable but below average for the *Y* variable.

Adding these lines to a scatter plot can be helpful for conceptualizing bivariate correlation. When there's a strong positive relationship between variables, such as in scatter plot A, most of the data points will be in the top-right and bottom-left quadrants. When there's a strong negative relationship, such as in scatter plot B, most of the data points will be in the top-left and bottom-right quadrants. When there's a weak relationship, or no relationship, between variables, such as in scatter plot C, the data points will be spread throughout each quadrant. Finally, when there's a perfect relationship (positive or negative), such as in scatter plot D, all data points will be in quadrants that are diagonal to each other (top-right and bottom-left or top-left and bottom-right).

This isn't a new concept, just another way to consider the consistency of the pattern of the deviations of the *X* and *Y* scores about their respective means, which contributes to the sum of products and therefore influences the correlation coefficient.

The coefficient of determination

When reporting the results of a correlation analysis, investigators will often report the coefficient of determination, which is simply the correlation coefficient, squared (r^2). In fact, the coefficient of determination is often referred to as the '*r*-squared'. The coefficient of determination describes the percentage of variance in one variable that's explained by the variance in the other variable and will range from 0.00 to 1.00 (or 0% to 100% if expressed as a percentage, which is common). It can also be thought of as the amount of shared variance between the variables. The stronger the correlation, the more variance explained, regardless of the direction of the relationship.

For example, as discussed earlier in this chapter, the correlation coefficient for the relationship between lower body strength and jump height was +0.76. In this case, 58% of the variation in jump height is explained by lower body strength ($0.76^2 = 0.58 \times 100 = 58\%$). Of course, this also means that factors other than strength contribute to jump height. The coefficient of determination is also a reflection of how well the line of best fit fits the data points. Chapter 9 includes additional discussion regarding the coefficient of determination.

Statistical significance

A correlation analysis is typically conducted using data from a sample in order to gain insight into the nature of the relationship in the population. However, it's important to recognize that a correlation coefficient based on sample data may not reflect the actual relationship between the variables in the population. For instance, even if there's truly no relationship between the *X* and *Y* variables in the population (population correlation coefficient = 0.00), the correlation coefficient from a sample will likely be non-zero because of sampling error. To address this, a test of statistical significance can be conducted to determine whether the observed correlation coefficient is sufficiently large in magnitude to infer that there's a relationship between the variables in the population. The null hypothesis for this test of statistical significance is that there's no relationship between the *X* and *Y* variables in the population (population correlation coefficient = 0). Essentially, the test is conducted to determine whether the sample correlation coefficient is significantly different from 0.

A *t*-test is typically used to test the statistical significance of a correlation coefficient (*t*-tests were discussed in Chapter 5). Equation 8.6 can be used to calculate a *t* statistic based on a correlation coefficient (*r*). The location of this *t* statistic within the *t* distribution is then used to determine the probability of observing a sample correlation coefficient of the given magnitude simply by chance, if the null hypothesis was true and the population correlation coefficient was 0. The stronger the sample correlation coefficient, the larger the *t* statistic and the more likely we are to reject the null hypothesis and conclude that there's a relationship in the population.

Equation 8.6

$$t \text{ statistic} = \frac{r\sqrt{n-2}}{\sqrt{1-r^2}}$$

In Equation 8.6, *n* is the number of *X/Y* pairs. Note that the sign of the *t* statistic is the same as the sign of the correlation coefficient (*r*).

If the *p*-value associated with the observed *t* statistic is less than our predefined alpha level (typically 0.05), we reject the null hypothesis and conclude that there's a statistically significant relationship between the variables. In other words, the evidence from our sample data is strong enough to conclude that there's a relationship between the variables in the population. Another way to think of it is that it would be very unlikely to observe a sample correlation coefficient of the given magnitude if there wasn't actually a relationship between the variables in the population.

In contrast, if the observed *p*-value is greater than our alpha level, we conclude that there's not a statistically significant relationship between the variables (i.e. we fail to reject the null hypothesis). In other words, the evidence from our sample data isn't strong enough to conclude that there's a relationship between the variables in the population.

Note: because the test of the statistical significance of a correlation coefficient is based on the *t* distribution, it's possible to conduct either a one- or two-tailed test; however, a two-tailed test is much more common. A two-tailed test will examine both sides of the distribution and can be used to detect both negative and positive relationships (Chapter 5 includes a more in-depth discussion of the *t*-distribution and one- and two-tailed tests).

Now let's revisit the data from our lower body strength and jump height example. The correlation coefficient for this relationship was +0.76. This can be tested to determine the probability of observing a correlation coefficient of this magnitude simply by chance if there was no relationship between these variables in the population. A two-tailed *t*-test of this correlation coefficient results in a *p*-value of 0.001 ($p = 0.001$). This essentially indicates that there would be a 0.1% chance of observing a sample correlation coefficient of at least 0.76 if the null hypothesis were true and there was no relationship between lower body strength and jump height in the population. Since this *p*-value is less than the conventional alpha level of 0.05, we would reject the null hypothesis and conclude that the relationship between lower body strength and jump height is statistically significant. In other words, the population correlation coefficient probably isn't 0.

The influence of sample size

It's critical to understand that statistical significance isn't a reflection of the strength of a relationship. As highlighted throughout this book, statistical significance is greatly influenced

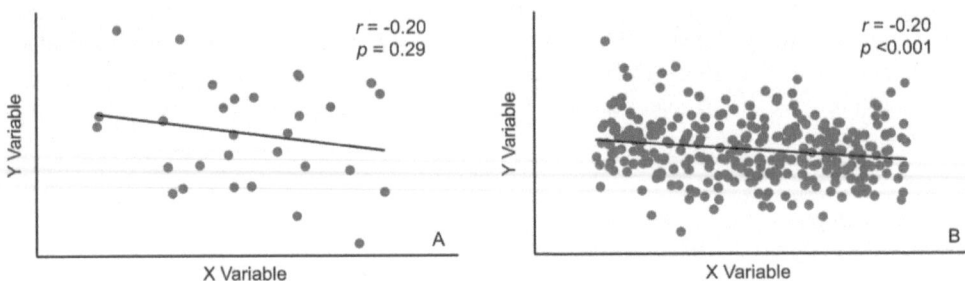

Figure 8.4 Example scatter plots for relationships with correlation coefficients (*r*) of –0.20. Scatter plot A (left) includes data from 30 subjects, and scatter plot B (right) includes data from 300 subjects. The plots also include *p*-values (*p*) based on tests of statistical significance of the correlation coefficients. Notice that the relationship isn't statistically significant for subplot A (*p* = 0.29); however, it is statistically significant for subplot B (*p* < 0.001), even though the correlation coefficients are equivalent.

by sample size. Therefore, there will be instances where weak relationships are statistically significant when the sample size is relatively large, as well as instances where moderate/strong relationships aren't statistically significant when the sample size is relatively small. For example, Figure 8.4 includes scatter plots for two different fictitious data sets (denoted A, B). In both cases, the correlation coefficient is –0.20; however, data set A includes 30 subjects, while data set B includes 300 subjects. The relationship isn't statistically significant (based on an alpha level of 0.05) for the sample with 30 subjects (*p* = 0.29); however, it is statistically significant for the sample with 300 subjects (*p* < 0.001). In this case, the strength of the relationship is the same, since the correlation coefficient is –0.20 in both instances; however, the statistical significance differs because of the difference in sample size. Again, this is meant to highlight that the strength of a relationship shouldn't be evaluated based on the results of a test of statistical significance.

Proceed with caution

While there are some instances where 'exploratory analyses' may be appropriate, in most cases, correlation analyses should only be conducted when there's a theoretical basis for the existence of a relationship between variables. Otherwise, there's the risk of falsely identifying a statistically significant relationship even when one doesn't truly exist. Remember, the risk of Type I error exists in any type of statistical test, including correlation. Not every significant relationship identified will be 'real'; therefore, testing relationships that have no basis should generally be avoided.

Confidence intervals for correlation coefficients

As discussed, the correlation coefficient from a sample won't perfectly reflect the correlation coefficient for the population because of sampling error. To account for this, we can use our sample data to estimate a range of values, or confidence interval, that's likely to include the population correlation coefficient.

Confidence intervals of 95% or 90% are commonly estimated. For a 95% confidence interval, there's a 95% probability that the population correlation coefficient falls within the lower and upper bounds of the interval. For example, the 95% confidence interval for the correlation coefficient based on the relationship between lower body strength and jump height is 0.55 (lower bound) to 0.92 (upper bound) [0.55, 0.92], indicating that there's a 95% probability that the correlation coefficient for the population falls within these bounds. Notice that 0 isn't located within this confidence interval, indicating that the population correlation coefficient probably isn't 0, which supports the existence of a relationship between lower body strength and jump height in the population. For a 90% confidence interval, the lower and upper bounds are 0.58 and 0.91, respectively [0.58, 0.91]. Notice that this range is narrower, and thus the estimate is more precise; however, we're less confident that the population correlation coefficient falls within this range.

The concept of confidence intervals vs. point estimates was first introduced in Chapter 4. Confidence intervals are also discussed in greater detail in Chapter 13 ('Effect Sizes and Confidence Intervals').

Correlations based on change scores

In some instances, correlation will involve change scores that represent the difference between an individual's baseline performance and their posttest performance. This can be used to examine factors that may influence the effectiveness of an intervention. For example, Yalamanchi et al. (2016) examined the extent to which fasting blood glucose levels influence the effects of exercise training on body composition in individuals with type 2 diabetes. Fasting blood glucose levels and body fat percentages were recorded for 50 individuals with type 2 diabetes at the beginning of the study (baseline). Participants then completed a 6-month training program that included resistance training and aerobic exercise. Body fat percentages were re-measured after completion of the program (posttest). The change in body fat percentage was calculated for each individual over the 6-month period by finding the difference between their body fat percentage at the baseline and posttest time points (change score). The investigators then examined the relationship between baseline fasting blood glucose and the change in body fat percentage. Interestingly, they found that individuals with higher baseline fasting blood glucose levels exhibited greater reductions in body fat percentage over the 6-month period.

Change scores can also be used to examine how changes in different factors may be related to one another. For example, Holm et al. (2010) examined percent changes in knee swelling and isometric knee extension strength, pre- vs. post-surgery, in 24 individuals who underwent total knee arthroplasty. These investigators observed a relationship between the changes in knee swelling and the changes in knee extension strength, indicating that individuals who exhibited a relatively large increase in knee swelling after surgery tended to also demonstrate a large reduction in knee extension strength.

Correlation vs. causation

If you've taken a statistics course, you've probably heard the axiom, 'correlation doesn't imply causation', or something along those lines. But what does this mean? Unfortunately, there are instances where there's an apparent relationship between two variables, but this relationship is the result of both variables being associated with another third variable (often described as the 'third variable problem'). An example commonly used in introductory statistics courses to highlight this issue is the positive correlation that's been observed between ice cream sales and drowning deaths. Obviously, an increase in ice cream sales isn't what causes the increase in drowning deaths or vice versa. Instead, both of these variables are related to temperature (third variable). As the temperature rises, more people buy ice cream cones and, unfortunately, more people drown since ice cream and swimming are both ways to deal with rising temperatures. As a result, ice cream sales and drowning deaths appear to be related because of their mutual correlation with the third variable (temperature in this case).

For a more clinically relevant example, consider the relationship that's been observed between handgrip strength and pulmonary function. Son et al. (2018) found that individuals with relatively poor grip strength also tend to exhibit relatively poor pulmonary function. In this case, this relationship between grip strength and pulmonary function is likely due to the fact that both variables are related to an individual's general conditioning. It seems unlikely that poor handgrip strength directly contributes to, or causes, poor pulmonary function, and we probably shouldn't expect to observe an improvement in a patient's pulmonary function simply by strengthening their grip.

These examples highlight the critical point that correlation doesn't imply causation. This is a fundamental concept of correlation, which shouldn't be overlooked. Establishing causation requires an experimental study, where investigators systematically manipulate one variable and examine the effect on the other variable.

Assumptions

This section highlights some of the key assumptions that should be met in order to conduct a Pearson product-moment correlation analysis.

1)   Both variables are continuous

This isn't an assumption that's tested statistically. Instead, it's related to the nature of the variables being measured.

Options if this assumption isn't met

Bivariate correlation is still possible with other types of variables. For example, Spearman's correlation is often used to analyze the relationship between pairs of ordinal variables or between one ordinal variable and another continuous variable. Spearman's correlation is a non-parametric test that relies on the rank ordering of the data instead of the actual values. Essentially, the analysis involves examining the relationship between the rank ordering of the values for the X and Y variables (e.g. with a positive relationship, subjects who are ranked relatively highly for variable X also tend to be ranked highly for variable Y). Fortunately, Spearman's correlation produces a correlation coefficient that's interpreted in the same manner as the Pearson product-moment correlation coefficient, so most of the concepts introduced in this chapter are relevant to both analyses. Spearman's correlation is discussed in Chapter 12 ('Non-Parametric Tests').

2)   There's a linear relationship between the variables

Pearson's product-moment correlation is only appropriate when there's a linear relationship between the variables. In some instances, variables are related to each other but in a nonlinear fashion. For example, age and bone mass exhibit a nonlinear relationship when examined across the lifespan, as individuals typically exhibit a rapid increase in bone mass during growth and development, a peak in bone mass between 20–30 years of age, and then a gradual decline (depicted in Figure 8.5). A straight line wouldn't fit this data very well, and thus, the strength of the relationship between age and bone mass would be underestimated. Examining a scatter plot is a simple way to determine if there's a linear relationship between the variables.

Options if this assumption isn't met

There are a few options if a nonlinear relationship is observed. First, you could attempt to fit a polynomial line to the data (depicted in Figure 8.5). You could also attempt to transform the data so that the relationship between the variables is more linear. Data transformation is discussed in Appendix B. Finally, you could use Spearman's correlation if the nonlinear relationship is monotonic, such as when there's an exponential increase in Y as X increases (see discussion of Spearman's correlation in Chapter 12).

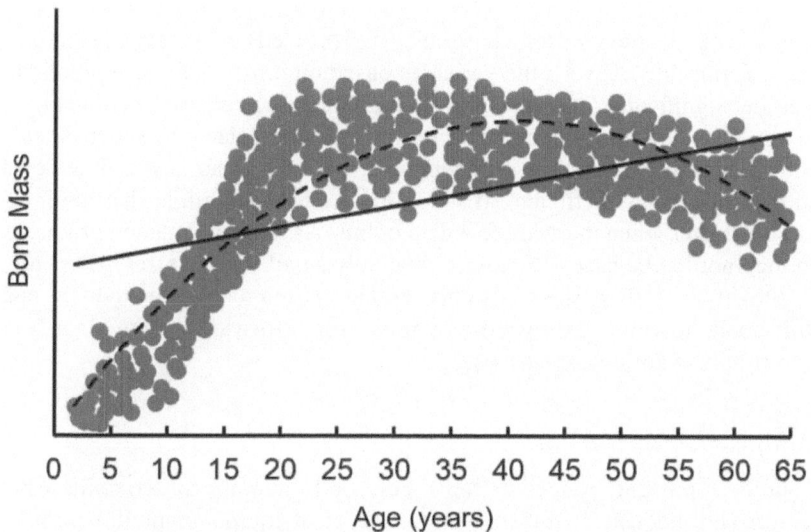

Figure 8.5 Scatter plot of the relationship between bone mass (y-axis) and age (x-axis). The solid line represents the linear line of best fit, and the dashed line represents a line of best fit based on a second-order polynomial. The coefficient of determination (r^2) for the linear and polynomial lines of best fit are 0.25 and 0.74, respectively, which highlights that the relationship between bone mass and age is better characterized by a curved line (i.e. nonlinear). Note: this is fictitious data generated as an example to highlight a nonlinear relationship.

3)   There are no major outliers

Outliers are data points that don't fit the same general pattern as the rest of the data and are far removed from the overall cluster of data points. Unfortunately, outliers can have a major influence on the Pearson product-moment correlation coefficient. For example, Figure 8.6

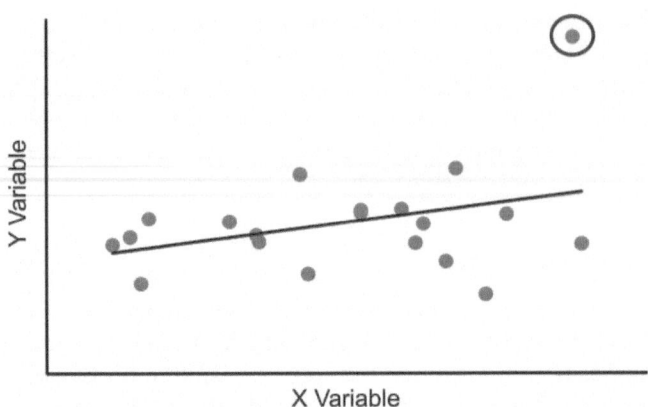

Figure 8.6 Example scatter plot with 20 data points, including one outlier (circled). The correlation coefficient without the outlier included is +0.10, whereas it is +0.35 with the outlier included.

includes a cluster of data points, along with an outlier (circled). As you can see, there appears to be no real relationship between the variables based on most of the data points; however, the single outlier significantly increases the strength of the correlation coefficient.

Outliers can have different effects on a correlation coefficient. In some cases, outliers increase the strength of the correlation coefficient, while in other cases, they decrease the strength of the correlation coefficient. It's also important to highlight that the influence of outliers will be greater when there are few data points. As a result, Pearson product-moment correlation may not be the best option with relatively small sample sizes. There are several ways to objectively identify outliers in a data set. Discussion of these methods is outside the scope of this book; however, the easiest and most straightforward way to identify potential outliers is to simply examine a scatter plot.

Options if this assumption isn't met

When an outlier is present, your first step should be to attempt to determine whether the data was entered erroneously or if there was some type of equipment malfunction that could explain the atypical observation. You should also consider whether the observed values are plausible (i.e. are the values within a range of what's likely to be humanly possible?). Outliers due to data entry errors, equipment miscalibration, and so on are easy to address by re-entering the correct data or removing data that's obviously erroneous.

When the reason for the outlier isn't clear, you need to carefully consider how to proceed. In some cases, investigators will remove the outlier from the analysis; however, this is generally discouraged when there's no obvious reason to believe that the data is erroneous. A better option is to report the results of the analysis both with the outlier included and with the outlier removed. This allows readers to appreciate how the outlier influenced the results of the analysis and make their own decision about how to interpret the study findings. Another option is to perform a Spearman's correlation instead of a Pearson product-moment correlation. Spearman's correlation is less affected by outliers since the analysis relies on rank ordering of the data and extreme scores won't have as great of an influence on the correlation coefficient.

4)   Normality

With Pearson product-moment correlation, both the X and Y variables should be approximately normally distributed. Appendix A discusses ways to assess normality. It should be noted that minor deviations from normality won't have a major influence on the results of a Pearson product-moment correlation analysis.

Options if this assumption isn't met

If the assumption of normality isn't met, you could attempt to transform your data so that it's more normally distributed (data transformation is discussed in Appendix B), or you could conduct a Spearman's correlation instead of a Pearson product-moment correlation (see discussion of Spearman's correlation in Chapter 12).

Application opportunity

Example data set

Madansingh et al. (2020) conducted a study to examine whether there's a relationship between lower body loading and hip bone mineral density. Their study included a sample of postmenopausal women, since they appear to be particularly susceptible to bone loss. Bone mineral density was measured using dual-energy x-ray absorptiometry (DEXA), and lower body loading was quantified over a 7-day period using a small sensor worn by the subjects around their ankle. The investigators generated a 'bone density index' metric for each subject, which captured the volume and intensity of lower body loading over the 7-day period. Higher bone density index values corresponded with a greater volume and intensity of lower body loading. The investigators hypothesized that greater lower body loading (higher bone density index values) would be associated with greater hip bone mineral density (positive relationship).

Note: the units for the bone density index ('Loading') are bodyweight$^{1/2}$, and the units for bone mineral density are g/cm^2.

Data files

BDI&BMD_data.xlsx – Excel file with bone density index values ('Loading') (first column) and bone mineral densities (BMD) (second column) for 68 subjects who participated in the study.

   BDI&BMD_data.sav – SPSS file with bone density index values ('Loading') (first column) and bone mineral densities (BMD) (second column) for 68 subjects who participated in the study.

Note: the values in this data set were extracted from a scatter plot included in the original publication; therefore, they may not exactly match the values in the original data set.

Video

Correlation.mp4 – video that includes a demonstration of how to create a scatter plot and conduct a Pearson product-moment correlation analysis using SPSS, as well as how to generate a Pearson product-moment correlation coefficient in Excel.

Sample write-up

A Pearson product-moment correlation analysis was conducted to examine the relationship between lower body loading (based on the bone density index) and hip bone mineral density for 68 postmenopausal women. The Pearson product-moment correlation coefficient was used to quantify the direction and strength of the relationship between the variables, and a two-tailed t-test, with an alpha of 0.05, was conducted to examine the statistical significance of the relationship.

There was a moderate, positive relationship between lower body loading and hip bone mineral density ($r = 0.44$; $p < .001$), indicating that subjects who demonstrated greater lower body loading (higher bone density index values) tended to exhibit greater hip bone mineral density. Lower body loading explained 19% of the variance in hip bone mineral density ($r^2 = 0.19$).

Answers to learning activity

Learning Activity 8.1

A: $r = -0.46$
B: $r = +0.94$
C: $r = +0.52$
D: $r = -0.81$
E: $r = -0.97$
F: $r = +0.07$

9 Simple linear regression

Chapter Objectives

The objectives of this chapter are to . . .

1) describe the general purpose of simple linear regression
2) provide examples of the types of clinical research questions that simple linear regression can be used to address
3) distinguish between the predictor variable and the outcome variable in a simple linear regression analysis
4) identify and describe the components of a regression equation
5) demonstrate how to generate a predicted value for the outcome variable based on a regression equation and calculate a residual
6) explain how a regression line is developed using the least squares method
7) describe how the standard error of the estimate and coefficient of determination can be used to assess goodness of fit
8) explain the basis for examining the statistical significance of a regression coefficient and constant
9) discuss generalizability in the context of simple linear regression
10) highlight the issue of extrapolation
11) describe key assumptions that should be met in order to conduct a simple linear regression analysis
12) demonstrate how to conduct a simple linear regression analysis using SPSS and the Excel Analysis Toolpak

Introduction

In general, regression involves developing a statistical model that can be used to make predictions or explain the nature of a relationship between variables. Simple linear regression is typically used to examine how well one continuous variable ('predictor variable') can predict another continuous variable ('outcome variable'). It's important to highlight that simple linear regression is really just an extension of bivariate correlation (discussed in Chapter 8). If you haven't done so already, it may be helpful to review Chapter 8 before proceeding, as many of the key concepts discussed in Chapter 8 will also be relevant to simple linear regression.

In order to conduct a simple linear regression analysis, data for both the predictor variable and the outcome variable is needed for each subject in the sample. With simple linear regression, the predictor variable (typically denoted X) and the outcome variable (typically

DOI: 10.4324/9781003179757-9

denoted *Y*) need to be designated, since the predictor variable is used to predict the outcome variable. Note that this is different from bivariate correlation (discussed in Chapter 8), where the variable denoted *X* vs. *Y* was typically arbitrary, since the intent of bivariate correlation is simply to determine whether the variables are related to one another, not to use one variable to predict the other. In the context of regression, you can also think of the predictor variable as the independent variable and the outcome variable as the dependent variable, since the assumption is that the independent variable potentially influences the dependent variable (i.e. the outcome variable 'depends' on the value of the independent variable). Again, this differs from bivariate correlation, where both variables are considered dependent on one another.

Now let's consider a couple examples of the types of questions that can be addressed using simple linear regression. When prescribing aerobic exercise, we may want a patient to work at a certain percentage of their maximal heart rate. This helps to ensure that the patient is exercising at an intensity that will promote cardiorespiratory gains without resulting in overexertion. Of course, this type of targeted exercise prescription requires knowledge of a patient's maximal heart rate. While it isn't feasible to conduct maximal exercise testing for every patient or client, investigators have used simple linear regression to examine whether maximal heart rate can be accurately predicted based on an individual's age (e.g. Tanaka et al., 2001). In this case, age is the predictor variable, and maximal heart rate is the outcome variable in the simple linear regression analysis. Investigators also commonly use simple linear regression to identify factors that can predict individuals' future performance or clinical outcomes. For instance, Tsang et al. (2004) used simple linear regression to examine whether performance on a test of seated postural control at the time of initial evaluation (predictor variable) could predict walking speed at discharge (outcome variable) in a group of patients who were referred to inpatient rehabilitation following a stroke. As you can probably imagine, the ability to identify factors that predict a patient's future performance can be tremendously beneficial when establishing a prognosis for recovery.

Basis for simple linear regression

A scatter plot is often used to display the two variables included in a simple linear regression analysis, with the predictor variable plotted along the *x*-axis (horizontal axis) and the outcome variable plotted along the *y*-axis (vertical axis). Each point on the scatter plot represents an individual subject's values for the predictor variable and the outcome variable (*X/Y* pair). As with bivariate correlation, a line is fit to this data that travels through the distribution of data points and gets as close as possible to each *X/Y* pair. This line is centered at the means of the predictor variable (*x*-axis) and the outcome variables (*y*-axis). In the context of bivariate correlation (Chapter 8), this line was referred to as the 'line of best fit' or 'trend line'; however, it's typically referred to as the 'regression line' when discussed in the context of regression.

The equation for the regression line ('regression equation') is fundamental to simple linear regression, as it's the basis for how the predictor variable (*X*) is used to estimate or predict the outcome variable (*Y*). Equation 9.1. includes the general form of the regression equation.

Equation 9.1

$$\hat{Y} = a + b\,(X)$$

You've probably seen this equation before in some form. It's simply the equation for a straight line, where *a* is the *y*-intercept and *b* is the slope. In the context of regression, the *y*-intercept is often referred to as the 'constant', and the slope is often referred to as the 'regression coefficient'. The variable $\hat{Y}$ (referred to as 'y-hat') is the predicted value for the outcome variable (Y), and the variable X is the observed value for the predictor variable (X). The regression constant (a) represents the value of $\hat{Y}$ when X is equal to 0, and the regression coefficient (b) represents the change in $\hat{Y}$ for each one-unit change in the X variable (think 'rise over run'). Note that when the regression coefficient is positive ($+b$), an increase in X will correspond with an increase in $\hat{Y}$, and when the regression coefficient is negative ($-b$), an increase in X will correspond with a decrease in $\hat{Y}$.

The regression equation serves as the statistical model that's used for prediction. Each subject's value for the predictor variable (X) is input into the regression equation (Equation 9.1) and used to generate a predicted value ($\hat{Y}$) for the outcome variable. These $\hat{Y}$ values fall directly on the regression line. Each $\hat{Y}$ is then compared to the actual value for the outcome variable. The differences between the predicted and actual values for the outcome variable ($Y - \hat{Y}$) are referred to as *residuals*. Residuals can be thought of as the errors in the predictions made using the regression model. The more accurate the predictions, the smaller the residuals. The residuals also reflect the vertical distances of the Y values from the regression line, since the $\hat{Y}$ values fall directly on the regression line.

Before moving on, let's consider an example. Kim et al. (2002) conducted a study to determine if the number of bench press repetitions that an individual can perform with a submaximal weight can be used to predict the maximum amount of weight they can bench press for a single repetition (one repetition maximum – 1RM). Their study included a group of 21 college-aged females. Each subject completed both submaximal bench press testing and 1RM bench press testing. For the submaximal testing, the subjects bench pressed a standard weight as many repetitions as possible, and for the 1RM testing, they bench pressed as much weight as possible for a single repetition. The investigators conducted a simple linear regression analysis where the number of repetitions completed during the submaximal testing was the predictor variable (X), and 1RM weight was the outcome variable (Y). The regression equation based on their analysis was $\hat{Y} = 19.2 + 0.31(X)$. In this case, X is the number of repetitions completed during the submaximal testing, and $\hat{Y}$ is the predicted 1RM weight. The constant (19.2 kg) represents the predicted 1RM weight if a subject couldn't complete any repetitions. The regression coefficient (0.31 kg) represents the amount of additional weight for the 1RM testing that a subject is predicted to be able to lift for each additional repetition completed during submaximal testing. For example, based on their regression equation, the predicted 1RM weight for a subject who completes 30 repetitions is 28.5 kg [$19.2 + 0.31(30) = 28.5$ kg]. In this example, the residuals are the differences between each subject's actual 1RM weight and their predicted 1RM weight. If a subject who completes 30 repetitions is able to bench press a 1RM weight of 30 kg, their residual would be 1.5 kg (30 kg – 28.5 kg). This would be a case where the regression equation underestimated the subject's 1RM weight (i.e. they could lift more weight than predicted). Learning Activity 9.1 includes another scenario where you can use a regression equation to make a prediction and calculate a residual.

Learning Activity 9.1

Tanaka et al. (2001) conducted a study to develop a regression equation to predict an individual's maximal heart rate (HR max) based on their age. Their study included 514 healthy adults between 18 and 81 years of age. Each subject's maximal heart rate was measured during a treadmill-based protocol where subjects walked or ran at a consistent speed and treadmill incline was increased 2.5% every 2 minutes until the subject reached exhaustion. The investigators then conducted a simple linear regression analysis to determine if age (predictor variable) could predict maximal heart rate (outcome variable). The regression equation that resulted from their analysis is included in the following:

HR max = 209 + –0.7(Age)

If one of the subjects who participated in the study was 63 years old and had an actual HR max of 170 beats/minute, what was the residual for their predicted HR max? Was their actual HR max overestimated or underestimated?
The answers are included at the end of the chapter.

Figure 9.1 includes a scatter plot based on the data reported by Kim et al. (2002). The predicted values for the 1RM weights lie directly on the regression line. The differences between each subject's actual 1RM weight and their predicted 1RM weight are the residuals. The residual for one subject has been highlighted in the scatter plot (Figure 9.1). In this case, the regression equation overestimated the subject's 1RM weight, as their predicted 1RM was 38 kg (19.2 + 0.31[60] = 38 kg); however, their actual 1RM weight was only 32 kg. As a result, the residual was –6 kg in this instance (32 kg – 38 kg). As you can see in the scatter plot, in other cases, the regression equation underestimated the actual 1RM weight. The sum of the residuals will always be 0, since the regression line is fit based on all the data points and negative residuals are canceled out by positive residuals. Establishing the regression line is discussed in the next subsection.

The accuracy of the predictions made using the regression model is dependent on the strength of the relationship between the variables. The stronger the relationship, the more

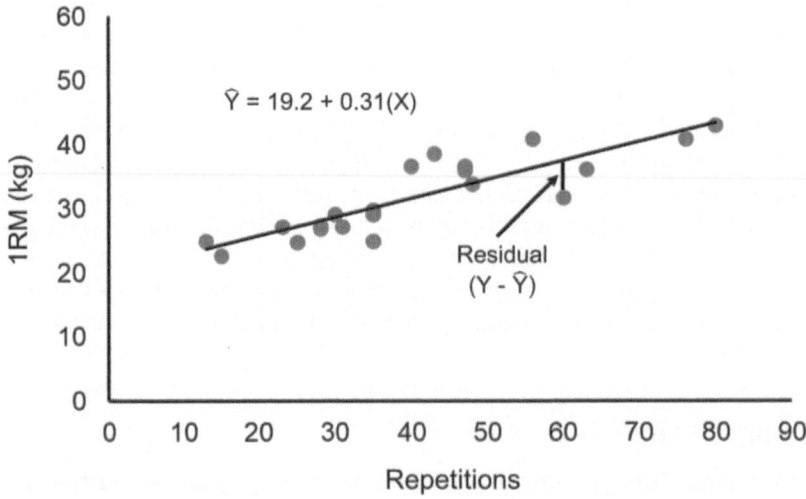

Figure 9.1 Scatter plot based on the number of repetitions completed during the submaximal bench press testing (*x*-axis) and the maximal one repetition maximum (1RM) bench press weights (*y*-axis) for 21 subjects who participated in the study conducted by Kim et al. (2002). The regression line is represented by the solid black line running diagonally through the data points. The regression equation is also included on the scatter plot. The residual is identified for one subject. The residuals represent the amount of error between the predicted and actual amount of weight lifted during the 1RM testing. The predicted 1RM values lie directly on the regression line.

accurate the predictions will be. In fact, when there's a perfect relationship between the variables ($r = \pm 1.00$), the predictor variable can be used to determine the outcome variable with no residuals or errors (i.e. perfect accuracy) (note: r represents the Pearson product-moment correlation coefficient discussed in Chapter 8). With imperfect relationships, the predictor variable can be used to estimate the outcome variable; however, the predictions aren't perfectly accurate (i.e. the true value of the outcome variable is overestimated in some instances and underestimated in others). This was the case for the regression model developed by Kim et al. (2002) to estimate 1RM weights. The relationship between the number of repetitions performed and the 1RM weights was strong ($r = +0.87$), and as a result, the predictions were fairly accurate; however, they weren't perfect, since the relationship wasn't perfect. When there's no relationship between the variables ($r = 0.00$), having information about the value of the predictor variable doesn't provide any insight into the value of the outcome variable.

Developing the regression line

As previously discussed, the regression line is the single line that 'best fits' the data (hence the terminology 'line of best fit'). But what does 'best fit' mean? The regression line 'best fits' the data in that it minimizes the residuals. In other words, it's the line that results in the most accurate prediction of Y based on X. Other straight lines could be fit to the data, but none would be as accurate in predicting the outcome variable (i.e. the residuals would be greater).

Now let's discuss more specifically how the parameters (constant and regression coefficient) for the regression equation can be derived. While the objective is to find the line that minimizes the residuals, we can't simply identify the line that produces the lowest total residuals. This is because the sum of the residuals for any line that passes through the center of the distribution of data points will be 0, regardless of how well it fits the data (demonstrated in Figure 9.2). As a result, there are an infinite number of lines that would satisfy the objective of minimizing the sum of the residuals, not only the regression line. To address this issue, the residuals can be squared [$(Y - \hat{Y})^2$] so that negative residuals become positive values. The sum (Σ) of these squared residuals will always be nonnegative, and there's only one line that best minimizes the residual sum of squares [$\Sigma(Y - \hat{Y})^2$], which is the regression

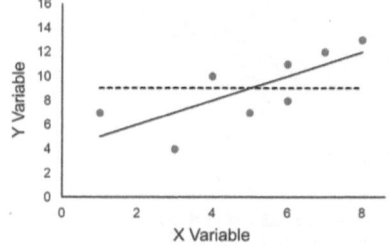

		$\hat{Y} = 4 + 1(X)$			$\hat{Y} = 9$		
X	Y	$\hat{Y}$	$(Y - \hat{Y})$	$(Y - \hat{Y})^2$	$\hat{Y}$	$(Y - \hat{Y})$	$(Y - \hat{Y})^2$
3	4	7	-3	9	9	-5	25
7	12	11	+1	1	9	+3	9
1	7	5	+2	4	9	-2	4
5	7	9	-2	4	9	-2	4
6	8	10	-2	4	9	-1	1
8	13	12	+1	1	9	+4	16
6	11	10	+1	1	9	+2	4
4	10	8	+2	2	9	+1	1
			Sum = 0	Sum = 28		Sum = 0	Sum = 64

Figure 9.2 Scatter plot with eight X/Y pairs and a regression line (solid black) with a regression equation of $\hat{Y} = 4 + 1(X)$. The plot also includes a horizontal line (dashed black) at the location of the mean for the Y variable, which is 9. The equation for this horizontal line is $\hat{Y} = 9$ since the regression coefficient is 0 (i.e. slope = 0). The table includes the values for the X and Y variables, the $\hat{Y}$ values based on the regression line and the horizontal line, the residuals for each line $(Y - \hat{Y})$, and the squared residuals $(Y - \hat{Y})^2$ for each line. Notice that the sum of the residuals equal 0 for both lines; however, the sum of the squared residuals is lower for the regression line vs. the horizontal line since it fits the data better. The objective of this 'least squares' method of regression is to identify the line that minimizes the sum of the squared residuals.

line. The parameters for the regression line (regression constant and regression coéfficient) can be estimated using Equations 9.2 and 9.3. Again, the constant and regression coefficient derived from these equations are the parameters for the unique line (regression line) that best minimizes the residual sum of squares. This approach to 'fitting' the regression line is typically referred to as the 'least squares method'.

Equation 9.2

$$b = \frac{\sum(X - \bar{X})(Y - \bar{Y})}{\sum(X - \bar{X})^2}$$

In Equation 9.2, X = the values for the predictor variable; $\bar{X}$ = the mean for the predictor variable; Y = the values for the outcome variable; $\bar{Y}$ = the mean for the outcome variable. Note that this equation involves dividing the sum of products for X and Y by the sum of squares for X.

Equation 9.3

$$a = \bar{Y} - b(\bar{X})$$

In Equation 9.3, $\bar{Y}$ = the mean for the outcome variable; $\bar{X}$ = the mean for the predictor variable; b = the regression coefficient for the regression line.

The regression coefficient (b) is closely related to the Pearson product-moment correlation coefficient (r) discussed in Chapter 8. When r is positive, b will also be positive; when r is negative, b will also be negative; and when r is 0, b will also be 0 (horizontal line). In fact, an alternative way of calculating b is to multiply r by the ratio of the standard deviations for the outcome variable (s_y) and the predictor variable (s_x) (Equation 9.4). Note that if the variables were standardized so that the means equaled 0 and the standard deviations equaled 1.0 (e.g. actual values converted to z-scores), then b and r would be equivalent. Another way to think of it is that standardizing the values essentially removes the constant from the regression equation. This is just another example of the close connection between bivariate correlation and simple linear regression.

Equation 9.4

$$b = r \times \frac{s_Y}{s_X}$$

It's critical to understand that the parameters for the regression equation will be different if X is used to predict Y compared to if Y is used to predict X. The denominator for Equation 9.2 helps to show why this is the case. When calculating the regression coefficient, if the X variable is used to predict the Y variable, the sum of products is divided by the sum of squares for X, whereas if the Y variable is used to predict the X variable, the sum of products is divided by the sum of squares for Y. As a result, the regression coefficient (and thus the constant) depends on which variable is designated as the predictor variable vs. the outcome variable. Therefore, the predictor variable and the outcome variable need to be defined for simple linear regression. This differs from bivariate correlation, where designation of a predictor variable and an outcome variable isn't necessary.

Assessing prediction accuracy

While the regression line best fits the data, this doesn't ensure that it's a particularly good fit, as the predictions of the outcome variable could be highly inaccurate. Therefore, once the regression model is developed, the accuracy of the predictions made by the model must be examined in order to determine how well the regression model fits the data. The standard error of the estimate and the coefficient of determination both provide an indication of the accuracy of a regression model, which is often referred to as the model's 'goodness of fit'.

Standard error of the estimate

The *standard error of the estimate* essentially represents the average degree of error in the predicted values of the outcome variable or, in other words, the average residual. The more accurate the regression model at predicting the outcome variable, the smaller the residuals and the lower the standard error of the estimate. In fact, the standard error of the estimate will be 0 if the model is perfectly accurate (i.e. no residuals).

The standard error of the estimate (SEE) can be calculated using Equation 9.5. The numerator in Equation 9.5 is the residual sum of squares [$\Sigma(Y - \hat{Y})^2$], which represents how the predicted values of Y ($\hat{Y}$) deviate from the actual values of Y. The residual sum of squares is then divided by its degrees of freedom ($n - 2$, where n is the number of X/Y pairs). The final step is to take the square root of this quotient so that the units for the standard error of the estimate revert back to the original units of the outcome variable. Notice how similar the equation for the standard error of the estimate is to the equation for calculating a standard deviation (Equation 9.6). The standard error of the estimate essentially reflects the standard deviation of the errors about the regression line. This is analogous to how the standard deviation reflects how individual values (X) deviate about the mean of these values ($\bar{X}$). A relatively large standard error of the estimate indicates that the Y values are dispersed widely about the regression line, which is reflective of a regression model with poor accuracy or, in other words, a regression line that's a poor fit to the data.

Equation 9.5

$$SEE = \sqrt{\frac{\sum \left(Y - \hat{Y}\right)^2}{n - 2}}$$

Equation 9.6

$$s = \sqrt{\frac{\sum \left(X - \bar{X}\right)^2}{n - 1}}$$

In Equation 9.6, s = sample standard deviation; X = the individual values for variable X; $\bar{X}$ = the mean of variable X; n = the number of observations; $n - 1$ = degrees of freedom.

Once the standard error of the estimate has been calculated, it's important to put the value into context by considering whether this degree of error is trivial or if it could result in erroneous decisions or place patients at risk. For example, Sarzynski et al. (2013) conducted a study to compare the accuracy of commonly used regression equations for predicting maximal heart rate based on age in a group of sedentary adults. They found the standard error of the estimate based on the regression equations they analyzed to be approximately 12 beats per minute. Once this information is available, clinicians need to consider whether this degree of error is acceptable.

Coefficient of determination (R²)

The coefficient of determination was first introduced in Chapter 8 when discussing bivariate correlation. Since simple linear regression only includes one predictor variable, the coefficient of determination is simply the Pearson product-moment correlation coefficient (r), squared. In the context of regression, the coefficient of determination is often denoted R^2 and referred to as the 'R-squared' (note: R^2 is typically used in the context of regression, while r^2 is typically used in the context of correlation, even though both represent the coefficient of determination). For simple linear regression, R^2 describes the percentage of variance in the outcome variable that's explained by the predictor variable and will range from 0.00 to 1.00 (or 0% to 100% if expressed as a percentage, which is common). The more accurate the predictions of the outcome variable, the larger R^2. If the outcome variable can be determined from the predictor variable without any errors or residuals ($r = \pm1.00$), then R^2 is 1.00 (or 100%).

Basis for R²

In order to calculate R^2, the total variation in the outcome variable must be partitioned into variation that's explained by the regression model and variation that isn't explained by the regression model. The sum of squares for Y captures the total variation in the outcome variable, since it quantifies how the Y values deviate about the mean of Y (Equation 9.7). In the context of regression, the sum of squares for Y is often referred to as the total sum of squares (SS_{Total}), since it represents the total variation in the outcome variable. In the example described earlier where 1RM bench press weights were predicted, the SS_{Total} captures the total variation in the 1RM bench press weights among the subjects or, in other words, the dispersion of the 1RM bench press weights about the mean ($\bar{Y}$). Some of the total sum of squares is explained by the regression model (unless $r = 0.00$) and some isn't (unless $r = \pm1.00$).

Equation 9.7

$$SS_{Total} = \sum \left(Y - \bar{Y}\right)^2$$

The residual sum of squares ($SS_{Residuals}$), which was discussed earlier in this chapter, captures the amount of variation that isn't explained by the regression model (Equation 9.8). Remember, $SS_{Residuals}$ represents the errors in the predictions made by the regression model [$\Sigma(Y - \hat{Y})^2$]. You can also think of $SS_{Residuals}$ as the variation that isn't accounted for by the regression model. In contrast, the variation that is explained by the regression model is captured by the sum of squares regression ($SS_{Regression}$). The $SS_{Regression}$ can be directly calculated by finding the sum of the squared differences between the mean of Y and the predicted values of Y (Equation 9.9). However, conceptually, it's easiest to think of the $SS_{Regression}$ as the difference between the total variation (SS_{Total}) and the unexplained variation ($SS_{Residuals}$), since $SS_{Total} = SS_{Regression} + SS_{Residuals}$ (i.e. total variation = explained variation + unexplained variation).

Equation 9.8

$$SS_{\text{Residuals}} = \sum \left(Y - \hat{Y} \right)^2$$

Equation 9.9

$$SS_{\text{Regression}} = \sum \left(\hat{Y} - \bar{Y} \right)^2$$

R^2 can be calculated by dividing the $SS_{\text{Regression}}$ by the SS_{Total} (Equation 9.10). Essentially, R^2 represents the proportion of the total variation in the outcome variable that can be explained by the regression model. Since the regression model only includes a single predictor variable in the case of simple linear regression, R^2 represents the amount of variation in the outcome variable that's explained by the predictor variable (i.e. the amount of variation in Y, explained by X). Conversely, the proportion of variation not explained by the model $(1 - R^2)$ can be calculated by dividing the $SS_{\text{Residuals}}$ by the SS_{Total} (Equation 9.11). This proportion of unexplained variation is often referred to as the 'coefficient of alienation'. You can think of this as the proportion of the total variation that isn't accounted for by the regression model. Figure 9.3 includes an example of how the proportion of total variation can be partitioned into unexplained and explained variation.

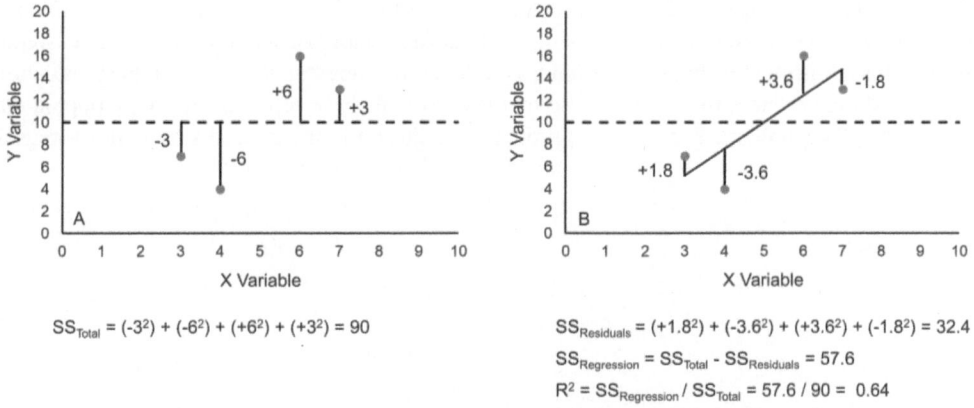

SS$_{\text{Total}}$ = (-3^2) + (-6^2) + (+6^2) + (+3^2) = 90

SS$_{\text{Residuals}}$ = (+1.8^2) + (-3.6^2) + (+3.6^2) + (-1.8^2) = 32.4

SS$_{\text{Regression}}$ = SS$_{\text{Total}}$ - SS$_{\text{Residuals}}$ = 57.6

R^2 = SS$_{\text{Regression}}$ / SS$_{\text{Total}}$ = 57.6 / 90 = 0.64

Figure 9.3 Scatter plots (A, B) with four *X/Y* pairs. Scatter plot A (left panel) demonstrates how the individual *Y* values deviate from the mean of *Y* (located at the horizontal dashed line). The total sum of squares (SS_{Total}) represents the total variation of the *Y* values about the mean of *Y*. Scatter plot B (right panel) shows how the residuals deviate from the regression line. The residual sum of squares ($SS_{\text{Residuals}}$) represents the variation not explained by the regression model, and the sum of squares regression ($SS_{\text{Regression}}$) represents the variation explained by the regression model. In this example, 64% of the total variation is explained by the regression model (57.6/90 = 0.64), and 36% of the total variation isn't explained by the regression model (32.4/90 = 0.36).

Equation 9.10

$$R^2 = \frac{SS_{\text{Regression}}}{SS_{\text{Total}}}$$

Or

$$R^2 = \frac{SS_{\text{Total}} - SS_{\text{Residuals}}}{SS_{\text{Total}}}$$

Equation 9.11

$$1 - R^2 = \frac{SS_{\text{Residuals}}}{SS_{\text{Total}}}$$

* **Note:** technically, R^2 represents how much the regression model improves prediction accuracy of the outcome variable, compared to the most basic predictor model which only incorporates the mean of the outcome variable (essentially, $\hat{Y} = \bar{Y}$). However, I think the description provided in this chapter allows for a better conceptual understanding of R^2.

Adjusted R²

Sometimes investigators will report an adjusted R^2 (R^2_{Adj}) instead of, or in addition to, the conventional R^2 already discussed. The adjustment to R^2 is based on the sample size and the number of predictor variables (one in the case of simple linear regression) (Equation 9.12). The reasoning behind this adjustment is that the R^2 from a sample likely overestimates the R^2 in the population. The adjustment reduces the sample R^2 so that it's more likely to represent R^2 in the population. Essentially, the smaller the sample, the more R^2 is adjusted in the case of simple linear regression. Note that the adjusted R^2 will always be lower than the unadjusted R^2.

Equation 9.12

$$R^2_{\text{Adj}} = 1 - (1 - R^2)\left(\frac{n-1}{n-k-1}\right)$$

In Equation 9.12, R^2 = unadjusted coefficient of determination; n = number of observations; k = number of predictor variables ($k = 1$ for simple linear regression).

Example of assessing model fit

Kim et al. (2002) reported that the unadjusted R^2 for the regression model they developed to predict 1RM weights was 0.76 ($r = +0.87$, $R^2 = 0.87^2 = 0.76$). This indicates that 76% of the variation in 1RM weights (outcome variable – Y) was explained by the number of repetitions completed during the submaximal bench press testing (predictor variable – X). Of course, this also means that 24% of the total variation in the outcome variable wasn't explained by the regression model $(1 - R^2)$. The standard error of the estimate for their regression model was 3.1 kg., which indicates that the typical magnitude of the residual was 3.1 kg. Again, it's important to consider whether an average error of 3.1 kg is acceptable when estimating 1RM weights.

Statistical significance

For regression, it's possible to test the statistical significance of the entire regression model, the regression coefficient(s) (slope – b), and the constant (y-intercept – a). An F-test is typically used to test the regression model, while t-tests are typically used to test the regression coefficient and constant (F-tests were introduced in Chapter 6, and t-tests were introduced in Chapter 5). For simple linear regression, testing the regression model and the regression coefficient is essentially equivalent since the model only includes a single predictor variable. Therefore, in this chapter, we'll only focus on the basis for testing the regression coefficient, since these results are more often reported than the results for the entire regression model in the case of simple linear regression. Testing the regression coefficient and the entire regression model aren't equivalent when the regression model is expanded to include multiple predictor variables ('Multiple Regression' – Chapter 10). Therefore, Chapter 10 includes an in-depth discussion of testing the statistical significance of the regression model.

Testing the regression coefficient

To reiterate, the regression coefficient (b) represents the amount of change in the predicted value of the outcome variable for each one-unit change in the predictor variable (i.e. the slope of the regression line, or the 'rise over run'). A regression coefficient equal to 0 indicates that the regression line runs horizontally through the mean of the outcome variable, and therefore, the predictor variable explains none of the total variation in the outcome variable since $SS_{Total} = SS_{Residuals}$ and $SS_{Regression} = 0$. In other words, the predictor variable has no influence on the outcome variable. Another way to think of it is that a regression coefficient equal to 0 indicates that using the predictor variable to estimate the outcome variable is no better than simply using the sample mean of the outcome variable for prediction (essentially $\hat{Y} = \bar{Y}$).

A t-test can be conducted to determine if the regression coefficient is significantly different from 0 (null hypothesis: regression coefficient = 0), with the t statistic calculated by dividing the regression coefficient by its standard error. When the magnitude of the t statistic is relatively large, it indicates that an observed non-zero regression coefficient is unlikely to be due to sampling error or 'chance'. Note that testing the regression coefficient is essentially equivalent to conducting a t-test to determine if the Pearson product-moment correlation coefficient (r) is significantly different from 0 (discussed in Chapter 8). If the p-value is less than our predefined alpha level (p-value < 0.05, assuming an alpha of 0.05), we conclude that the regression coefficient is 'statistically significant' (i.e. the predictor variable is a predictor of the outcome variable in the population). If the p-value is greater than or equal to the alpha level, we conclude that the regression coefficient isn't statistically significant.

As an example, the regression coefficient in the model developed by Kim et al. (2002) was 0.31 kg. This indicates that the predicted 1RM weight increases by 0.31 kg for each additional repetition completed during the submaximal testing. The results of a t-test of the regression coefficient indicated that the regression coefficient was significantly different from 0 (p-value < 0.05). In other words, the number of repetitions completed during submaximal testing was a significant predictor of 1RM weight.

Testing the constant

As highlighted earlier in this chapter, the constant (*a*) represents the predicted value of the outcome variable when the predictor variable is 0 (i.e. the *y*-intercept of the regression line). As with the regression coefficient, a *t*-test can be conducted to determine if the constant is significantly different from 0. The null hypothesis for this test of statistical significance is that the constant = 0. Therefore, if the *p*-value is less than our predefined alpha level (*p*-value < 0.05, assuming an alpha of 0.05), we conclude that the regression constant is significantly different from 0. For example, the constant in the regression model developed by Kim et al. (2002) was 19.2 kg. The results of a *t*-test indicated that this regression constant was significantly different from 0 (*p*-value < 0.05). Of course, this isn't surprising, since we would expect apparently healthy, college-aged individuals to be able to bench press at least some weight (>0 kg) for a single repetition, even if they couldn't complete any repetitions at the standard weight used in the study.

While there are instances where testing the statistical significance of the constant is of interest, most of the time, it's of little relevance, partly because in many cases, a value of 0 for the predictor variable isn't plausible. For example, consider a simple linear regression analysis conducted to determine if waist-to-hip circumference ratio (predictor variable) predicts cholesterol level (outcome variable). In this case, a waist-to-hip circumference ratio of 0 isn't possible, since it would mean that the circumference of an individual's waist and/ or hips are 0. This limits the relevance of testing the constant. Regardless, most statistical analysis software packages automatically test the constant in addition to testing the entire regression model and the regression coefficient. Therefore, it's good to be familiar with the conceptual basis for testing the constant.

A word of caution

Tests of statistical significance aren't particularly good indicators of how well a regression model fits the data, since regression models that are statistically significant may still be inaccurate and explain very little of the overall variance in the outcome variable. This is analogous to a correlation that's weak but statistically significant (discussed in Chapter 8). The R^2 and standard error of the estimate provide greater insight into the goodness of fit of a regression model. Tests of statistical significance are also not very helpful in deciding if a regression model should be used to make predictions in clinical practice. Instead, decisions about whether to use a regression model in clinical practice should ultimately depend on the usefulness of the regression model and the level of risk that errors present. In the end, common sense and clinical intuition can't be replaced by a test of statistical significance.

Confidence intervals

The regression coefficient derived from sample data is typically meant to represent the regression coefficient for the regression line in the population. However, the regression coefficient from a sample won't perfectly reflect that of the population because of sampling error. To account for this, we can estimate a range of values, or confidence interval, in which the regression coefficient is expected to be located within. If 0 doesn't fall within this confidence interval, we have some degree of confidence that the regression coefficient for the population isn't 0 (i.e. *X* is a significant predictor of *Y* in the population). Conceptually, this is the same as creating a confidence interval for a correlation coefficient, which was discussed in Chapter 8.

Confidence intervals of 95% or 90% are commonly estimated, although any confidence interval can be generated. For a 95% confidence interval, there's a 95% probability that the regression coefficient for the population falls within the lower and upper bounds of the confidence interval. With a lower confidence interval (e.g. 90%), the interval is narrower, and thus more precise; however, we're less confident that the value falls within the bounds of the confidence interval. The concept of confidence intervals vs. point estimates was introduced in Chapter 4. Confidence intervals are also discussed in greater detail in Chapter 13 ('Effect Sizes and Confidence Intervals').

Note: a confidence interval can also be generated for the constant; however, this is of little relevance in most cases.

Generalizability

As we've already discussed, a regression model is optimized to fit the data from which it is derived. However, the accuracy of a regression model will typically deteriorate to some extent when applied to a new data set from a different sample, since the regression model wasn't optimized to fit this new data set. Sometimes the reduction in accuracy is trivial; however, in other cases, it may be substantial (i.e. poor generalizability). This creates issues, especially if the goal is to use a regression model to make future predictions for individuals not included in the original sample (e.g. future patients). We can explore this potential issue by examining whether our regression model still maintains acceptable accuracy in a new sample, which is typically referred to as model validation. Regression model validation is discussed in greater detail in Chapter 10. Regardless, it's important to remember that the results of a regression analysis really represent the best-case scenario regarding the accuracy of a regression model.

Extrapolation

When applying a regression model to make predictions, it's important to consider the range of predictor values that were used to derive the regression model. For example, Tanaka et al. (2001) included subjects who ranged from 18 to 81 years of age when developing their regression model to predict maximal heart rate based on age. As a result, it may not be appropriate to apply this regression model to individuals who are outside of this age range, since the accuracy of the regression model for individuals younger than 18 years of age or older than 81 years of age is unknown. Making predictions based on values not included in the range of predictor values used to develop the regression model is referred to as extrapolation. Figure 9.4 highlights the potential issue created by extrapolation.

A final note regarding correlation vs. simple linear regression

Chapters 8 and 9 clearly distinguish between bivariate correlation and simple linear regression, as Chapter 8 explains that bivariate correlation is used to examine relationships between variables, while Chapter 9 explains that simple linear regression involves developing an equation by which one variable can be used to predict another. However, the distinction between bivariate correlation and simple linear regression is much less clear in the literature. Investigators will often use simple linear regression to examine relationships between variables, even if their goal isn't to develop a predictive model (since r and b are so closely

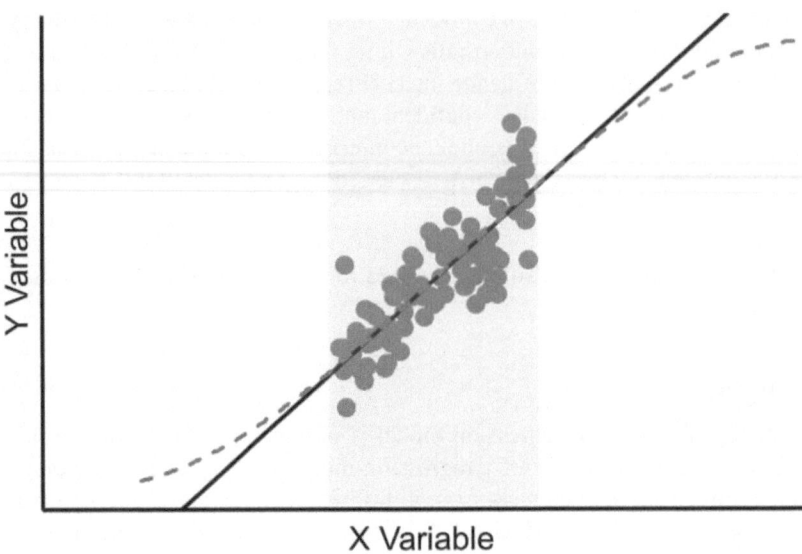

Figure 9.4 Example scatter plot with 100 *X/Y* pairs. The shaded region highlights the range of *X* values from which the regression line (solid black line) was derived. The predicted values of *Y* lie directly on the regression line. The dashed gray line characterizes the actual relationship between the *X* and *Y* variables. Notice that the predicted values for *Y* become less accurate above and below the range of *X* values that were used to develop the regression model. More specifically, the model tends to underestimate *Y* when *X* is below the minimum value from the sample and overestimate *Y* when *X* is above the maximum value from the sample.

related). This use of simple linear regression is more common when the investigators can make an argument about the directional nature of the relationship or, in other words, that the predictor variable (or independent variable) influences the outcome variable (or dependent variable). However, I would contend that correlation is usually a better approach whenever the objective of the analysis doesn't involve developing a predictive model, since with correlation, the direction and strength of the relationship can be captured by a single value (the correlation coefficient – *r*) and there's no need to differentiate between a predictor variable and an outcome variable.

Note: there's also a statistical basis for the difference between bivariate correlation and simple linear regression, which is related to the nature of the variables (bivariate correlation involves two random variables, while simple linear regression involves one random variable and one fixed variable); however, this distinction is largely theoretical.

Assumptions

This section highlights some of the key assumptions that should be met in order to conduct a simple linear regression analysis. Most of the assumptions are the same as those associated with Pearson product-moment correlation (Chapter 8); however, some are unique to simple linear regression.

1) Both variables are continuous

This isn't an assumption that's tested statistically. Instead, it's related to the nature of the variables being measured.

Options if this assumption isn't met

There are different types of regression analyses that can be used with ordinal data (e.g. ordinal regression). Discussion of these analyses is outside the scope of this book; however, many of the general concepts covered in this chapter still apply.

2) There's a linear relationship between the variables

Simple linear regression is only appropriate when there's a fairly linear relationship between the predictor variable and the outcome variable (i.e. the relationship between the variables would be characterized well by a straight line). Examining a scatter plot is an easy way to determine if there's a linear relationship between the variables. The assumption of linearity is discussed in greater detail in Chapter 8, since it's also an assumption for Pearson product-moment correlation.

Options if this assumption isn't met

There are a couple options if a nonlinear relationship is observed. First, you could attempt to transform your data so that the relationship between variables is more linear. Data transformation is discussed in Appendix B. You could also run different types of regression analyses that can be applied when the relationship between variables is nonlinear (e.g. polynomial regression, nonlinear regression). Discussion of these alternative analyses is outside the scope of this book.

3) There are no major outliers

Outliers are data points that don't fit the same general pattern as the rest of the data. Unfortunately, outliers can have a major influence on the regression equation and thus the accuracy of the regression model. There are several ways to objectively identify outliers in a data set. Discussion of these various methods is outside the scope of this book; however, the easiest and most straightforward way to identify potential outliers is to simply examine a scatter plot.

Options if this assumption isn't met

When an outlier is present, your first step should be to attempt to determine whether the data was entered erroneously or there was some type of equipment malfunction that could explain the atypical observation. You should also consider whether the value for the outcome variable is plausible (i.e. is the value within a range of what's likely to be humanly possible?). Outliers due to data entry errors, equipment miscalibration, and so on are easy to address by re-entering the correct data or removing data that's obviously erroneous.

When the reason for the outlier isn't clear, you need to carefully consider how to proceed. In some cases, investigators will remove the outlier from the analysis; however, this is generally discouraged when there's no obvious reason to believe that the data is erroneous.

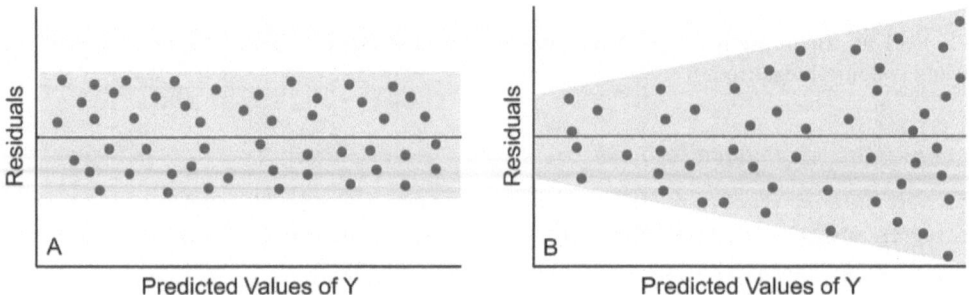

Figure 9.5 Example scatter plots with the predicted values of *Y* plotted on the *x*-axis and the residuals plotted on the *y*-axis. Scatter plot A (left panel) exhibits homoscedasticity, as the residuals are consistent across the entire range of predicted values of *Y*. Scatter plot B (right panel) exhibits heteroscedasticity, as the magnitude of the residuals differ across the range of predicted values of *Y*.

A better option is to report the results of the analysis both with the outlier included and with the outlier removed. This allows readers to appreciate how the outlier influenced the results of the analysis and make their own decision about how to interpret and apply the results.

4)   Homoscedasticity

For simple linear regression, it's assumed that the variance of the residuals is fairly uniform across all of the values for the predictor variable (*homoscedasticity*). In other words, the accuracy of the regression model is consistent over the entire range of predictor values. The assumption of homoscedasticity is typically checked by examining a plot of the residuals (*y*-axis) and the predicted values of the outcome variable ($\hat{y}$) (*x*-axis). The assumption of homoscedasticity is met if the spread of the residuals remains consistent over the range of $\hat{Y}$ values. If the residuals tend to increase or decrease when moving along the *x*-axis of the plot, then the data violates this assumption and is described as exhibiting heteroscedasticity. One simple check is to draw an outline around the data points included in the scatter plot. If the outline is rectangular, the assumption of homoscedasticity is likely met; however, if the outline takes on more a funnel shape, the assumption of homoscedasticity is likely not met. Figure 9.5 includes plots of data that meet the assumption of homoscedasticity (subplot A) and data that doesn't meet the assumption of homoscedasticity (subplot B). Notice that in subplot A, the residuals are fairly consistent across the entire range of the $\hat{Y}$ values, whereas in subplot B, the residuals become larger as the $\hat{Y}$ values increase (described as heteroscedasticity).

Options if this assumption isn't met

If the assumption of homoscedasticity is violated, you could attempt to transform your data. Data transformation is discussed in Appendix B. You could also consider running different types of regression analyses that don't require the assumption of homoscedasticity to be met (e.g. weighted least-squares regression). Discussion of these alternative analyses is outside the scope of this book.

5) Normality of the residuals

For simple linear regression, the residuals should be approximately normally distributed. Appendix A describes ways to assess normality.

Options if this assumption isn't met

If the assumption of normality isn't met, you could attempt to transform the outcome variable so that it's more normally distributed (data transformation is discussed in Appendix B).

Application opportunity

Example data set

Hsu et al. (2005) conducted a study to examine whether pre-operative sensitivity to pressure predicts post-operative analgesic consumption in patients undergoing abdominal total hysterectomy or myomectomy surgery. The study included a sample of 40 women. An algometer was used to measure pain pressure tolerance immediately prior to surgery. Pain pressure tolerance reflects the amount of pressure that a patient can tolerate before it produces pain that's too much to bear (note: lower pain pressure tolerance values are indicative of greater sensitivity to pressure). Pressure was applied to the patient's finger for the pain pressure tolerance testing. Postoperatively, patients were provided with a patient-controlled analgesia (PCA) pump that delivered morphine (an opioid analgesic) as requested by the patient. The PCA pump recorded the amount of morphine each patient consumed in the first 24 hours after surgery. The objective of this analysis is to determine if pre-operative pain pressure tolerance predicts post-operative morphine consumption.

Note: the units for the pain pressure tolerance (*PPT*) variable are kilopascals (kPa) and the units for morphine consumption are mg.

Data files

PPT&Morphine_data.xlsx – Excel file with pain pressure tolerance ('PPT') (first column) and morphine consumption (Morphine) (second column) values for 40 subjects who participated in the study.
   PPT&Morphine_data.sav – SPSS file with pain pressure tolerance ('PPT') (first column) and morphine consumption (Morphine) (second column) values for 40 subjects who participated in the study.

Note: the values in this data set were extracted from a scatter plot included in the original publication; therefore, they may not exactly match the values in the original data set.

Video

SimpleLinearRegression.mp4 – video that includes a demonstration of how to conduct a simple linear regression analysis using SPSS and the Excel Analysis Toolpak.

Sample write-up

Simple linear regression was used to examine whether pre-operative pain pressure toler-ance predicts post-operative morphine consumption in women undergoing abdominal total hysterectomy or myomectomy surgery. The statistical significance of the slope of the regres-sion coefficient was examined using a *t*-test with an alpha level of 0.05. The coefficient of determination (R^2) was calculated to represent the percentage of variation in post-operative morphine consumption, explained by pre-operative pain pressure tolerance.

Pre-operative pain pressure tolerance was a significant predictor of post-operative mor-phine consumption ($b = -0.05$; $p < 0.001$) and explained 34.7% of the variance in post-operative morphine consumption ($R^2 = 0.347$). The regression equation developed based on the analysis was: predicted morphine consumption (mg) = 33.31 − 0.05 × (pain pressure tolerance).

Answers to learning activity

Learning Activity 9.1

Answer:

Predicted HR max = 209 + −0.7(63) = 165 beats/minute
Residual = 170 beats/minute − 165 beats/minute = +5 beats/minute
The subject's HR max was underestimated by 5 beats/minute

10 Multiple regression

Chapter Objectives

The objectives of this chapter are to . . .

1) describe the general purpose of multiple regression
2) provide examples of the types of clinical research questions that multiple regression can be used to address
3) identify and describe the components of a regression equation that includes multiple predictor variables
4) demonstrate how to generate a predicted value for an outcome variable based on a multiple regression equation and calculate a residual
5) explain how a multiple regression model is developed using the least squares method
6) highlight how dummy coding can be used to incorporate categorical predictor variables into a multiple regression model
7) describe how the standard error of the estimate and coefficient of multiple determination can be used to assess the goodness of fit of a multiple regression model
8) differentiate between unstandardized and standardized regression coefficients and discuss what information each provide
9) explain the basis for examining the statistical significance of the regression model, regression coefficients, and constant
10) provide an overview of commonly used variable selection methods
11) discuss generalizability and cross-validation in the context of multiple regression
12) highlight key assumptions that should be met in order to conduct a multiple regression analysis
13) demonstrate how to conduct a multiple regression analysis using SPSS and the Excel Analysis Toolpak

Introduction

Chapter 9 introduced simple linear regression, which involves examining the extent to which one continuous 'predictor' variable (or 'independent' variable) can predict another continuous 'outcome' variable (or 'dependent' variable). Multiple regression is an extension of simple linear regression, where multiple predictor variables are used to predict an outcome variable (note: multiple regression is also referred to as multiple *linear* regression). With multiple regression, the outcome variable is still continuous; however, the predictor variables can be continuous or categorical. If you haven't done so already, it may be helpful to review Chapter 9 before proceeding.

DOI: 10.4324/9781003179757-10

First, let's consider some examples of the types of clinical research questions that can be addressed using multiple regression. Wee and Hopman (2005) conducted a study to identify factors that predicted length of stay in an inpatient rehabilitation facility for a cohort of older adults who had suffered a stroke. The objectives of their study were to determine which factors have the greatest influence on length of stay and to develop a model that could potentially be used to predict length of stay in future patients. Their study included 313 patients who were admitted to an inpatient rehabilitation facility shortly after experiencing a stroke. An examination of each patient was conducted at the time of admission in order to identify their motor and cognitive impairments. The investigators also recorded additional factors that they believed could influence length of stay, such as presence of family or caregiver support at home. They then conducted a multiple regression analysis to create a combination of these factors to predict length of stay (length of stay = the number of days spent in the inpatient rehabilitation facility from admission to discharge). Their results indicated that poorer balance, a greater number of physical impairments, presence of aphasia, and lack of support at home were associated with a greater length of stay. Multiple regression is commonly used for this purpose of identifying factors that influence, or predict, the extent or timeline of recovery.

Multiple regression can also be used to examine how a combination of inter-related factors (i.e. predictor variables) relate to, or explain variance in, an outcome variable. For example, Mangione et al. (2008), used multiple regression to explore how various demographic factors, physical characteristics, psychological factors, and overall general health (predictor variables) related to gait speed (outcome variable) in a sample of older adults who had sustained a hip fracture. Their results indicated that individuals with greater lower body strength, better overall general health, and more confidence in their balance tended to exhibit a faster gait speed.

The key benefit of multiple regression when compared to simple linear regression is that including more than one predictor variable allows for a more accurate prediction of the outcome variable. In other words, the additional predictor variables help to explain a greater proportion of variance in the outcome variable. Not surprisingly, a single variable will typically not accurately predict something as multifaceted as the length of stay in a rehabilitation facility. This is true for a lot of research questions related to health, medicine, and rehabilitation. However, with multiple regression, a combination of factors from different domains can be combined, allowing for a more complete and accurate predictive model. To put this into a more clinical context, think about how you typically predict a patient's prognosis for recovery. In most cases, you're probably not basing your patient's prognosis on a single factor, such as their age or the type of procedure they had (analogous to simple linear regression). Instead, you likely consider the totality of their condition, physical factors, personal factors, environmental factors, and so on (analogous to multiple regression). This is a good way to think about multiple regression. We're essentially incorporating more information into the model so that we can gain greater insight instead of only relying on a single factor or characteristic.

Basis for multiple regression

Chapter 9 introduced the regression equation as the basis for how a predictor variable (X) is used to estimate or predict an outcome variable (Y) in a simple linear regression analysis. Equation 10.1. includes the general form of the regression equation for simple linear regression, where a is the y-intercept, b is the slope, $\hat{Y}$ (referred to as 'y-hat') is the predicted value of the outcome variable, and X is the observed value of the predictor variable. In this regression equation, the constant (a) represents the value of $\hat{Y}$ when X is equal to 0, and the regression coefficient (*b*) represents the change in $\hat{Y}$ for each one-unit change in the *X* variable ('rise over run').

Equation 10.1

$$\hat{Y} = a + b(X)$$

In the case of multiple regression, the equation is expanded to include multiple predictor variables (Equation 10.2). In Equation 10.2, b_1 represents the regression coefficient for the first predictor variable, X_1 represents the value of *X* for the first predictor variable, b_2 represents the regression coefficient for the second predictor variable, and X_2 represents the value of *X* for the second predictor variable. Additional regression coefficients are added to the equation for each predictor variable (b_1 to b_k, where *k* represents the total number of predictor variables). There's no limit to the number of predictor variables that can be added to a regression equation.

Equation 10.2

$$\hat{Y} = a + b_1(X_1) + b_2(X_2) \ldots + b_k(X_k)$$

The multiple regression equation serves as the statistical model that's used for prediction of the outcome variable. Each subject's values for the predictor variables (X_1 to X_k) are input into the regression equation (Equation 10.2) and used to generate a predicted value for the outcome variable ($\hat{Y}$). The differences between the predicted and actual values for the outcome variable ($Y - \hat{Y}$) are the *residuals*. Note that this is no different than simple linear regression, except now the model includes multiple predictor variables.

The regression coefficients in a multiple regression model represent the change in $\hat{Y}$ for each one-unit change in the value of *X* for the specific predictor variable of interest when the values of the other predictor variables are held constant (i.e. remain unchanged). Regression coefficients in a multiple regression model can be any combination of positive and negative values. When a regression coefficient is positive, higher values of *X* for the predictor variable of interest contribute to higher values of $\hat{Y}$. When a regression coefficient is negative, higher values of *X* for the predictor variable of interest contribute to lower values of $\hat{Y}$. The constant (*a*) in a multiple regression equation represents the value of $\hat{Y}$ when the values for each of the predictor variables (X_1 to X_k) are equal to 0.

Before moving forward, let's revisit an earlier example. The final regression model reported by Wee and Hopman (2005) for predicting inpatient rehabilitation length of stay included four predictor variables: 1) Berg Balance Scale (BBS) score (higher scores reflect better balance) (Berg et al., 1989), 2) presence of aphasia (categorized as yes or no), 3) the number of impairments identified during the patient's exam (count from 0 to 10), and 4) the presence of support at home (categorized as yes or no). As you can see, their regression model included a mix of ordinal and nominal variables (nominal variables – presence of aphasia, presence of home support).*

* **Note:** in order to include nominal variables in the analysis, the investigators needed to assign a value of 1 or 0 to represent each patient's status (yes = 1, no = 0). The process for incorporating these types of categorical variables into a multiple regression analysis will be described in a following subsection titled 'Dummy Coding'.

The regression equation based on their analysis was:

$$\hat{Y} = 67.16 + -0.75(\text{BBS}) + 7.33(\text{aphasia} - 1/0) + 1.30(\text{impairments}) + -4.21(\text{home support} - 1/0)$$

The constant in the regression equation ($a = 67.16$) represents the predicted length of stay if the values for all predictor variables were 0. In this case, the predicted length of stay for a patient with a Berg Balance Scale score of 0, who did not exhibit aphasia, had no impairments identified during their physical exam, and had no home support would be 67.16 days. The signs of the regression coefficients indicate how each predictor variable influences the predicted length of stay. In this example, some factors increased the predicted length of stay and others decreased the predicted length of stay. You can think of the constant as a starting point for predicting length of stay, which gets modified based on each patient's status for the predictor variables. The regression coefficient for the Berg Balance Scale variable is –0.75, which indicates that each 1-point increase in a patient's Berg Balance Scale score corresponds with a reduction in their predicted length of stay by 0.75 days (assuming all other predictor variables are held constant). This makes sense, since higher Berg Balance Scale scores reflect better balance. Essentially, having better balance (i.e. a higher Berg Balance Scale score) reduces the predicted length of stay. The regression coefficient for the presence of aphasia variable was 7.33. This nominal variable was coded as 1 or 0, with 1 indicating that the patient exhibited aphasia. In this case, the predicted length of stay increases by 7.33 days if a patient exhibits aphasia. The regression coefficient for the number of impairments variable was +1.30, which indicates that each additional impairment identified during the patient exam increases the predicted length of stay by 1.30 days. Finally, the regression coefficient for the presence of home support variable was –4.21. This nominal variable was coded as 1 or 0, with 1 indicating that the patient had support at home. Therefore, having home support decreases the predicted length of stay by 4.21 days.

Not surprisingly, the predicted length of stay for each patient didn't perfectly match their actual length of stay. Some patients were discharged earlier than expected (i.e. the regression model overestimated their length of stay), while others were discharged later than expected (i.e. the regression model underestimated their length of stay). The differences between the actual and predicted lengths of stay for each patient are the residuals ('errors') in this example. Learning Activity 10.1 provides an opportunity for you to use a regression equation to generate a predicted length of stay and calculate a residual.

Learning Activity 10.1

Based on the regression equation developed by Wee and Hopman (2005), what is the predicted length of stay for a patient with a Berg Balance Scale score of 44 out of 56, who doesn't exhibit aphasia, has six noted impairments, and has support from a family member at home? If this patient spent 36 days in the inpatient rehabilitation facility, what was their residual?

The answers are included at the end of the chapter.

Deriving the regression model

Chapter 9 included an in-depth discussion of how a regression equation is developed when there's a single predictor variable (simple linear regression). Developing a regression equation with multiple predictor variables (multiple regression) involves the same process;

however, the focus of this chapter will be more conceptual, since the math gets a bit more cumbersome as additional predictors are added.

For multiple regression, the objective is to create a combination of the predictor variables that minimizes the sum of the squared residuals or the 'residual sum of squares' $[\Sigma(Y - \hat{Y})^2]$. In other words, the predictor variables are combined in a manner that produces the most accurate prediction of the outcome variable. No other set of regression coefficients would produce more accurate predictions of the outcome variable. Note that the objective of minimizing the sum of the squared residuals is the same as for simple linear regression, except now multiple predictor variables are combined to generate the predicted values of the outcome variable.

Conceptualizing multiple regression

There are several different ways to conceptualize multiple regression; however, I'll describe the one that I find easiest to understand. In multiple regression, the variables are combined to create predicted values for the outcome variable ($\hat{Y}$s). These $\hat{Y}$ values are essentially a weighted combination of all the predictor variables included in the regression model. As a result, you can think of multiple regression as a way of combining the values for the predictor variables into a new composite variable ($\hat{Y}$) that captures multiple pieces of information.

We can then examine the correlation between this composite variable ($\hat{Y}$ values) and the actual outcome variable (Y values) to determine how the multiple predictor variables included in the regression model are related to the outcome variable. In this case, the Pearson product-moment correlation coefficient captures the strength of the relationship between the composite variable ($\hat{Y}$ values), which is composed of the multiple predictor variables included in the regression model and the actual values for the outcome variable (Y values). In multiple regression, this Pearson product-moment correlation coefficient is referred to as the 'multiple correlation coefficient' and is denoted as R; however, it's no different than the Pearson product-moment correlation coefficient (r value) described in Chapter 8.

The multiple correlation coefficient will always be positive, which makes sense since we'd expect to observe a positive relationship between the predicted and actual values of the outcome variable. While the multiple correlation coefficient typically isn't reported, it's standard output when running multiple regression using most statistical analysis software packages, including SPSS.

Again, this is just one of several ways of thinking about multiple regression; however, I've found it to be fairly easy to grasp conceptually.

Dummy coding*

As discussed earlier in this chapter, multiple regression can accommodate categorical predictor variables (e.g. presence of aphasia, home support) in addition to continuous predictor variables. *Dummy coding* is a method that's commonly used to incorporate categorical variables into a multiple regression model. Dummy coding involves creating *dummy variables* where 1s and 0s are used to represent each subject's status for the categorical variable of interest. In general, the minimum number of dummy variables needed to capture each level of a categorical variable is the number of levels for the categorical variable minus 1.

For example, Wee and Hopman (2005) created a dummy variable to capture patient home support status when predicting inpatient rehabilitation length of stay. Each subject's status for this dummy variable was coded as 1 or 0, with 1 indicating that the patient had support at home and 0 indicating that the patient didn't have support at home. In the regression equation, the regression coefficient for the home support variable was $b = -4.21$, indicating that having home support ($X = 1$) decreased the predicted length of stay by 4.21 days. Another way to think of it is that if two patients had exactly the same Berg Balance Scale scores, both exhibited aphasia and presented with the same number of impairments, but one patient had home support ($X = 1$) and the other didn't ($X = 0$), the predicted length of stay for the patient with home support would be 4.21 days less than the patient without home support.

In the home support example, the categorical predictor variable only had two levels (home support, no home support), so only one dummy variable needed to be created (2 levels – 1 = 1 dummy variable). However, in some cases, a categorical variable will include more than two levels. For example, imagine that we're developing a multiple regression model to predict clinicians' salaries and we decide to include the highest level of degree earned (3 levels – bachelor's, master's, or doctorate). In this case, we could create two dummy variables (3 levels – 1 = 2 dummy variables). One dummy variable (denoted *MS*) could be coded as 1 for those whose highest degree earned was a master's (0 otherwise), and the other dummy variable (denoted *DR*) could be coded as 1 for those whose highest degree earned was a doctorate (0 otherwise). In this case, we wouldn't need to create a third dummy variable since 0s for the *MS* and *DR* variables already indicates that the highest degree earned was a bachelor's. The group with all 0s (bachelor's recipients in this example) serves as the reference category. The regression coefficients for the dummy variables can be examined to see how the other levels of the categorical variable compare to the reference category. For this example, the regression coefficients for the *MS* and *DR* variables would reflect how holding a master's or a doctorate degree affects salary, compared to holding a bachelor's degree (reference category).

* Note: this is intended to be a general overview of dummy coding. If you're planning to include a categorical variable with more than two levels in your regression analysis, it may be a good idea to consult a more advanced resource, especially if you're planning to interpret the regression coefficients for the dummy variables.

Assessing prediction accuracy

As we've already discussed, the regression model combines the predictor variables in a manner that produces the most accurate predictions of the outcome variable. However, this doesn't ensure that the regression model is a particularly good fit, as the predictions of the outcome variable could be highly inaccurate. It's important to remember that even the 'best' combination of the predictor variables could be quite poor. Therefore, once the multiple regression model is developed, the accuracy of the predictions made by the model must be examined in order to determine how well the regression model fits the data. The standard error of the estimate and the coefficient of multiple determination both provide an indication of the accuracy of a multiple regression model, which is often referred to as the model's 'goodness of fit'.

Standard error of the estimate

The standard error of the estimate essentially represents the average degree of error in the predicted values of the outcome variable or, in other words, the average residual. The more accurate the multiple regression model is at predicting the outcome variable, the smaller the residuals and the lower the standard error of the estimate. In fact, the standard error of the estimate will be 0 if the model is perfectly accurate (i.e. no residuals). The standard error of the estimate can be calculated using Equation 10.3.

Equation 10.3

$$SEE = \sqrt{\frac{\sum \left(Y - \hat{Y} \right)^2}{n-2}}$$

In Equation 10.3, Y = the actual values for the Y variable; $\hat{Y}$ = the predicted values for the Y variable; n = the number of observations; $n - 2$ = the degrees of freedom.

Once the standard error of the estimate has been calculated, it's important to put the value into context. For example, the standard error of the estimate for the study conducted by Wee and Hopman (2005) would represent the average degree of error in the predicted inpatient rehabilitation length of stay for the individuals in their sample.

Coefficient of multiple determination (R^2)

The coefficient of determination was first introduced in Chapter 8 ('Correlation') and was discussed in detail in Chapter 9 ('Simple Linear Regression'). In the case of simple linear regression, where there's only one predictor variable, the coefficient of determination represents the proportion of variation in the outcome variable that's explained by the predictor variable. In multiple regression, the terminology *coefficient of multiple determination* is typically used instead of *coefficient of determination*; however, these are conceptually the same, and both are typically denoted as R^2. I'll use R^2 throughout the rest of the chapter to minimize confusion.

In the case of multiple regression, where there are multiple predictor variables, R^2 represents the proportion of variation in the outcome variable that's explained by the entire regression model. R^2 ranges from 0.00 to 1.00 (or 0% to 100% if expressed as a percentage, which is common), with larger values reflecting a greater proportion of explained variation. In simple linear regression, R^2 is equal to the Pearson product-moment correlation coefficient squared. For multiple regression, R^2 is equal to the multiple correlation coefficient squared.

Basis for R^2

Chapter 9 included an in-depth discussion of how calculating R^2 involves partitioning the total variation in the outcome variable into variation that's explained by the regression model and variation that isn't explained by the regression model. This process is the same for multiple regression. The total sum of squares (SS_{Total}) captures the total variation in the outcome variable (Equation 10.4), since it represents how the Y values deviate about their mean, and the residual sum of squares ($SS_{Residuals}$) captures the variation in the outcome variable that isn't explained by the regression model (Equation 10.5). The $SS_{Regression}$ can be calculated by finding the difference between the total variation (SS_{Total}) and the unexplained variation ($SS_{Residuals}$), since $SS_{Total} = SS_{Regression} + SS_{Residuals}$ (i.e. total variation = explained variation + unexplained variation). Finally, R^2 can be calculated by dividing the $SS_{Regression}$ by the SS_{Total} (Equation 10.6). Again, R^2 represents the proportion of the total variation in the outcome variable that's explained by the regression model. Conversely, the proportion of variation not explained by the model ($1 - R^2$)

can be calculated by dividing the $SS_{\text{Residuals}}$ by the SS_{Total} (Equation 10.7). This proportion of unexplained variation is typically referred to as the 'coefficient of alienation'.

Equation 10.4

$$SS_{\text{Total}} = \sum \left(Y - \bar{Y} \right)^2$$

Equation 10.5

$$SS_{\text{Residuals}} = \sum \left(Y - \hat{Y} \right)^2$$

Equation 10.6

$$R^2 = \frac{SS_{\text{Regression}}}{SS_{\text{Total}}}$$

Or

$$R^2 = \frac{SS_{\text{Total}} - SS_{\text{Residuals}}}{SS_{\text{Total}}}$$

Equation 10.7

$$1 - R^2 = \frac{SS_{\text{Residuals}}}{SS_{\text{Total}}}$$

Another way of conceptualizing R^2

In Chapter 9, I alluded to the fact that R^2 can also be thought of as representing how much the regression model improves prediction of the outcome variable, compared to the most basic predictor model, which only incorporates the mean of the outcome variable. I'll elaborate on this idea a bit more in this chapter to provide you with another way of conceptualizing R^2. In the end, you can choose which way of thinking about R^2 makes the most sense to you.

Without a regression model, our 'best guess' of each subject's value for the outcome variable would simply be the mean from the entire sample. For example, if attempting to predict length of stay in an inpatient rehabilitation facility without incorporating information about patients' balance, number of impairments, presence of aphasia, or home support status, our best prediction would be the average length of stay for the entire sample. This prediction based on the sample mean represents the most basic predictive model (essentially, $\hat{Y} = \bar{Y}$). With this most basic predictive model, SS_{Total} and $SS_{\text{Residuals}}$ are equal, since both capture how the actual values of Y deviate about the mean of Y, and therefore, $SS_{\text{Regression}}$ equals 0.

Once the more advanced regression model is applied, we can examine the change in $SS_{\text{Residuals}}$ to get an impression of how much better the regression model is at explaining variation in the outcome variable compared to just using the sample mean for prediction. In this context, R^2 represents the improvement in prediction accuracy when the regression model is used or, in other words, the extent to which the regression model informs us of the value of the outcome variable compared to just knowing the average for the outcome variable. Again, this isn't a new concept, just another way of thinking about R^2.

Adjusted R^2

As discussed in Chapter 9, sometimes investigators will report an adjusted R^2 (R^2_{Adj}) instead of, or in addition to, the conventional R^2 already discussed. The adjustment to R^2 is based on the sample size and the number of predictor variables (Equation 10.8). The reasoning behind this adjustment is that the R^2 from a sample likely overestimates R^2 in the population. This is especially true with a small sample size and/or a large number of predictor variables. The adjustment reduces ('adjusts') R^2 so that it's more likely to represent R^2 in the population (i.e. it's a less biased estimate). Essentially, the smaller the sample and the greater the number of predictor variables, the more R^2 is adjusted. Note that the adjusted R^2 will always be lower than the unadjusted R^2.

Equation 10.8

$$R^2_{\text{Adj}} = 1 - (1 - R^2)\left(\frac{n-1}{n-k-1}\right)$$

For Equation 10.8, R^2 = unadjusted coefficient of multiple determination; n = number of observations; k = number of predictor variables.

R^2 *example*

Wee and Hopman (2005) reported that the unadjusted R^2 associated with their regression model to predict inpatient rehabilitation length of stay was 0.318 ($R^2 = 0.318$). This indicates that 31.8% of the variation in length of stay was explained by a regression model that included factors related to patients' balance, aphasia status, number of impairments, and home support. In this case, it's perhaps more interesting to note the amount of variation that wasn't explained by the regression model ($1 - R^2 = 68.2\%$), as this speaks to the complex nature of the rehabilitation timeline.

Standardized regression coefficients

In addition to examining the entire regression model, we may also be interested in examining the individual predictor variables in order to determine which predictor variables are most influential or, in other words, which of the predictor variables contribute most to prediction of the outcome variable. While it's tempting to simply compare the magnitudes of the regression coefficients, this is deceiving, since the predictor variables typically have different measurement scales or units. For example, if developing a model to predict maximal oxygen consumption based on age and 6 Minute Walk Test distance, the influence of a 1-unit increase in age (1 year) shouldn't be compared directly to the influence of a 1-unit increase in walk distance (1 meter), since walk distances will likely vary much more than ages simply because of the nature of the measurements. Obviously, we wouldn't expect an increase in walk distance of 1 meter to have the same influence on the outcome variable as an increase in age of 1 year. However, if the variables are standardized, it allows for a more direct, 'apples to apples' comparison. Once standardized, the regression coefficients represent the change in the predicted value of the outcome variable (in units of standard deviations) for each one standard deviation increase in the predictor variable (note: the 'units' for the variables are standard deviations once standardized). Essentially, the standardized regression coefficients capture the relationship between the predictor variable and the outcome variable independently of the other predictor variables in the model.

The magnitudes of the standardized regression coefficients can be compared to get a general impression of the relative importance of the predictor variables in the model. Predictor variables with standardized regression coefficients that are relatively large in magnitude generally contribute more to the prediction of the outcome variable compared to predictor variables with relatively small standardized regression coefficients closer to 0. Standardized regression coefficients are typically referred to as 'betas' (β_1 to β_k). Both unstandardized and standardized regression coefficients are generated by most statistical analysis software packages, and both are often reported. Learning Activity 10.2 provides you with an opportunity to compare the influence of different predictor variables based on their standardized regression coefficients.

Learning Activity 10.2

The Timed Up and Go (TUG) test is commonly used to assess functional mobility (Podsiadlo & Richardson, 1991). For the TUG test, the patient rises from a chair, walks around a cone positioned 3 m away, and then returns to the chair and sits. A clinician records the time required to complete the TUG test with a stopwatch. A shorter TUG time reflects better functional mobility. Kwan et al. (2011) used multiple regression to examine how various physical and psychological factors influenced TUG performance in a group of 280 community-dwelling older adults. Their regression model included nine predictor variables, which explained 43.5% of the variance in TUG performance. The standardized regression coefficients (betas – βs) for four of the predictor variables are included in the following. Which of these four variables had the greatest influence on TUG performance?

Postural sway: $\beta = 0.178$
Knee extension strength: $\beta = -0.223$
Age: $\beta = 0.203$
Cognitive function: $\beta = -0.108$
The answer is included at the end of the chapter.

Statistical significance

For regression, it's possible to test the statistical significance of the entire regression model, the regression coefficients (slopes – bs), and the constant (y-intercept – a). An F-test is typically used to test the regression model, while t-tests are typically used to test the regression coefficients and constant (F-tests were first introduced in Chapter 6, and t-tests were first introduced in Chapter 5). In the following subsections, the conceptual basis for testing the entire regression model, the regression coefficients, and the constant are discussed.

Testing the regression model

Testing the statistical significance of the regression model involves examining the amount of the variance explained by the regression model relative to the amount of unexplained variance. As discussed earlier, $SS_{\text{Regression}}$ captures the variation explained by the regression model, and $SS_{\text{Residuals}}$ captures the variation not explained by the regression model. An F statistic can be calculated to capture the ratio of the explained variance relative to the unexplained variance (Equation 10.10). When a large proportion of the total variance is explained by the regression model, the F statistic will be relatively large. In contrast, if the regression model doesn't explain any variance in the outcome variable, the F statistic will be 0.

Equation 10.10

$$F \text{ statistic} = \frac{\text{Explained Variance}}{\text{Unexplained Variance}}$$

Or

$$F \text{ statistic} = \frac{\dfrac{SS_{\text{Regression}}}{k}}{\dfrac{SS_{\text{Residuals}}}{n-k-1}}$$

In Equation 10.10, k = the number of predictor variables; n = the number of observations (i.e. subjects in the sample). Dividing the sums of squares by their corresponding degrees of freedom (k; $n - k - 1$) results in the average sum of squares (mean squares) for the $SS_{\text{Regression}}$ and $SS_{\text{Residuals}}$.

The location of the F statistic within the F distribution can be used to determine the probability (p-value) of observing an F statistic of the given magnitude simply by chance (F-test). The null hypothesis for this test of statistical significance is that the regression model doesn't explain any variance in the outcome variable ($R^2 = 0$). If our observed p-value is less than our predefined alpha level (p-value < 0.05, assuming an alpha level of 0.05), we conclude that the regression model explains a significant proportion of the variance in the outcome variable. When the p-value is greater than or equal to our alpha level (p-value ≥ 0.05), we conclude that the regression model doesn't explain a significant proportion of the variance in the outcome variable.

It should be noted that technically, testing the statistical significance of the regression model involves determining whether the regression model predicts the outcome variable with better accuracy than the most basic predictor model ($\hat{Y} = \bar{Y}$), which doesn't include any predictor variables. However, I've found this to be difficult for most to conceptualize. Therefore, I've presented what I feel to be a more intuitive explanation.

Testing the regression coefficients

In addition to testing the entire regression model, it's also common to test the statistical significance of the individual predictor variables by examining the magnitude of the regression coefficients. A regression coefficient equal to 0 indicates that the predictor variable doesn't make a unique contribution to predicting the outcome variable. Note that by 'unique', I mean beyond the contributions from the other variables in the model. A t-test can be conducted to determine if the regression coefficient is significantly different from 0 (null hypothesis: regression coefficient = 0), where the t statistic is the regression coefficient divided by its standard error. When the magnitude of the t statistic is relatively large, it indicates that the observed non-zero regression coefficient is unlikely to be due to sampling error or 'chance'.

If the p-value associated with a t-test of the regression coefficient is less than our predefined alpha level (p-value < 0.05, assuming an alpha of 0.05), we conclude that the regression coefficient is significantly different from 0. In other words, the predictor variable makes a significant contribution to predicting the outcome variable. In contrast, if the p-value is greater than or equal to our alpha level, we conclude that the regression coefficient isn't significantly different from 0. In other words, the predictor variable doesn't make a significant contribution to predicting the outcome variable.

In most cases, we examine the statistical significance of the entire regression model and then follow this up by examining the individual predictor variables. Confidence intervals can also be generated for the regression coefficients. Chapter 9 included an in-depth discussion of confidence intervals in the context of regression coefficients.

Testing the constant

A t-test can be conducted to determine if the constant is significantly different from 0. The null hypothesis for this test of statistical significance is that the constant = 0. Therefore, if the p-value is less than our alpha level (p-value < 0.05, assuming an alpha of 0.05), we conclude that the constant is significantly different from 0. The conceptual basis for testing the constant was discussed in greater detail in Chapter 9; however, in most cases, the results of the t-test of the constant are of little relevance.

A word of caution

Tests of statistical significance aren't particularly good indicators of how well a regression model fits the data, since regression models that are statistically significant may still explain very little of the overall variance in the outcome variable. R^2 and the standard error of the estimate are better indicators of the goodness of fit of a regression model.

Variable selection methods

In many cases, not all predictor variables will make a unique contribution in a regression model. As a result, we may attempt to develop a more 'efficient' or 'parsimonious' model that can explain a comparable amount of variance with fewer variables. For example, Mangione et al. (2008) initially started with 24 predictor variables that they believed could potentially influence gait speed in individuals who had sustained a hip fracture; however, their final regression model was narrowed down to 3 predictor variables (lower body strength, general health, balance confidence) that explained 71.7% of the variance in gait speed ($R^2 = 0.717$).

While they could have included more, or all, of the original 24 predictor variables in their final regression model, including these additional variables wouldn't have dramatically improved prediction accuracy. In other words, the additional variance explained by including more predictor variables in the final regression model would have been trivial. The general process of identifying a subset of predictor variables from a larger set of possible predictor variables is referred to as *variable selection.*

In the following subsections, I provide a general overview of some common variable selection methods. I don't go into specific details about these procedures, since variable selection is somewhat of an advanced topic that's outside the scope of this book. However, it's good to be familiar with the general idea.

Forward selection method

With the forward selection method, an initial model is created that only includes a constant. Then, the predictor variable that exhibits the strongest correlation with the outcome variable is added to the model. You can think of this as adding the predictor variable that individually explains the greatest amount of variance in the outcome variable. If adding this predictor variable significantly improves the regression model, the variable is retained and the process continues. Next, the predictor variable that explains the greatest amount of remaining unexplained variance is identified. For example, if the first predictor variable explained 40% of the variance in the outcome variable, forward selection would identify the predictor variable that explains the greatest amount of the remaining 60% of the variance. This second variable is then added to the regression model. If the model improves significantly with the addition of this second predictor variable, this variable is retained. This process continues until adding another predictor variable no longer significantly improves accuracy of the regression model. The predictor variables included in the model up to this point make up the final subset of predictor variables.

Stepwise method

The stepwise method is similar to the forward method, with one subtle difference. With the forward method, once a predictor variable is added to the regression model, it won't be removed. Conversely, with the stepwise method, the entire set of predictor variables in the regression model are re-evaluated each time a new predictor variable is added. If a predictor variable that was previously added to the model no longer makes a unique contribution, it's removed. Therefore, with the stepwise method, predictor variables can be added and retained in one step and then removed from the regression model in a subsequent step.

Backward selection method

The backward selection method is essentially the opposite of the forward selection method. With backward selection, a regression model is developed with all of the predictor variables included. The predictor variable that contributes least to the regression model is identified and analyzed to determine if it makes a significant contribution (note: the contributions of the individual predictor variables are typically based on t-tests of the regression coefficients). If the predictor variable doesn't make a significant contribution, it's removed, and the regression analysis is re-run with the remaining predictor variables. This process continues until the predictor variable that contributes least still makes a significant contribution to the regression model (i.e. all predictor variables contribute significantly). The variables that weren't removed from the regression model make up the final subset of predictor variables. Another way you can think of this backward selection process is that predictor variables are deleted one at a time until the point where significant predictor variables would start being removed from the model. Again, this is conceptually the same as the forward selection procedure, but in reverse.

Final thoughts on variable selection

Software packages such as SPSS offer a lot of different options for variable selection. If you're considering using variable selection, you should attempt to fully understand the details and potential limitations of the various options before deciding which specific method best meets your needs. That said, this isn't the book to learn some of the subtle nuances of different variable selection methods.

It should also be noted that variable selection methods are based solely on statistical criteria, not theory or previous research. This is one of many reasons why the use of these methods is controversial. My advice is to proceed with caution if attempting to use variable selection methods and to avoid including potential predictor variables that aren't strongly supported by theory or prior research. In the end, if the predictor variables included in the final regression model 'make sense' based on theory or past research, the variable selection process probably worked well. However, if the predictor variables included (or not included) in the final regression model are surprising, it's probably a good idea to dig deeper into the data and investigate more.

Hierarchical regression

While in most cases, all of the predictor variables are entered into a regression model simultaneously (referred to as the 'enter method'), it's also possible to select the order in which predictor variables, or groups of predictor variables, are entered into the regression model. This is generally referred to as *hierarchical regression*. In most cases, hierarchical regression is used when investigators have a reason to specify the order in which the variables are entered into the regression model. The change in R^2 can be examined as each new set of predictor variables are added to the regression model.

For example, Falvo and Earhart (2009) used hierarchical regression when predicting 6 Minute Walk Test distances in individuals with Parkinson's disease. They first entered a block of predictor variables that were related to the stage and severity of the patient's Parkinson's disease (block 1). They then entered a second block of predictor variables that were related to the patient's balance and mobility (block 2). The variables entered in block 1 explained 19.6% of the variance in walk distance ($R^2 = 19.6\%$), while the variables entered in block 2 explained an additional 35.5% of the variance in walk distance (change in $R^2 = 35.5\%$). As a result, the final model (block 1 and block 2) explained a total of 55.1% of the variance in walk distance (19.6% + 35.5% = 55.1%). Based on these results, the investigators concluded that balance and mobility explained additional variance beyond what could be explained solely based on the stage and severity of a patient's Parkinson's disease.

Generalizability and cross-validation

Although a regression model is almost always developed based on sample data, the objective is typically to approximate the model in the population or, in other words, to generalize the results of the regression analysis from a sample to the entire population. We can get an impression of the generalizability of a regression model by examining the accuracy of the model when it's applied to a different sample from the same population. If a regression model is generalizable, there shouldn't be a major dropoff in prediction accuracy when the model is applied to a new sample. However, a substantial reduction in the accuracy of the regression model when applied to a new sample indicates that the model may be unique to the sample data from which it was derived (i.e. poor generalizability). The process of examining the accuracy of a regression model in a new sample is referred to as *cross-validation*.

One common method of cross-validation is to split the sample data into two separate subsets. One subset is used to develop the regression model (often referred to as the *training set*). Once the model is developed, it's then applied to the other subset (often referred to as the *validation set*). If the accuracy of the regression model is similar when applied to the valida-tion set (i.e. minimal reduction in R^2), then the model likely generalizes beyond the data set from which it was derived and therefore to the population. However, if there's a substantial reduction in prediction accuracy (e.g. large reduction in R^2) when applied to the validation set, then generalizability is likely poor. In many cases, investigators will use a greater propor-tion of their sample to develop the model (e.g. 70% of the entire sample) and then attempt to validate their model using a smaller subset of their sample (e.g. 30% of the entire sample). Regardless, this approach still requires a relatively large sample, since only some of the data set will be used to develop the regression model.

Another approach that's becoming increasingly popular as computer computational power continues to improve is referred to as *leave-one-out* cross-validation. I won't discuss this pro-cedure in depth but will attempt to explain the general concept. The leave-one-out approach involves developing a regression model based on data from all subjects in the sample, except one (i.e. this subject's data is 'left out' when deriving the model). Once the regression model is developed, it's applied to predict the value of the outcome variable for the subject who was left out during model development. The difference between the predicted value and the actual value of the outcome variable for this subject is the residual (i.e. error). This process continues iteratively until each subject's data has been left out during model development. For example, if a sample included data from 1000 subjects, 1000 regression models would be developed based on data from 999 subjects, with data from a different subject left out in each iteration. You can imagine the amount of 'computational horsepower' required to do this in a timely manner. The average degree of error based on the residuals across the multiple itera-tions can be used to gauge the generalizability of the regression model. Essentially, this is a way to use one data set to both derive and validate a regression model. There are also other variations of this general method.

Overfitting a regression model

In general, our objective is typically to develop a regression model that explains a substan-tial proportion of the variance in the outcome variable. One way to increase R^2 is to include additional predictor variables in the regression model, since adding a predictor variable will never decrease, and in most cases will increase, R^2. However, including too many predictor variables may result in *overfitting* of the regression model, which occurs when the model starts to explain random variation (or 'noise') in the data set rather than real relationships between the predictor variables and the outcome variable. When a regression model is over-fit, R^2 starts to become inflated (i.e. it drastically overestimates R^2 in the population), and the model becomes less generalizable, since different data sets will likely have their own unique 'noise'. In general, only a limited number of predictor variables that can be supported by theory and/or prior research should be included in a regression model. Although tempt-ing, it's important to avoid attempting to increase R^2 by indiscriminately adding predictor variables to a regression model. In the end, there will always be some variance that remains unexplained, no matter how many predictor variables are included in the model.

Earlier in this chapter, we discussed how R^2 can be adjusted based on the number of predictor variables included in the regression model (Equation 10.8). This adjustment to R^2 essentially penalizes a model (by reducing R^2) that includes predictor variables which explain a trivial amount of variance in the outcome variable. If there's a major difference between the unadjusted and adjusted R^2, it likely means that not all predictor variables are contributing.

Sample size

In general, multiple regression tends to require a much larger sample size than many of the other analyses discussed in this book. But how many subjects are enough? While there isn't a clear answer regarding the minimum sample size for multiple regression, there are many different rules of thumb (Green, 1991). For example, one commonly referenced rule of thumb is that there should be a minimum of ten subjects for each predictor variable in the model. This would mean that data from 100 subjects, at minimum, is required for a regression model that includes ten predictor variables. Another commonly used rule of thumb suggests that the minimum sample size should be 50 subjects, plus 8 times the number of predictor variables. This equates to a sample size of 74 if there are three predictor variables ($50 + 3 \times 8 = 74$ subjects). These are just two of many of these types of rules of thumb, which highlights the fact that these are not strict rules. It's also possible to conduct a sample size estimate to determine a minimum sample size based on the anticipated strength of the relationship between the predictor variables and the outcome variable. The concept of sample size estimation is discussed in Chapter 14 ('Sample Size Estimation').

Regardless, it's good to appreciate that, in general, the larger the sample, the better when it comes to multiple regression. It's also important to note that in many cases, we must consider whether it's feasible to collect data from a large enough sample to conduct a multiple regression analysis. There are many excellent clinical research questions that could be effectively addressed with multiple regression, but the limiting factor is the feasibility of collecting data from a sufficiently large sample.

Final thoughts on multiple regression

Multiple regression is a tremendously useful tool that can address a wide variety of important clinical research questions. However, it's a relatively advanced analysis compared to many of the others discussed in this book. While this book is a good starting point for learning multiple regression, I encourage you to consult more advanced resources if you're planning to use multiple regression for your own research.

Assumptions

This section highlights some of the key assumptions that should be met in order to conduct a multiple regression analysis. Most of the assumptions for multiple regression are the same as those for simple linear regression (Chapter 9). Therefore, I only briefly revisit the assumptions (1–4) that were already discussed in Chapter 9.

1) There's a linear relationship between the individual predictor variables and the outcome variable and the combination of the predictor variables and the outcome variable

Multiple regression is only appropriate when there's a fairly linear relationship between each of the predictor variables and the outcome variable. In addition, there should also be a linear relationship between the predictor variables collectively and the outcome variable. The predicted values of the outcome variable ($\hat{Y}$ values) represent the combination of the predictor variables. Examining scatter plots is an easy way to determine if there are linear relationships between the predictor variables and the outcome variable and the $\hat{Y}$ values and the outcome variable.

2)   There are no major outliers

Outliers are cases that don't fit the same general pattern as the rest of the data. Unfortunately, outliers can have a major influence on a regression model. There are several ways to objectively identify outliers in a data set. While discussion of these various methods is outside the scope of this book, most rely on identifying residuals that are relatively extreme.

3)   Homoscedasticity

For multiple regression, it's assumed that the variance of the residuals is fairly uniform across the predicted values of the outcome variable ($\hat{Y}$ values) (i.e. homoscedasticity). In other words, the accuracy of the regression model is consistent over the entire range of predicted values. The assumption of homoscedasticity is typically checked by examining a plot of the residuals (y-axis) and the $\hat{Y}$ values (x-axis). The assumption of homoscedasticity is met if the spread of the residuals remains consistent over the range of $\hat{Y}$ values. If the residuals tend to increase or decrease when moving along the x-axis of the plot, then the data violates this assumption and is described as exhibiting heteroscedasticity. Figure 9.5 in Chapter 9 ('Simple Linear Regression') includes plots of data that meets the assumption of homoscedasticity (subplot A) and don't meet the assumption of homoscedasticity (subplot B).

4)   Normality of the residuals

For multiple regression, the residuals should be approximately normally distributed. Appendix A ('Assessing Normality') describes ways to assess normality.

5)   No evidence of multicollinearity

One of the key assumptions for multiple regression is that the data doesn't show evidence of *multicollinearity*. Multicollinearity occurs when some, or all, of the predictor variables are strongly correlated with each other. Predictor variables are often correlated with each other to some extent, which isn't surprising since they likely have at least some relationship with the outcome variable (otherwise, why are they in the model?). However, when the correlations among the predictor variables are too strong, it creates a number of issues. Note that we didn't have to worry about multicollinearity in simple linear regression, since the regression model only included a single predictor variable.

Examining the correlations among the predictor variables is a good starting point for identifying multicollinearity. If there's a strong relationship (e.g. $r \geq 0.80$) between any pair of predictor variables, it may be worth omitting one of these predictor variables from the model, since having both variables provides little unique information (i.e. the variables are somewhat redundant). It's also important to avoid the extreme case where variables are completely redundant or where one predictor variable is simply a combination of other predictor variables in the model. For example, you wouldn't want to include body mass, height, and body mass index as predictor variables in a multiple regression model, since body mass index is a combination of body mass and height (body mass index = body mass/height^2). In addition, if you had data from a questionnaire with different subscales, you wouldn't want to include the scores from the individual subscales and the total score (sum of all subscales) as predictor variables.

Software packages such as SPSS provide additional metrics, such as the variance inflation factor and tolerance, which are worth exploring if you have concerns about the potential for multicollinearity.

Application opportunity

Example data set

This example is based on a data set published by Terradas-Monllor et al. (2020) (DOI: 10.7717/peerj.9903/supp-2), which includes data for 59 subjects who had undergone knee arthroplasty. The predictor variables in the data set include sex, age, lower body strength, knee passive range of motion, and pain during walking, while the outcome variable is gait speed. Lower extremity strength was assessed using the 30-Second Chair Stand test, where the number of times a subject can sit-to-stand over a 30-second period is recorded (more repetitions reflects greater lower body strength). Knee passive range of motion reflected the total amount of passive motion the subject exhibited for knee flexion/extension. Pain during walking was based on self-reported pain on a 0–10 scale (0 – no pain, 10 – worst pain imaginable). The purpose of this analysis is to examine the relationship between this collection of predictor variables and an individual's gait speed following knee arthroplasty. All data was recorded 6 months after the knee arthroplasty procedure.

Data files

KA_GaitSpeed_data.xlsx – Excel file with the predictor variables Sex (male = 0, female = 1), Age (years), Strength (30-Second Chair Stand repetitions), Knee_motion (total knee passive range of motion), and Pain (0–10) and the outcome variable Gait_speed included in separate columns.

    KA_GaitSpeed_data.sav – SPSS file with the predictor variables Sex (male = 0, female = 1), Age (years), Strength (30-Second Chair Stand repetitions), Knee_motion (total knee passive range of motion), and Pain (0–10) and the outcome variable Gait_speed included in separate columns.

Video

MultipleRegression.mp4 – video that includes a demonstration of how to conduct a multiple regression analysis using SPSS and the Excel Analysis Toolpak.

Sample write-up

Multiple regression was used to examine the extent to which a model composed of the variables sex, age, lower body strength, knee motion, and pain during walking predicted gait speed in individuals who had undergone knee arthroplasty. An F-test was conducted to assess the statistical significance of the entire regression model, while t-tests of the regression coefficients were conducted to assess the statistical significance of the individual predictor variables. An alpha level of 0.05 was used for all tests of statistical significance.

    The regression model was statistically significant ($F(5, 53) = 4.99$; $p < 0.001$) and explained 58.6% of the variance in gait speed ($R^2 = 0.586$). The variables sex (<0.001, $\beta = -0.338$), lower body strength ($p < 0.001$, $\beta = 0.447$), knee motion ($p = 0.006$, $\beta = 0.257$), and pain during walking ($p = 0.007$; $\beta = -0.276$) made significant contributions to predicting gait speed, while age ($p = 0.092$; $\beta = -0.156$) did not make a significant contribution.

Notes: F is the F statistic, with its corresponding degrees of freedom (5, 53). p are the p-values associated with F-test and t-tests.

Answers to learning activities

Learning Activity 10.1

Answer:

Predicted length of stay = $67.16 + -0.75(44) + 7.33(0) + 1.30(6) + -4.21(1)$
= 37.75 or ~38 days
Residual = 36 days – 38 days = –2 days
The patient's length of stay was overestimated by 2 days

Learning Activity 10.2

Answer:

Knee extension strength: $\beta = -0.223$

11 Logistic regression

Chapter Objectives

The objectives of this chapter are to . . .

1) describe the general purpose of logistic regression
2) provide examples of the types of clinical research questions that logistic regression can be used to address
3) identify and describe the components of a logistic regression model
4) explain how to interpret the regression coefficients and odds ratios associated with a set of predictor variables
5) describe how the results of a logistic regression analysis can be used for classification
6) introduce commonly reported pseudo R^2 metrics
7) explain the basis for examining the statistical significance of a regression model and the regression coefficients
8) describe how variable selection methods are commonly used in logistic regression
9) discuss generalizability and cross-validation in the context of logistic regression
10) demonstrate how to conduct a binary logistic regression analysis using SPSS

Introduction

Chapters 9 and 10 discussed linear regression, which involves using a single predictor variable (simple linear regression – Chapter 9) or a combination of predictor variables (multiple regression – Chapter 10) to predict the value of a continuous outcome variable. In contrast, logistic regression is used when the outcome variable is a categorical variable with discrete categories or levels. In the simplest form of logistic regression, the categorical outcome variable is dichotomous, with two discrete categories. This is referred to as binary logistic regression. Binary logistic regression will be the primary focus of this chapter. However, logistic regression can also include an outcome variable with more than two categories, which is typically referred to as multinomial logistic regression.*

* **Note:** the general principles are the same for binary logistic regression and multinomial logistic regression.

Before moving forward, it's important to note that logistic regression is one of the most advanced topics covered in this book. While this chapter introduces some key concepts, I encourage you to seek out additional resources or consult with a statistician if you're planning to use logistic regression for your own research. That said, it's critical for clinicians to

DOI: 10.4324/9781003179757-11

have at least a basic understanding of logistic regression, since it's commonly used in health-related research.

Logistic regression is tremendously useful for addressing clinical research questions for a couple of reasons. First, many health-related outcomes are naturally categorical (e.g. presence or absence of disease). In addition, much like multiple regression, the logistic regression model can include any combination of continuous and categorical predictor variables, which allows for flexibility in the types of 'clinical data' that can be incorporated into the model. As a result, logistic regression has been used to address a wide range of clinical research questions. For example, logistic regression has been used to identify factors that contribute to falls in older adults (e.g. Tiedemann et al., 2008), knee injuries in athletes (e.g. Vacek et al., 2016), deep vein thrombosis (DVT) following surgery (e.g. Shimoyama et al., 2012), and pressure ulcers in hospitalized patients (Delmore et al., 2015). In each of these examples, the outcome variable was naturally dichotomous (i.e. fall or no fall, injury or no injury, DVT or no DVT, ulcer or no ulcer), making these questions conducive to binary logistic regression.

Let's take a closer look at another example. Pereira et al. (2014) used binary logistic regression to predict the discharge locations of individuals who had been admitted to a rehabilitation unit following a stroke. Their regression model included the patient's age, total Functional Independence Measure (FIM) score at the time of admission, and caregiver availability as predictor variables. The FIM is a measure that quantifies a patient's level of function and independence, with higher scores reflecting greater function and more independence (Granger et al., 1986). In the regression model, caregiver availability was a dichotomous predictor variable that was coded as 1 if a patient had caregiver support at home or 0 if not. For the outcome variable (discharge location), patients were categorized as either being discharged to home (coded 1) or to a long-term care facility (coded 0) (notice the 'binary' nature of this outcome variable, hence the terminology *binary* logistic regression). Interestingly, the investigators found that their three-factor model accurately predicted the discharge location (home vs. long-term care facility) for 87.8% of the 189 patients enrolled in the study. Their results indicated that the odds of being discharged to home were greater for patients who were younger, had higher FIM scores at admission (i.e. greater levels of function and more independence), and had caregiver support at home.

As you can see from this example, there are a lot of similarities between multiple regression and logistic regression. If you haven't done so already, it may be helpful to review Chapter 10 before proceeding, as many of the general concepts of multiple regression will also be relevant to logistic regression. A brief review of linear regression is also included in the next section. You may also want to review the concepts of probability and odds, which were introduced in Chapter 4, since they are also critical to logistic regression.

Basis for binary logistic regression

The following subsections will discuss the basis for binary logistic regression. Many subtle details are omitted in an attempt to promote a more conceptual understanding of the analysis. Detailed discussions of the theoretical basis and components of the logistic regression model can be found in more advanced textbooks.

Linear regression

First, let's quickly review the general concepts of linear regression. Chapters 9 and 10 introduced the regression equation as the basis for how predictor variables (X_1 to X_k) are combined to predict a continuous outcome variable. The general form of the multiple regression equation is presented in Equation 11.1. In this equation, the bs (b_1 to b_k) represent the regression coefficients associated with the predictor variables included in the model, the Xs (X_1 to X_k) represent the values for the predictor variables, and $\hat{Y}$ represents the predicted values of the continuous outcome variable. The regression equation combines the variables in a manner that minimizes the residuals, or errors, in the predictions of the outcome variable. For example, Chapter 10 described a study by Wee and Hopman (2005) where multiple regression was used to develop a model to predict length of stay in an inpatient rehabilitation facility for patients who had experienced a stroke. In this case, the outcome variable, length of stay, was continuous.

Equation 11.1

$$\hat{Y} = a + b_1(X_1) + b_2(X_2)\ldots + b_k(X_k$$

While linear regression works well for predicting a continuous outcome variable, it's not particularly well suited for predicting a dichotomous outcome. One reason is that the predictor variables aren't linearly related to a dichotomous outcome variable, making a linear model a poor fit for this type of data. In the logistic model, the outcome variable essentially undergoes a logarithmic transformation to linearize the relationship between the predictor variables and the dichotomous outcome variable. This helps to make the logistic model a better fit in cases where the outcome variable is categorical.

Binary logistic regression

Binary logistic regression still relies on a linear combination of the predictor variables; however, the model is no longer predicting the value of a continuous outcome variable. Instead, the model estimates the probability that a subject is a member of a certain category of the outcome variable. In most cases, it's helpful to think of this as predicting the probability of an event. The term 'event' is used quite liberally, as it could mean experiencing a fall, sustaining an injury, developing a DVT, or achieving a certain clinical outcome. The outcome variable can be coded so that 1 indicates that the subject experienced the event ($Y = 1$) and 0 indicates that the subject didn't experience the event ($Y = 0$). For each subject, the logistic regression model will estimate the probability that the subject experienced the event, based on their values for the predictor variables. In other words, the predictor variables are used to estimate the probability that $Y = 1$. Probabilities can range between 0 and 1. The closer the probability is to 1, the more likely it is that the event occurred (i.e. $Y = 1$).

Let's revisit the example introduced earlier in this chapter. Pereira et al. (2014) used age, FIM score, and caregiver availability to predict discharge locations in a group of older adults who had been admitted to a rehabilitation unit following a stroke. They coded discharge to home as 1 and discharge to a long-term care facility as 0. In this case, the 'event' was discharge to home. Therefore, the probabilities estimated by their model reflected the probability that the patient would be discharged to home. A probability closer to 1 indicated that the patient was more likely to be discharged to home ($Y = 1$), whereas a probability closer to 0 indicated that the patient was more likely to be discharged to a long-term care facility ($Y = 0$). A patient with a probability of 0.5 would be just as likely to be discharged to home ($Y = 1$) as to a long-term care facility ($Y = 0$). Again, these estimated probabilities are based on a linear combination of the patient's age, FIM score, and caregiver availability.

The logistic regression model

The logistic regression model is a bit more complex than the linear regression model since it incorporates a logarithmic transformation to link the predictor variables to the outcome variable. However, there are a lot of similarities between the logistic and linear models. Equation 11.2 includes the general form of the logistic regression model. The output, $p(Y = 1)$, is the probability that $Y = 1$ (i.e. the probability of the event), and e is the base of natural logarithms. Notice that the logistic regression model incorporates a linear combination of the predictor variables (exponent of e), where the bs (b_1 to b_k) represent the regression coefficients associated with the predictor variables, the Xs (X_1 to X_k) represent the values for the predictor variables, and a is the constant. Essentially, the linear model is built in as a component of the logistic model. Much like the linear model predicts the value of Y for any combination of the predictor variables, the logistic regression model estimates the probability of an event ($Y = 1$) for any combination of the predictor variables.

Equation 11.2

$$p(Y = 1) = \frac{1}{1 + e^{-[a + b_1(X_1) + b_2(X_2)\ldots + b_k(X_k)]}}$$

Plotting the logistic regression function

Let's explore the logistic model a bit more with a simple example. Suppose we're trying to develop a model to estimate the probability that an individual will experience a complication following surgery based on their age (single predictor variable). For this example, I created a data set that included ages and surgical outcomes for a sample of fictitious patients. Subjects were coded as 1 if they experienced a complication and 0 if not. I developed both a logistic model $[p(Y = 1) = \frac{1}{1 + e^{-[a+b(age)]}}]$ and a linear model $[\hat{Y} = a + b(age)]$ based on this data in an attempt to map the probabilities of experiencing a complication across the age range. Figure 11.1 includes plots of these logistic and linear functions. Age is plotted along on the x-axis and the estimated probability of experiencing a complication ($Y = 1$) is plotted along the y-axis. The plot includes data points for those who experienced a complication (gray diamonds: $Y = 1$) and those who didn't experience a complication (gray circles: $Y = 0$). The black S-shaped curve shows the estimated probability of a complication as function of age based on the logistic model. Note that each point along this curve represents the probability of experiencing a complication, for a given age. This curve approaches the bounds of 0 and 1 but never exceeds them. Therefore, the estimated probability will always fall between 0 and 1, obeying the rules of probability. Based on the plot, it appears that the probability of a complication tends to increase as age increases. It also appears that the probability of experiencing a complication (p) becomes greater than the probability of not experiencing a complication ($1 - p$) around 74 years of age (odds > 1) (note: remember, this is based on a fictitious data set that I generated as an example).

The straight gray line in Figure 11.1 is based on the linear model. Notice that this linear regression line doesn't fit the dichotomous data as closely as the S-shaped logistic curve. Also notice that the predicted values of Y aren't contained between the limits of 0 and 1, which also makes the linear model poorly suited for estimating the probability of an event. For example, based on the linear model, the estimated probability of experiencing a surgical

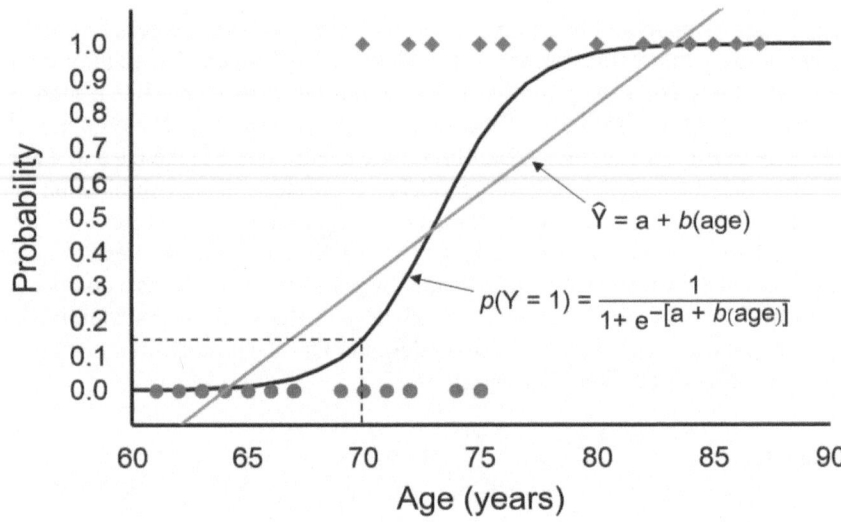

Figure 11.1 Logistic model curve (black) and linear model line (gray) for estimating the probability of a surgical complication (*y*-axis) as a function of age (*x*-axis). The plot includes data points for patients who experienced a complication (gray diamonds: $Y = 1$) and those who didn't experience a complication (gray circles: $Y = 0$). Notice that based on the logistic model curve, the estimated probability of a complication would be approximately 0.15 for a patient who was 70 years of age (black dashed lines). Note that this figure is based on fictitious data and is only intended to serve as an example.

complication for an individual who is 62 years of age would be approximately –0.10. Obviously, a negative probability doesn't make sense. Again, these are just some of the reasons a linear regression model isn't optimal with a dichotomous outcome variable (which is why we use a logistic model instead).

Estimating the regression coefficients

In multiple regression, regression coefficients are typically derived using the least-squares method, which involves finding the combination of regression coefficients that minimizes the residuals, or errors, in the predicted values of the continuous outcome variable. Logistic regression involves a different process, referred to as maximum likelihood estimation. Essentially, maximum likelihood estimation involves finding the combination of regression coefficients that produces the closest match to the observed outcome data. The process involves an initial 'best guess' at the solution, which is then evaluated, refined, and re-evaluated. This iterative process ends when the model can no longer be refined (i.e. the model has 'converged'). Maximum likelihood estimation is a sophisticated process that requires a fairly powerful software package, such as SPSS.

Regression coefficients and odds ratios

The regression coefficients in a logistic regression model represent the change in the natural log of the odds ('log-odds') of the event occurring for each one-unit change in the value of the predictor variable of interest, holding all other predictor variables in the model constant.

Obviously, this is challenging to conceptualize, since the log-odds unit is hard to put into context. However, a regression coefficient (*b*) can be converted to an odds ratio by raising *e* to the power *b* (e^b). Remember, odds represent the probability of the event occurring (*p*) relative to the probability of the event not occurring $(1 - p)$ (odds $= \dfrac{p}{1-p}$). In this case, the odds ratio represents the change in odds. In the context of logistic regression, the odds ratio associated with each predictor variable represents the change in the odds of the event for each one-unit increase in the value of the predictor variable of interest (e.g. X_1), holding all other predictor variables (X_{2-k}) in the model constant. An odds ratio greater than 1.0 indicates that an increase in the value of *X* tends to increase the odds of the event, while an odds ratio less than 1.0 indicates that an increase in the value of *X* tends to decrease the odds of the event.

As an example, let's examine some of the odds ratios for the model developed by Pereira et al. (2014). Their regression model included the predictor variables age, FIM score, and caregiver availability. The odds ratio for the FIM score predictor variable was 1.08 ($e^b = e^{0.075} = 1.08$), which indicates that for each 1-point increase in the FIM score, the odds of being discharged to home increased by a factor of 1.08 (again, assuming all other variables in the model are held constant or remain unchanged). In other words, each 1-point increase in the FIM score corresponded with an 8% increase in the odds of being discharged to home. This makes sense, since higher FIM scores reflect greater function and more independence. The odds ratio for the age predictor variable was 0.87 ($e^b = e^{-0.137} = 0.87$), which indicates that each 1-year increase in age corresponded with a 13% reduction in the odds of being discharged to home.

Classification

The probabilities that are generated by logistic regression can be used to predict a subject's category for the outcome variable. The accuracy of these model-based predictions can then be compared to the subjects' actual outcomes. For example, Pereira et al. (2014) estimated the probability of a patient being discharged to home based on their age, FIM score, and caregiver availability. Subjects with a probability greater than or equal to 0.50 were classified as likely to be discharged to home, while subjects with a probability less than 0.50 were classified as unlikely to be discharged home (i.e. likely to be discharged to a long-term care facility). You can think of 0.50 as the threshold or cutoff point for classifying patients or predicting their outcome. The investigators found that 93.5% of subjects who were predicted to be discharged to home actually were discharged to home, while 76.9% of subjects who were predicted to be discharged to a long-term care facility actually were discharged to a

Table 11.1 Classification table based on results reported by Pereira et al. (2014).

Observed	Predicted		Percentage correct
	LTC	*Home*	
LTC (*n* = 65)	50	15	76.9%
Home (*n* = 124)	8	116	93.5%
Overall			87.8%

Observed column – actual discharge locations; *n* = number of patients.
Predicted – discharge locations predicted by the model.
Home – discharged to home; LTC – discharged to a long-term care facility.
93.5% = percentage accurately predicted to be discharged to home.
76.9% = percentage accurately predicted to be discharged to a long-term care facility.
87.8% = overall percentage of patients whose discharge location was accurately predicted.

long-term care facility. Table 11.1 includes a classification table based on their results. This is a common way to present the classification accuracy of a model. Learning Activity 11.1 provides an opportunity for you to classify patients based on their estimated probabilities.

Learning Activity 11.1

The following table includes ages, FIM scores, and caregiver support availability statuses for four hypothetical patients admitted to a rehabilitation unit following a stroke. The probabilities of being discharged to home (coded 1) are also included in the table. These probabilities are based on the model developed by Pereira et al. (2014). Based on the model output, which patients are predicted to be discharged to home?

Patient	Age	FIM score	Caregiver	p(Y = 1)
1	68	50	1	0.91
2	71	77	0	0.11
3	88	48	1	0.37
4	76	47	1	0.74

Age – age in years
FIM score – total Functional Independence Measure score at admission
Caregiver available at home – 1 = yes, 0 = no
$p(Y = 1)$ – probability that $Y = 1$

$$p(Y = 1) = \frac{1}{1 + e^{-[1.874 + -0.137(age) + 0.075(FIM\ score) + 6.064(caregiver)]}}$$

The answer is included at the end of the chapter.

While a 0.50 probability cutoff is logical in many cases and is the default in SPSS, it's important to consider how a model will be utilized and the risks/costs associated with the different misclassifications when deciding on a threshold for classification. For example, if a model is intended to be used to identify patients with a significant medical condition that requires urgent care, it may be prudent to use a lower probability threshold in order to reduce the number of patients who are classified as not having the condition when they actually do (false negatives). A receiver operating characteristic (ROC) curve can be used to help identify an 'optimal' threshold for classification by illustrating the tradeoff between sensitivity (true positives/total positives) and specificity (true negatives/total negatives) over the range of probabilities. While this application of ROC analysis is beyond the scope of this book, it's worth exploring if you're interested in using logistic regression for classification as part of your own research.

Pseudo R^2 measures

For linear models, R^2 ('R-squared') represents the proportion of variation in the outcome variable that's explained by the regression model. R^2 can range from 0 to 1, with higher values reflecting better model fit. This conventional R^2 is not very informative when the outcome variable is categorical. However, comparable metrics have been developed for use in logistic regression. These metrics are generally referred to as *pseudo R^2* measures. There are a lot of different methods for deriving these pseudo R^2 values and little consensus regarding which is best. One commonly reported pseudo R^2 metric was proposed by Cox and Snell (1989). Like the conventional R^2 metric used in linear regression, this pseudo R^2 metric is meant to capture the amount of variation explained by the model, with values closer to 1 reflecting better model fit. However, a limitation of Cox and Snell's pseudo R^2 is that it will never reach a value of 1, even in the case of perfect model fit. To account for this, Nagelkerke (1991) developed an adjusted version of Cox and Snell's pseudo R^2, which ranges from 0 to 1 like the conventional R^2. Both Cox and Snell's and Nagelkerke's pseudo R^2 measures are output by SPSS. Again, these metrics are generally interpreted in the same way as the conventional R^2, with values closer to 1 reflecting better model fit.

Statistical significance

For logistic regression, the statistical significance of the entire regression model and the individual regression coefficients can be tested. The following subsections discuss the conceptual basis for testing the entire regression model and the regression coefficients.

Note: the constant can also be tested; however, it's typically not pertinent.

Testing the regression model

Before taking the predictor variables into account, our 'best guess' for each subject's outcome would be whichever category was most frequently observed. For example, Pereira et al. (2014) found that 124 of the 189 patients in their sample were discharged to home. Therefore, our best guess across the entire sample would be to simply predict that everyone was discharged to home. In other words, since most patients were discharged to home, we would just predict that everyone was discharged to home, regardless of their age, FIM score, or caregiver availability. You can think of this as the most basic predictive model, which only includes a constant and no predictor variables.

Next, we consider whether a model that includes the predictor variables results in better prediction accuracy. In other words, does knowing a patient's age, FIM score, and caregiver availability help to predict their discharge location more accurately? A chi-squared test can be conducted to determine the extent to which the full model improves prediction accuracy compared to the most basic model. This chi-squared test involves calculating a chi-square statistic and then determining where this statistic falls within the chi-square distribution. This chi-square test is analogous to how the F-test is used to test a linear model (discussed in Chapter 10). If the p-value associated with the chi-square test is less than our predefined alpha level (p-value < 0.05, assuming an alpha of 0.05), we conclude that the model significantly predicts the outcome. In other words, the model makes significantly better predictions than the most basic predictive model, which doesn't include any predictor variables. When the p-value is greater than or equal to our alpha level (p-value ≥ 0.05), we conclude that the model isn't significantly better than the most basic model. This chi-square test can also be used to compare different models, for example, a model that includes the full set of predictor variables and a model that includes a subset of predictor variables.

Note: the Hosmer-Lemeshow test is also commonly used to assess the goodness of fit of a logistic regression model. For this test, a significant result (p-value $<$ alpha) indicates that the model is a poor fit to the data. Note that this is a bit counterintuitive, since we are typically expecting (and perhaps hoping) to observe a non-significant result for the Hosmer-Lemeshow test, as this indicates that the regression model fit our data at least fairly well.

Testing the regression coefficients

In addition to testing the entire regression model, it's also common to test the statistical significance of the individual predictor variables by examining the magnitudes of the regression coefficients. A regression coefficient equal to 0 indicates that the predictor variable didn't make a unique contribution to predicting the outcome. By 'unique', I mean beyond the contributions from the other variables in the model. Note that this is conceptually the same as testing the regression coefficients in a linear model (Chapter 10).

In linear regression, a t-test is typically conducted to determine if a regression coefficient is significantly different from 0. In logistic regression a Wald test (or z-test) is conducted instead; however, it's conceptually the same as the t-test used in linear regression. If the p-value is less than our alpha level (p-value < 0.05, assuming an alpha of 0.05), we conclude that the regression coefficient is significantly different from 0, which suggests that the predictor variable made a significant contribution. If the p-value is greater than or equal to our alpha level, we conclude that the predictor variable didn't make a significant contribution. In most cases, investigators examine the statistical significance of the entire regression model and then follow this up by examining the statistical significance of the individual predictor variables.

Variable selection

Variable selection methods are often incorporated in logistic regression. These procedures involve using statistical criteria to identify a subset of predictor variables from a larger set of possible predictor variables. The purpose of these procedures is to develop a more 'efficient' or 'parsimonious' model or, in other words, to develop a model that can accurately predict the outcome with as few variables as possible. Common variable selection procedures include the forward and backward selection methods. The forward selection method starts with an initial model that only includes a constant. Then variables are incrementally added until the point when adding another predictor variable no longer significantly improves the model. The predictor variables included in the model up to this point constitute the final subset of predictor variables. The backward selection method starts with all of the predictor variables included in the model. Then predictor variables are incrementally removed from the model until the point when variables making significant contributions to the model would begin to be removed. The variables remaining in the model up to this point make up the final subset of predictor variables. Variable selection methods are discussed in greater detail in Chapter 10, since they're also commonly used in multiple regression.

Clinical prediction rules

If you're a clinician or future clinician, you're likely familiar with *clinical prediction rules*. Clinical prediction rules are clusters of 'clinical data' (i.e. patient attributes, examination findings, subjective information, etc.) that can be combined to diagnose a condition or predict a clinical outcome (Jewell, 2018). Logistic regression is typically used to derive these clinical prediction rules, and variable selection methods are often applied to identify a subset of key clinical findings.

For example, Wainner et al. (2003) used a forward selection method when developing a clinical prediction rule to diagnose or rule out cervical radiculopathy. Their analysis initially included 11 potential predictor variables. The predictor variables included a combination of examination findings (e.g. special test results, cervical spine range of motion, sensory/reflex testing results) and subjective information reported by the patient. Forward selection helped to narrow this down to a subset of four predictor variables that could accurately diagnose cervical radiculopathy. These four predictor variables made up the clinical prediction rule.

Generalizability and cross-validation

Although a regression model is almost always developed based on sample data, the objective is typically to approximate the model in the population or, in other words, to generalize the results of the regression analysis from a sample to the entire population. We can get an impression of the generalizability of a regression model by examining the accuracy of the model when it's applied to a different sample from the same population. If a regression model is generalizable, there shouldn't be a major dropoff in prediction accuracy when the model is applied to a new sample. However, a substantial reduction in the accuracy of the regression model when applied to a new sample indicates that the model may be unique to the sample data from which it was derived (i.e. poor generalizability). The process of examining the accuracy of a regression model in a new sample is referred to as *cross-validation*.

One common method of cross-validation is to split the sample data into two separate subsets. One subset is used to develop the regression model (often referred to as the *training set*). Once the model is developed, it's then applied to the other subset (often referred to as the *validation set*). If the accuracy of the regression model is similar when applied to the validation set, then the model likely generalizes beyond the data set from which it was derived and therefore to the population. However, if there's a substantial reduction in prediction accuracy when applied to the validation set, then generalizability is likely poor.

In many cases, investigators will use a greater proportion of their sample to develop their model and then attempt to validate in a smaller subset of the data set. For example, Delmore et al. (2015) used this approach when developing a model to predict heel pressure ulcers in hospitalized patients. They derived their model using data from 337 patients (training set) and then applied the model to a separate group of 80 patients (validation set). The overall classification accuracy of their model was 76.0% in the training set and 72.5% in the validation set, indicating that model accuracy was maintained fairly well in the new sample.

Sample size

Both linear and logistic regression tend to require relatively large sample sizes. While there isn't a clear answer regarding the minimum sample size needed for regression, there are many different rules of thumb (Green, 1991). Some common rules of thumb were discussed in Chapter 10. Regardless, it's important to appreciate that in general, the larger the sample, the better when it comes to regression.

Application opportunity

Example data set

This example is based on a data set published by Chen et al. (2020) (DOI: 10.7717/peerj.8793/supp-1), which includes data for 137 patients who underwent surgery to repair a patellar fracture. Investigators followed up with patients to determine whether they had ($Y = 1$) or hadn't ($Y = 0$) developed sarcopenia (note: 'sarcopenia' is characterized by a loss of muscle mass and strength). The median follow-up time was 3.7 years post-surgery. At follow-up,

45 patients exhibited signs of sarcopenia, and 92 didn't. The data set includes four predictor variables (Sex, Age, Diabetes, and Exercise). The objective of this analysis is to examine how well this four-factor model predicts the development of sarcopenia.

Note: the investigators included additional predictor variables in their model; however, I selected a subset of predictor variables to simplify this example.

Data files

Fracture&Sarcopenia_data.sav – SPSS files with the predictor variables Sex (Male = 0, Female = 1), Age (years), Diabetes (No = 0, Yes = 1), and Exercise (0 = ≤2 hours/week; 1 = >2 hours/week), and the outcome variable Sarcopenia (0 = No; 1 = Yes), included in separate columns.

Video

LogisticRegression.mp4 – video that includes a demonstration of how to conduct a binary logistic regression analysis using SPSS.

Sample write-up

Binary logistic regression was used to determine the extent to which sex, age, diabetes history, and weekly exercise time predict the development of sarcopenia following surgical repair of a patellar fracture. A chi-square test was conducted to assess the statistical significance of the entire regression model, and Wald tests were conducted to assess the statistical significance of the individual predictor variables. An alpha of 0.05 was used for all tests of statistical significance.

The regression model was statistically significant ($p < 0.001$; Nagelkerke's $R^2 = 0.309$). The model accurately predicted 89.1% of the cases where patients did not develop sarcopenia but only 51.1% of the cases where the patients did develop sarcopenia (overall accuracy = 76.6%). The variables age (p = 0.001), diabetes history ($p = 0.008$), and exercise ($p = 0.001$) made significant contributions to the model, while sex did not ($p = 0.101$). More advanced age (odds ratio = 1.086) and having diabetes (odds ratio = 3.147) increased the odds of developing sarcopenia, while exercising more than 2 hours per week reduced the odds of developing sarcopenia (odds ratio = 0.222).

Answers to learning activity

Learning Activity 11.1

Answer:

Patient 1 and patient 4

12 Non-parametric tests

Chapter Objectives

The objectives of this chapter are to . . .

1) describe the general purpose and basis for non-parametric tests
2) discuss instances where non-parametric tests may be appropriate
3) differentiate between parametric and non-parametric tests
4) provide examples of commonly used non-parametric tests
5) discuss the limitations of non-parametric tests

Introduction

Most of this book has focused on what are referred to as *parametric tests* (e.g. *t*-tests, analysis of variance, Pearson product-moment correlation). Parametric tests require certain distribution-related assumptions to be met (e.g. scores are approximately normally distributed) and are appropriate when dealing with variables measured on an interval or ratio scale. In contrast, *non-parametric tests* are used when the assumptions associated with parametric tests aren't met and/or when working with nominal or ordinal data.

In general, non-parametric tests are based on the rank ordering of the scores, not the actual values. As a result, non-parametric tests may also be more appropriate when there are notable outliers in the data, since these relatively 'extreme' values will have less of an impact when only their rank is considered. This is especially true when working with relatively small samples, since outliers tend to have a disproportionate influence on the results of an analysis when there are a limited number of observations in a data set.

Non-parametric analogs

For each parametric test discussed in this book, there's a comparable non-parametric test, which can be used to address similar types of questions. In this chapter, we'll discuss three commonly used non-parametric tests: the Mann-Whitney *U* test, the Wilcoxon signed-rank test, and Spearman's rho correlation. These tests are analogous to the independent *t*-test (Chapter 5), paired *t*-test (Chapter 5), and Pearson product-moment correlation (Chapter 8), which were discussed earlier in this book.

Table 12.1 includes a more comprehensive list of non-parametric analogs. While it's worth exploring some of these other non-parametric tests, understanding the conceptual basis for the three tests discussed in this chapter should give you an idea of how non-parametric tests tend to function.

DOI: 10.4324/9781003179757-12

Table 12.1 Parametric tests and examples of their non-parametric analogs.

Parametric test (chapter discussed)	Non-parametric analog(s)	General objective
Independent *t*-test (Ch. 5)	Mann-Whitney *U* test or Wilcoxon rank-sum test	Compare two independent groups
Paired *t*-test (Ch. 5)	Wilcoxon signed-rank test	Compare two time points or conditions for a single group
One-way ANOVA (Ch. 6)	Kruskal-Wallis test	Compare three or more independent groups
Repeated-measures ANOVA (Ch. 6)	Friedman test	Compare three or more time points or conditions for a single group
Pearson product-moment correlation (Ch. 8)	Spearman's correlation	Examine the relationship between two variables

Note: this isn't an exhaustive list of all non-parametric tests; however, it does include the most commonly used non-parametric tests.

The Mann-Whitney *U* test

The Mann-Whitney *U* test is used to compare two distinct groups, or independent samples, of subjects. It's the non-parametric analog of the independent *t*-test, which was discussed in Chapter 5. The Mann-Whitney *U* test is often used when working with ordinal data, when certain assumptions associated with the independent *t*-test aren't met and/or when sample sizes are relatively small. The null hypothesis associated with the Mann-Whitney *U* test is that the samples were taken from populations with identical distributions. In other words, any observed differences in the groups are due to chance.

General procedure

The Mann-Whitney *U* test involves rank ordering all subjects' scores from lowest to highest, regardless of their group membership. The subject with the lowest score receives the rank of 1, the subject with the second-lowest score receives the rank of 2, and so on, until all scores have been ranked. Then the rankings of the two groups are averaged ('mean rank') and the average rankings of the groups are compared.

Now, consider what would happen if the null hypothesis were true and there was no difference between the populations of interest. In this case, both groups would tend to include a mix of relatively high and low ranks, and therefore, there would be minimal difference between the groups' mean ranks. Conversely, if the null hypothesis were false, one of the groups would likely exhibit appreciably lower rankings than the other group, resulting in a more notable difference in the mean ranks. The Mann-Whitney *U* test essentially involves comparison of the mean ranks of the groups. The greater the difference in the mean ranks, the more likely we are to reject the null hypothesis.

Like the independent *t*-test, the Mann-Whitney *U* test produces a *p*-value which represents the probability of obtaining the observed results if the null hypothesis were true. If this *p*-value is less than our predefined alpha level (which is conventionally 0.05), we reject the null hypothesis and conclude that there's a statistically significant difference between the populations of interest.

Table 12.2 Hypothetical data set of Berg Balance Scale (BBS) scores for a group of ten older adults who had experienced a recent fall ('Fallers') and a group of ten older adults who hadn't recently fallen ('Non-Fallers').

	Fallers			Non-fallers	
Subject	BBS score	Rank	Subject	BBS score	Rank
1	20	1	1	52	19
2	47	14	2	40	7
3	34	2	3	43	10
4	45	12	4	48	15.5
5	36	4	5	44	11
6	37	5	6	49	17
7	41	8	7	51	18
8	46	13	8	54	20
9	35	3	9	48	15.5
10	42	9	10	38	6
Rank sum = 71			Rank sum = 139		
Mean rank = 7.1			Mean rank = 13.9		

Notice that Subject 1 in the Fallers group had the lowest BBS score (rank = 1), while Subject 8 in the Non-Fallers group had the highest BBS score (rank = 20). Subjects 4 and 9 in the Non-Fallers group both had a BBS score of 48. In this case, their ranks were averaged and both subjects received the average ranking [(15 + 16)/2 = 15.5]. This is one way to handle these types of 'ties'.

As you can see, the non-fallers tended to have higher rankings than the fallers (mean rank = 13.9 vs. 7.1), which is why the null hypothesis was rejected.

It's also important to appreciate how relatively 'extreme' scores in the data set are less influential when only their rank is considered. For example, notice that Subject 1 in the Fallers group performed quite a bit worse than the rest of the subjects in the study (BBS score = 20/56). However, since only their rank is considered, their relatively extreme score doesn't have a greater impact than the other scores in the data set.

Mann-Whitney U example

Now let's consider an example. Imagine that we conduct a study to compare the balance of older adults who have recently experienced a fall ('fallers') and older adults who haven't recently fallen ('non-fallers').

Table 12.2 includes a hypothetical data set of Berg Balance Scale scores for ten fallers and ten non-fallers. The Berg Balance Scale is a commonly used balance assessment, where individuals are asked to perform 14 different tasks and a clinician rates their performance on a scale of 0–4, with 0 representing the lowest level of balance performance and 4 representing the highest level of balance performance (Berg et al., 1989). The overall Berg Balance Scale score can range from 0 to 56 (14 items × 4 = 56). Since the Berg Balance Scale is based on an ordinal scale, a non-parametric test, such as the Mann-Whitney *U* test, is appropriate.

Within Table 12.2, each subject's Berg Balance Scale score is ranked from 1 to 20. The subject with the lowest score (Subject 1, Fallers; BBS score = 20) received the rank of 1, while the subject with the highest score (Subject 8, Non-Fallers; BBS score = 54) received the rank of 20. The ranks of the two groups are summed (rank sum) and then averaged (mean rank). Notice that, in general, the non-fallers tended to outperform the fallers, as the mean rank for the non-fallers group was 13.9, compared to 7.1 for the fallers group. Of course, we want to know whether this observed group difference is greater than what would likely occur by chance alone. To address this question, we could conduct a Mann-Whitney *U* test.

For this example, the null hypothesis associated with the test is that there's no difference in Berg Balance Scale performance between fallers and non-fallers. A Mann-Whitney U test comparing the fallers and non-fallers results in a p-value of 0.009 ($p = 0.009$), which is less than the conventional alpha level of 0.05. Therefore, in this case, we would reject the null hypothesis and conclude that non-fallers perform significantly better on the Berg Balance Scale compared to fallers. Of course, it's important to remember that this is just a hypothetical data set.

Wilcoxon signed-rank test

The Wilcoxon signed-rank test is used to compare two sets of scores within a single group of individuals, such as when patients are assessed before and after treatment (post vs. pre) or tested in two different conditions. It's the non-parametric analog of the paired t-test, which was discussed in Chapter 5. The Wilcoxon signed-rank test is often used with ordinal data, when certain assumptions associated with the paired t-test aren't met, and/or when working with a relatively small sample.

The null hypothesis associated with the Wilcoxon signed-rank test is that there's no difference between the two time points or conditions of interest. More specifically, it states that the median of the differences is 0 for the population.

General procedure

The Wilcoxon signed-rank test involves finding the difference between the scores for the two time points or conditions of interest.* These differences are then ranked from smallest to largest, regardless of their sign. The ranks for those that exhibited positive differences and negative differences are then summed separately, ignoring differences of 0 (i.e. no change).

* **Note:** remember that the paired t-test was also based on analysis of the differences between time points or conditions. This should help you appreciate the degree of similarity between the paired t-test and Wilcoxon signed-rank test. The main difference is that the differences aren't rank ordered for the paired t-test, as they are for the Wilcoxon signed-rank text.

Now, consider what would happen if the null hypothesis were true. In this case, some subjects' performance would improve, others would get worse, and some wouldn't change at all. In the end, the totals of the ranks for the positive and negative differences would be comparable. Essentially, there would be no systematic pattern to the changes between time points or conditions. Conversely, if the null hypothesis were false, there would be a tendency for the ranks of the positive and negative differences to differ. For example, if most subjects tended to improve after training, then the total of the rankings for the positive differences would exceed the total of the rankings for the negative differences. The Wilcoxon-signed rank test is based on analysis of the summed ranks associated with the positive and negative differences. The greater the difference in the totals for the positive and negative differences, the more likely we are to reject the null hypothesis.

Like the paired t-test, the Wilcoxon signed-rank test results in a p-value that represents the probability of obtaining the observed results if the null hypothesis were true. If this p-value is less than our predefined alpha level (conventionally 0.05), we reject the null hypothesis and conclude that there's a statistically significant difference between the time points or conditions.

Wilcoxon signed-rank example

Let's consider another example. Imagine that as a follow-up study, we have the individuals in the fallers group complete a general strength training program. Table 12.3 includes a set

Table 12.3 Hypothetical data set of Berg Balance Scale (BBS) scores recorded before (baseline) and after (post) completion of a general strength training program.

Subject	BBS scores		Difference	Rank	Positive differences	Negative differences
	Baseline	Post				
1	20	36	+16	9	9	
2	47	47	0	—		
3	34	41	+7	8	8	
4	45	43	−2	2.5		2.5
5	36	41	+5	6	6	
6	37	31	−6	7		7
7	41	45	+4	5	5	
8	46	43	−3	4		4
9	35	37	+2	2.5	2.5	
10	42	41	−1	1		1
					Sum = 30.5	Sum = 14.5

The values in the Difference column represent the changes in BBS scores from baseline to post, with positive values reflecting improved balance. These differences are ranked based on their magnitude.

The Wilcoxon sign-rank test is based on comparison of the rank totals for the positive and negative differences. Notice that in this case, BBS scores tended to improve after training, as the sum of the rankings for the positive differences (30.5) exceeded the sum for the rankings for the negative differences (14.5); however, the results of the Wilcoxon signed-rank test indicate that the change in BBS scores isn't statistically significant ($p = 0.34$).

of hypothetical Berg Balance Scale scores recorded before (baseline) and after (post) completion of the training program. In this case, our null hypothesis is that the strength training program has no effect on Berg Balance Scale performance.

Notice that the differences in Berg Balance Scale scores from baseline to post-training have been calculated (Difference column) and then ranked (Rank column) in Table 12.3. Five subjects exhibited an increase ('positive difference') in their Berg Balance Scale score (Subjects 1, 3, 5, 7, 9), four subjects exhibited a decrease ('negative difference') in their Berg Balance Scale score (Subjects 4, 6, 8, 10), and one subject demonstrated no change (Subject 2). Notice that the sum of the ranks of the positive differences (30.5) exceeds the sum of the ranks of the negative differences (14.5), which suggests that Berg Balance Scale performance tended to improve following training. The Wilcoxon signed-rank test will tell us whether this observed difference is statistically significant – in other words, whether the observed improvements are greater than what's likely to occur by chance alone.

The *p*-value associated with a Wilcoxon signed-rank test comparing the baseline and post time points is 0.34 ($p = 0.34$). Since this *p*-value is greater than the conventional alpha level of 0.05, we would conclude that there wasn't a statistically significant change in Berg Balance Scale performance. In other words, the evidence wasn't strong enough to reject the null hypothesis.

Note: both the Mann-Whitney *U* test and the Wilcoxon signed-rank test are included as part of the SPSS 'Nonparametric Tests' package.

Spearman's correlation

Spearman's correlation (also referred to as Spearman's rank-order correlation) is used to examine the relationship between two variables (bivariate correlation), often denoted *X* and *Y*. It's the non-parametric analog to Pearson product-moment correlation, which was discussed in Chapter 8. Spearman's correlation is often used when working with ordinal data, when the assumptions associated with Pearson's product-moment correlation aren't met, and/or when the sample is relatively small.*

* Note: some suggest using Spearman's correlation instead of Pearson product-moment correlation when the sample size is approximately 30 or less; however, this is more of a general guideline than a hard rule.

Spearman's rho

Spearman's correlation results in a correlation coefficient referred to as Spearman's rho (often denoted r_s or ρ), which reflects the direction and strength of the relationship between the two variables of interest. Spearman's rho is interpreted in the same manner as the Pearson product-moment correlation coefficient, with the sign indicating the direction of the relationship (positive or negative) and the magnitude reflecting the strength of the relationship, with values ranging from -1.00 (perfect negative relationship) to $+1.00$ (perfect positive relationship). The closer the value to ± 1.00, the stronger the relationship. Table 12.4 includes proposed guidelines for interpreting Spearman's rho. Notice that these are the same guidelines provided in Chapter 8 for interpreting the Pearson product-moment correlation coefficient.

General procedure

Spearman's rho is essentially equivalent to the Pearson product-moment correlation coefficient, except it's based on the rankings of the scores for the X and Y variables instead of the actual values.

A positive Spearman's correlation coefficient indicates that individuals with relatively high ranks for variable X tend to have relatively high ranks for variable Y, while individuals with relatively low ranks for variable X tend to have relatively low ranks for variable Y. In fact, in the case of a perfect positive relationship (Spearman's rho = $+1.00$), there's perfect agreement between the ranks for the two variables (i.e. the individual with the highest score for variable X also has the highest score for variable Y, the individual with the second-highest score for variable X also has the second-highest score for variable Y, and so on).

Table 12.4 Proposed guidelines for interpreting the Spearman's rho correlation coefficient (r_s).

Positive r_s value	Interpretation	Negative r_s value	Interpretation
0 to 0.25	Little or no relationship	0 to −0.25	Little or no relationship
0.25 to 0.50	Weak, positive relationship	−0.25 to −0.50	Weak, negative relationship
0.50 to 0.75	Moderate, positive relationship	−0.50 to −0.75	Moderate, negative relationship
≥0.75	Strong, positive relationship	≤−0.75	Strong, negative relationship

Note the overlap between categories; this is meant to highlight that these are general guidelines, not strict cutoff points.
Guidelines proposed by Portney (2020).

A negative Spearman's correlation coefficient indicates that individuals with relatively high ranks for variable X tend to have relatively low ranks for variable Y, while individuals with relatively low ranks for variable X tend to have relatively high ranks for variable Y. In the case of a perfect negative relationship (Spearman's rho = −1.00), the rank orders are completely reversed (i.e. the individual with the highest score for variable X has the lowest score for variable Y, the individual with the second-highest score for variable X has the second-lowest score for variable Y, and so on).

As you can see, Spearman's rho is conceptually the same as the Pearson product-moment correlation coefficient, except it deals with rankings instead of actual values. In fact, Spearman's rho is equivalent to the Pearson product-moment correlation coefficient when the variable ranks are correlated. In other words, if you want to find Spearman's rho, simply convert the values to ranks (rank from 1 to n, where n is the number of X/Y pairs) and perform a Pearson product-moment correlation using the rankings. The result will be Spearman's rho.

Note: Table 12.5 includes example data and an equation that's useful when calculating Spearman's rho by hand.

Statistical significance

As with the Pearson product-moment correlation coefficient, Spearman's rho can be converted to a t statistic and a t-test can be conducted to determine if the relationship between the variables is statistically significant. The null hypothesis associated with this test is that there's no relationship between the variables of interest (Spearman's rho = 0). The more Spearman's rho deviates from 0, the stronger the evidence against the null hypothesis. Again, this is conceptually equivalent to testing the statistical significance of the Pearson product-moment correlation coefficient.

Spearman's correlation example

As an example, imagine that we conduct a study to examine the relationship between performance on the 2 Minute Walk Test and the 6 Minute Walk Test. The 2 Minute Walk Test and 6 Minute Walk Test are both tests of aerobic capacity and endurance (Butland et al., 1982). For the 2 Minute Walk Test, individuals walk for 2 minutes, and their total walk distance is recorded at the end of the 2-minute period. The 6 Minute Walk Test is the same, except individuals walk for 6 minutes. For both tests, longer walk distances reflect better aerobic capacity and endurance. While the 6 Minute Walk Test is more commonly utilized, the 2 Minute Walk Test has the advantage of being easier to implement because of its shorter duration. Let's say that our study objective is to examine the relationship between 2 Minute Walk Test performance and 6 Minute Walk Test performance in order to determine whether the 2 Minute Walk Test could potentially serve as a useful alternative to the 6 Minute Walk Test.

Table 12.5 includes a hypothetical data set of 2 Minute Walk Test distances and 6 Minute Walk Test distances for 15 subjects. The table also includes each subject's rank on the 2 Minute Walk Test and the 6 Minute Walk Test. Notice that, in general, subjects who performed well on the 2 Minute Walk Test also tended to perform well on the 6 Minute Walk Test (i.e. high ranks for the 2 Minute Walk Test tended to correspond with high ranks for the 6 Minute Walk Test). For instance, Subject 1 had the longest walk distance for the 2 Minute Walk Test (rank = 15) and the second-longest walk distance for the 6 Minute Walk Test (rank = 14). Also notice that subjects who performed relatively poorly on the 2 Minute Walk Test tended

Table 12.5 Hypothetical data set of 2 Minute Walk Test (2MWT) distances and 6 Minute Walk Test (6MWT) distances for 15 older adults.

Subject	2MWT distances	6MWT distances	2MWT ranks	6MWT ranks	d	d²
1	114	303	15	14	1	1
2	63	85	5	1	4	16
3	96	262	10	11	−1	1
4	97	274	11	12	−1	1
5	44	160	2	4	−2	4
6	88	291	9	13	−4	16
7	37	94	1	2	−1	1
8	82	186	6	6	0	0
9	107	311	14	15	−1	1
10	60	170	4	5	−1	1
11	52	145	3	3	0	0
12	86	232	8	7	1	1
13	106	248	13	9	4	16
14	85	236	7	8	−1	1
15	99	257	12	10	2	4
						$\sum d^2 = 64$

Column *d* includes the differences in the ranks for the 2MWT and the 6MWT (2MWT rank − 6MWT rank), while column *d²* includes the squared differences. The following equation can be used to calculate Spearman's rho (r_s); within this equation, $\sum d^2$ is the sum of the squared differences in ranks, and *n* is the number of *X/Y* pairs.

$$r_s = 1 - \frac{6\sum d^2}{n(n^2-1)} = 1 - \frac{6(64)}{15(15^2-1)} = 0.89 \text{ (strong, positive relationship)}$$

r_s can be converted to a *t*-statistic using the equation:

$$t = r_s \sqrt{\frac{n-2}{1-r_s^2}}$$

This *t*-statistic is used to test the statistical significance of the relationship.

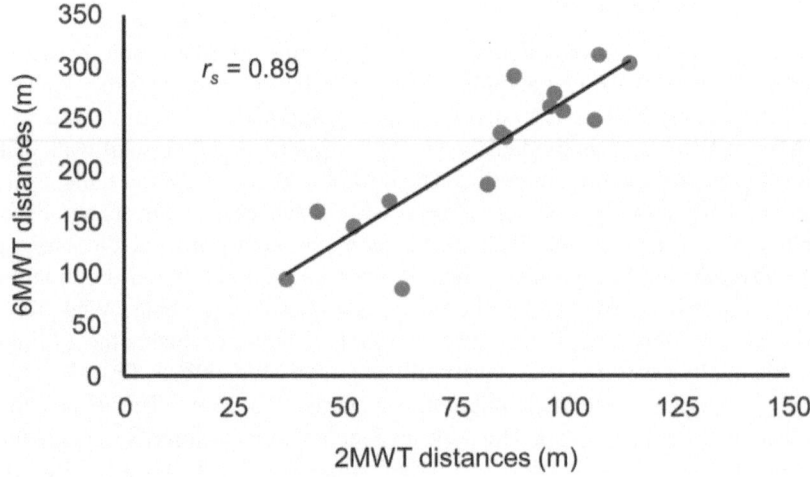

Scatter plot of the 2MWT distances and 6MWT distances.

to perform relatively poorly on the 6 Minute Walk Test (i.e. low ranks for the 2 Minute Walk Test tended to correspond with low ranks for the 6 Minute Walk Test). For example, Subject 7 had the shortest walk distance for the 2 Minute Walk Test (rank = 1) and the second-shortest walk distance for the 6 Minute Walk Test (rank = 2). This general pattern reflects a positive relationship between the variables (i.e. high performance on the 2 Minute Walk Test tends to correspond with high performance on the 6 Minute Walk Test, and vice versa).

The Spearman's rho correlation coefficient associated with the walk distances in Table 12.5 is 0.89, which represents a strong, positive relationship between the variables (based on the guidelines proposed in Table 12.4). A two-tailed *t*-test of the Spearman's rho correlation coefficient results in a *p*-value of less than 0.001 ($p < 0.001$). Since this *p*-value is less than the conventional alpha level of 0.05, we would conclude that the relationship between performance on the 2 Minute Walk Test and the 6 Minute Walk Test is statistically significant. Again, this is just hypothetical data; however, I'd suspect that these results are close to what we'd actually observe if we conducted this study.

Note: SPSS gives you the options for Pearson's product-moment correlation or Spearman's correlation as part of its Bivariate Correlation package (introduced in Chapter 8). There's also the option to run another type of non-parametric correlation analysis (Kendall's tau-b).

Note: it's important to note that, like Pearson product-moment correlation, Spearman's correlation is only appropriate when there's a monotonic relationship between the variables (i.e. as one variable increases, so does the other, or as one variable increases, the other tends to decrease). Other types of correlation analyses should be used when there's a non-monotonic relationship between variables. A scatter plot can help you determine whether the relationship between variables is monotonic.

Why not always use non-parametric tests?

As we've discussed, non-parametric tests require fewer assumptions to be met and can address similar questions to the parametric tests described throughout this book. As a result, you're probably asking yourself, 'Why not just always use non-parametric tests?' The main reason is that parametric tests tend to be more powerful than their non-parametric counterparts, as long as certain assumptions are met. As a result, parametric tests generally have less risk of Type II error. In addition, parametric tests tend to be easier to interpret, since they deal with means, variances, and other values derived from actual quantities, instead of ranks.

Final thoughts

If you're planning to conduct your own research, it's worth exploring non-parametric statistics in more detail. There are entire textbooks devoted to the topic. That said, this chapter should give you a general understanding of the basis for non-parametric tests and an appreciation for when they may be appropriate.

13 Effect sizes and confidence intervals

Chapter Objectives

The objectives of this chapter are to . . .

1) discuss some of the limitations and criticisms of null hypothesis significance testing
2) describe the concept of effect size
3) introduce some commonly used standardized effect size measures
4) discuss the benefits of reporting confidence intervals

Introduction

Much of this book has focused on null hypothesis significance testing; however, as noted in Chapter 4, this conventional approach has some significant limitations and many vocal critics. In fact, some have even proposed completely abandoning null hypothesis significance testing (e.g. McShane et al., 2019), and even those who think null hypothesis significance testing has its place tend to agree that it's probably overused and perhaps misused in many cases. One of the main limitations of conventional null hypothesis significance testing is that it encourages 'black-or-white' thinking, where findings are either statistically significant ($p < \alpha$) or they aren't ($p \geq \alpha$), depending on how a p-value compares to a somewhat arbitrarily defined alpha level. As the psychologists Ralph Rosnow and Robert Rosenthal once wrote, 'surely God loves 0.06 nearly as much as 0.05' (1989), meaning that there isn't much of a difference between p-values of 0.05 and 0.06, even though these results often lead to completely different conclusions.

Critics of null hypothesis significance testing also correctly point out that p-values are heavily influenced by sample size (whereas effect sizes aren't, or at least not to the same extent). Therefore, larger samples will produce lower p-values compared to smaller samples, even if the magnitude of the effect is the same. The result is that small, and perhaps trivial, effects may be statistically significant when samples are large, while large, and potentially meaningful, effects may not be statistically significant when samples are small. For example, imagine that two different studies (Study A, Study B) examine the relationship between a pair of variables. Both studies produce correlation coefficients of 0.10; however, Study A includes 500 subjects, while study B only includes 50 subjects. In this case, tests of the statistical significance of the correlation coefficients for Study A and Study B would result in p-values of 0.03 ($p = 0.03$) and 0.49 ($p = 0.49$), respectively. Therefore, we would likely conclude that the relationship is statistically significant ($p < 0.05$) for Study A, but not statistically significant ($p > 0.05$) for study B, even though the correlation coefficients are equivalent. Again, opponents of null hypothesis significance testing often point out that the singular focus on p-values is somewhat illogical, and I tend to agree.

DOI: 10.4324/9781003179757-13

Many argue that it's more appropriate to consider effects on a continuum instead of simply reaching a dichotomous conclusion of statistically significant ($p < \alpha$) or not statistically significant ($p \geq \alpha$). This sentiment has led to a more universal agreement that there's a need to move beyond just considering and reporting p-values. In fact, many journals have begun to recommend, or even require, that the results of null hypothesis significance tests be supplemented by effect sizes and/or confidence intervals. For example, many of the primary journals in the areas of physical and occupational therapy (e.g. *Physical Therapy, American Journal of Occupational Therapy*) stipulate in their instructions to authors that reporting p-values alone is insufficient when submitting an article for review. Moving forward, I think you can expect more consistent reporting of effect sizes and confidence intervals along with, or instead of, p-values. Therefore, it's important to have an appreciation for what effects sizes and confidence intervals represent.

In this chapter, we'll discuss the general logic of effect sizes and confidence intervals, explain how they can supplement the results of a null hypothesis significance test, and highlight some commonly used effect size metrics.

General concept of effect size

In general, an effect size quantifies the extent to which our observed results deviate from what's expected based on the null hypothesis or, in other words, the degree to which the null hypothesis is false. Notice the words *extent* and *degree*, which imply more of a continuum, instead of the dichotomous result of 'reject' or 'fail to reject' a null hypothesis.

An effect size can be as simple as the difference between means. For instance, imagine that we conduct a study to compare the finger dexterity of individuals with Parkinson's disease (PD group) and individuals without Parkinson's disease (control group). As part of the study, subjects complete the Nine-Hole Peg Test, which is commonly used to assess finger dexterity (Mathiowetz et al., 1985). For the Nine-Hole Peg Test, individuals are asked to pick up pegs from a container and place them into holes on a board, one by one, as quickly as possible. Once all the pegs are placed, the individual removes them from the holes and places them back in the container. Performance is based on the time needed to complete the task (shorter time reflects better performance). In this case, the null hypothesis would state that there's no difference in finger dexterity between individuals with Parkinson's disease and individuals without Parkinson's disease. In other words, the mean Nine-Hole Peg Test times are equivalent for the populations of individuals with and without Parkinson's disease (H_0: $\mu_{PD} = \mu_{Control}$).

Now, let's say that on average, the control group performed the test in 20 seconds ($\bar{X}_{Control} = 20$ s), while the PD group performed the test in 25 seconds ($\bar{X}_{PD} = 25$ s). In this case, the 5-second difference in test performance would be considered an effect size since it reflects how the observed results (mean difference = 5 seconds) differed from what was expected based on the null hypothesis (mean difference = 0). Notice that in this case, the greater the difference between the groups, the larger the effect size. Also note that this effect size is independent of the sample size. For instance, the difference in the sample means would still be 5 seconds regardless of whether the groups included 10 subjects or 1000 subjects.

While the mean difference can serve as a measure of the effect size, we typically work with effect sizes that have been standardized in some way. Standardization allows for more uniform interpretation and easier comparisons among studies; especially studies that rely on different measures. For example, without standardization, it would be difficult to directly compare the results of our study to those of other studies that used different measures of finger dexterity. In most cases, standardization also incorporates the variability within groups or conditions, which is also important to consider.

Standardized effect sizes

There are many different types of standardized effect sizes. However, most can be grouped into one of two general categories: 1) standardized mean differences (the '*d*' family) or 2) measures related to the variance explained (the '*r*' family).

Standardized mean differences

Standardized mean differences are typically used when comparing two means, either from independent groups or across different time points or conditions. A metric referred to as Cohen's *d* is a very commonly reported effect size from the standardized mean differences family.* Cohen's *d* expresses the differences between means in terms of standard deviations. It often accompanies the results of a *t*-test.

* **Note:** Cohen's *d* is named after Dr. Jacob Cohen, who was a psychologist and statistician. Dr. Cohen did very influential work in the areas of effect sizes and statistical power. He was also a staunch critic of null hypothesis significance testing [for an example, read Cohen, 1994 – *The Earth is Round (p < .05)*].

There are different ways of calculating Cohen's *d*, depending on whether the data comes from independent samples (Group A, Group B) or a single sample (condition A vs. condition B). However, the general concept is the same, regardless of how Cohen's *d* is calculated. Equation 13.1 includes a general form of the equation for calculating Cohen's *d* when comparing the means of two groups of equal size ($n_1 = n_2$). Notice that in this case, calculating Cohen's *d* simply involves dividing the mean difference ($\bar{X}_1 - \bar{X}_2$) by the average of the standard deviations [$(s_1 + s_2)/2$]. Equation 13.2 includes a different form of the equation that can be used when group sizes differ ($n_1 \neq n_2$). Again, the specifics for calculating Cohen's *d* will depend on the nature of the study, but this should give you a general idea of what Cohen's *d* represents. A paper by Lakens (2013) includes a more in-depth discussion of the different variations of Cohen's *d* in case you're interested (included in the references section).

Equation 13.1

$$\text{Cohen's } d = \frac{\bar{X}_1 - \bar{X}_2}{(s_1 + s_2)/2}$$

Equation 13.2

$$\text{Cohen's } d = \frac{\bar{X}_1 - \bar{X}_2}{s_{\text{pooled}}}$$

$$s_{\text{pooled}} = \sqrt{\frac{(n_1 - 1)s_1^2 + (n_2 - 1)s_2^2}{n_1 + n_2 - 2}}$$

In Equation 13.2, s_{pooled} is the 'pooled standard deviation', which accounts for the difference in sample sizes (n_1, n_2). It's essentially a weighted average of the standard deviations (s_1, s_2), based on sample size.

As you can see, Cohen's *d* expresses the difference between means in terms of standard deviations. For instance, a Cohen's *d* of 2.0 would indicate that the means are two standard deviations apart (which most would consider a large degree of separation). There's no limit to the magnitude of Cohen's *d*; it can range from 0 to ±infinity, with the sign depending on the order in which the means are subtracted (although most tend to report the absolute value of Cohen's *d* and simply describe the direction of the effect). It's also important to note that Cohen's *d* is a unitless metric since the means and standard deviations have the same units and therefore cancel each other out. This allows for direct comparison of the effects across studies, even if they used different outcome measures.

Guidelines for interpreting Cohen's *d*

Cohen himself proposed the following general rules of thumb for interpreting Cohen's *d*: 0.20 = 'small effect', 0.50 = 'moderate effect', and 0.80 = 'large effect' (1988). However, it's important to note that these are just points along a continuum. Treating these guidelines as strict cutoffs presents much the same problem as blindly interpreting *p*-values based on their relationship to an alpha level. Even Cohen cautioned against considering his guidelines as strict rules for interpretation. As Dr. Bruce Thompson once wrote, 'if people interpreted effect sizes with the same rigidity with which $\alpha = .05$ has been used in statistical testing, we would merely be stupid in another metric' (2001).

Learning Activity 13.1 provides an opportunity for you to calculate and interpret a Cohen's *d* effect size statistic.

Learning Activity 13.1

Mistry et al. (2021) conducted a study to compare the maximal grip strength of women with upper extremity lymphedema due to breast cancer ('cases') and women without lymphedema or a history of breast cancer ('controls'). Their study included 31 women in the cases group and 31 women in the controls group. The mean (±standard deviation) grip strength for the cases and controls were 24.42 ± 9.87 kg and 29.26 ± 7.09 kg, respectively. Calculate a Cohen's *d* effect size statistic based on these sample statistics and interpret based on the guidelines provided in the chapter. The answer is provided at the end of the chapter.

Note: this example is based on the data set described in Chapter 5 ('Application Opportunities – Example Data Set #1').

Measures related to the variance explained

Correlation coefficient (r)

In the case of bivariate correlation, the Pearson product-moment correlation coefficient (*r*) is typically reported as a measure of the effect size. Remember that *r* captures the strength of the relationship between two variables (discussed in Chapter 8). The more *r* deviates from 0, the stronger the relationship between variables (guidelines for interpreting *r* are included in Chapter 8 – Table 8.1). It's critical to report the value of r and not just whether the relationship was statistically significant. Remember that testing the statistical significance of r only tells us whether the evidence from our sample is sufficient to conclude that there's a correlation for the population (i.e. whether the correlation coefficient for the population is likely non-zero). It doesn't really tell us anything about the strength of the relationship. As we've already discussed, weak relationships can be statistically significant if the sample size is sufficiently large, while strong relationships may not be statistically significant if the sample size is small.

R^2

The coefficient of determination (R^2) is commonly reported as an effect size for regression analyses (R^2 was discussed in detail in Chapters 8–10). R^2 represents the proportion of variation in the outcome variable that's explained by the predictor variable(s). The larger R^2, the more variance the regression model explains. Remember that even a poor model can be statistically significant (i.e. better than no model at all), which is why it's important to examine metrics such as R^2 and not just rely on the results of a null hypothesis significance test.

Eta squared

Eta squared (η^2) is an effect size metric that's typically used when conducting a single-factor analysis of variance (discussed in Chapter 6). η^2 is the ratio of the sum of squares associated with the factor of interest (SS_{Factor}), relative to the total sum of squares (SS_{Total}) (Equation 13.3). Therefore, η^2 can range from 0 to 1; the closer η^2 gets to 1, the greater the proportion of the total variation explained by the factor of interest. Notice that η^2 is very similar to R^2 from a conceptual standpoint, as it expresses the proportion, or percentage, of explained variation.

Equation 13.3

$$\eta^2 = \frac{SS_{Factor}}{SS_{Total}}$$

As an example, let's revisit a study discussed in Chapter 6 ('Application Opportunities – Example Data Set #1'), which was based on a data set published by Jerez-Mayorga et al. (2019). For this example, the results of a one-way analysis of variance indicated that there was a statistically significant difference in Sit-to-Stand test performance among groups of older adults with hip osteoarthritis ('OA group'), older adults without hip osteoarthritis ('older group'), and younger adults without hip osteoarthritis ('younger group') ($p < 0.001$). What this indicates is that there's likely some difference in Sit-to-Stand test performance among these distinct populations; however, the ANOVA results don't provide any indication of the magnitude of the difference among the groups. In this case, η^2 would reflect the ratio of the between-groups sum of squares ($SS_{Between}$ or more generally SS_{Factor}), relative to the total sum of squares (SS_{Total}). For the study comparing Sit-to-Stand test performance, $SS_{Between}$ was 158.59, while SS_{Total} was 302.48, resulting in an η^2 of 0.52 ($\eta^2 = \dfrac{158.59}{302.48} = 0.52$). In other words, 52% of the variation in Sit-to-Stand test performance was explained by the factor 'group'.

Cohen also proposed guidelines for interpreting η^2. As a rule of thumb, η^2 values of 0.01, 0.06, and 0.14 are considered to represent 'small', 'medium', and 'large' effects, respectively. Again, these are just guidelines, not strict rules for interpretation.

Note: there's also a similar effect size metric referred to as partial eta squared (η_p^2), which is commonly used with factorial designs. For single-factor studies, η^2 and η_p^2 are equivalent; however, this isn't the case for studies which incorporate multiple factors.

Effect size as an indicator of clinical significance?

You'll often hear effect sizes discussed in relation to 'clinical significance' (or 'practical significance'). The general premise is that moderate or large effects are inherently clinically significant in some way. I've always found this a bit illogical. To me, clinical significance is something beyond what's represented by most effect size metrics, and the results of a study should only be considered 'clinically significant' if the observed effects are sufficient to influence patient outcomes, risk of injury/illness, how a disease/disorder is managed, cost, and so on. There are certainly instances where large effects have little relevance to patient care, which I would contend is 'clinically insignificant'. The opposite is also true, as some effects may influence clinical practice, even if they are small in magnitude. To me, judgments regarding clinical significance should be based on clinical judgment, not an effect size measure (at least not entirely).

Confidence intervals

We've discussed confidence intervals in different contexts throughout this book. For example, we discussed confidence intervals for mean differences in Chapter 5, correlation coefficients in Chapter 8, and regression coefficients in Chapter 9. Remember, regardless of the context, a confidence interval is a range of values that's likely to include the population parameter of interest, whether it's a mean difference, correlation coefficient, regression coefficient, or some other parameter.

The key benefit of confidence intervals is that they provide some indication of the precision of our estimate of the effect. Consider the following example. Imagine that we've conducted a study to examine the effects of trigger point dry needling on shoulder range of motion in individuals with adhesive capsulitis. As part of the study, we record shoulder range of motion before (baseline) and after (post) treatment. Let's say that we observe an increase in shoulder flexion range motion from baseline to post-treatment that's considered statistically significant based on the results of a paired t-test ($p < 0.05$). What this tells us is that the observed change in shoulder motion is unlikely to be due to chance alone. While this is interesting to some extent, it really doesn't provide much insight.

Now let's say that we also calculate a 95% confidence interval ($CI_{95\%}$) based on our observed change in shoulder flexion range of motion (post-baseline) and that the lower bound and upper bound of this confidence interval are 0.5 and 20.5, respectively ($CI_{95\%} = [0.5, 20.5]$). What this indicates is that the true change in shoulder flexion range of motion for the population is likely to fall within a range of 0.5° to 20.5°. Essentially, what we've found is that while the change in shoulder flexion motion probably isn't 0°, our estimate of the effect is somewhat imprecise, and the true effect may not be very large at all. In fact, it could plausibly be as low as 0.5°, which is hardly enough to affect shoulder function. Note that this presents a more complete picture compared to simply reporting that *there was a statistically significant increase in shoulder flexion range of motion (p < 0.05)*.

While confidence intervals are still underutilized, their use appears to be increasing steadily over time (Freire et al., 2019). Therefore, it's important for you to be comfortable interpreting confidence intervals and reporting them if conducting your own research.

Note: a paper by Kamper (2019) nicely highlights the insights that can be gained by examining confidence intervals. I've included this paper in the references section in case you're interested in reading more on this topic.

Final thoughts

In my opinion, the most important thing to take away from this chapter is that statistical significance is only a small part of the story, and in most cases, it's the least interesting part. There's so much more to learn from our data. As consumers of the literature, it's important for us to consider more than just whether an effect was statistically significant, and as investigators, we should work to ensure that we're reporting our results in a manner that promotes transparency. Understanding and consistently reporting effect sizes and confidence intervals certainly helps in this regard.

Answers to Learning Activity 13.1

$$\text{Cohen's } d = \frac{\overline{X}_{\text{Cases}} - \overline{X}_{\text{Controls}}}{\left(s_{\text{Cases}} + s_{\text{Controls}}\right)/2} = \frac{24.42 - 29.29}{(9.87 + 7.09)/2} = -0.57 \text{ (moderate-large difference)}$$

Note: the sign of Cohen's *d* depends on the order in which the means are subtracted. In this case, Cohen's *d* is negative, since the mean grip strength was lower for the cases compared to the controls.

14 Sample size estimation

Chapter Objectives

The objectives of this chapter are to . . .

1) introduce the general concept of sample size estimation
2) provide an overview of the process involved in sample size estimation
3) describe different approaches used to estimate an effect size
4) introduce different tools available for sample size estimation, including G*Power software
5) work through an example of how to generate a sample size estimate
6) highlight the tradeoff between effect size and sample size

Introduction

A common question that must be addressed by investigators is, 'How many subjects do I need for my study?' The answer to this question depends on a number of different factors, including the nature of the study, the analysis that'll be performed, the anticipated effect size, and the desired level of statistical power. While in some cases, investigators will simply propose a sample size they deem sufficient and/or feasible, it's becoming increasingly common for investigators to complete a more formal quantitative analysis to derive the sample size needed for their study. This process is generally referred to as sample size estimation or 'power analysis'. In general, sample size estimation involves conducting an analysis before a study is initiated to determine the minimum number of subjects needed for the anticipated effect (i.e. the effect we expect to observe) to be considered statistically significant. Or, more formally stated, the minimum number of subjects needed to correctly reject the null hypothesis. Sample size estimation is essentially a preliminary step to reduce the risk of Type II error, which occurs when we incorrectly fail to reject the null hypothesis.

While sample size estimation was rare at one point, it's becoming increasingly common for funding agencies, such as the National Institutes of Health, to require (or at least strongly encourage) that a sample size estimate be included as part of a grant proposal. It makes sense; nobody wants to waste precious research funding on a project that's 'underpowered'. It's also common for journal editors and reviewers to ask investigators to justify their sample size, especially if they're reporting non-significant findings, where there's a risk of Type II error. Many times, details regarding sample size estimation are included in the methods

DOI: 10.4324/9781003179757-14

section of a research article. You've probably already read papers where the authors describe the steps involved in coming up with their target sample size.

Note: Chapter 4 discusses the concept of statistical power, and Chapter 13 discusses the concept of effect size. It may be helpful to review these chapters if you need a refresher before moving forward.

General overview

As discussed in Chapter 4, statistical power is a function of the effect size, alpha level, and sample size. We can make use of the relationships among these four variables (statistical power, effect size, alpha level, sample size) to come up with a sample size estimate. To do so, we simply specify our desired level of statistical power (typically 0.80), the alpha level we plan to use (typically 0.05), and the effect size we expect to observe. Once these variables are specified, the only remaining unknown is sample size, and therefore, we can determine the value of this single unknown parameter.

The sample size value we derive represents the minimum number of subjects needed to reach our desired level of statistical power. In most cases, investigators will enroll at least a few additional subjects in their study so that they'll be sufficiently powered to detect somewhat smaller effects than what's anticipated or to account for potential dropouts, missing data, and so on.

Although there are additional details to consider depending on the type of analysis to be conducted, this is the general process involved in sample size estimation. Essentially, it involves specifying the desired statistical power and alpha level, estimating the effect size that will be observed, and then deriving the necessary sample size for this effect to be considered statistically significant.

Estimating the effect size

A key aspect of sample size estimation is developing a reasonable estimate of the effect size (i.e. Cohen's d, η^2, r, R^2, etc.) that will be observed. You can think of this as making a 'best guess' at the results of a study before it's even started. While we never know how a study will turn out, projecting what we expect to observe can help to ensure that our study isn't 'doomed from the start' because of inadequate statistical power resulting from too small of a sample.

But the question becomes, how can we come up with an estimate of the effect size? Coming up with a reasonable effect size is probably the biggest challenge involved in sample size estimation. The three most common approaches are to estimate an effect size based on prior research, to conduct a preliminary 'pilot study' to generate an effect size, or to simply use an effect size that's considered somewhat 'meaningful' or reasonable to expect based on intuition or experience. The benefits and drawbacks of these approaches are discussed in the following subsections.

Estimating an effect size based on prior research

In most cases, investigators will estimate an effect size based on the results of previous research which is comparable to the study they plan to conduct. For example, imagine that we're planning to conduct a study to examine the effects of a balance training program on postural control in individuals with multiple sclerosis and that we want to determine the minimum number of subjects needed for our study to be 'adequately powered'. To do so, we need to come up with a reasonable estimate of the effect size that we expect to observe. Let's say that a previous study examined the effects of a similar balance training program on postural control in older adults and reported a moderate effect size for the change in postural control from baseline to post-training. If we anticipate that individuals with multiple sclerosis will respond in a similar manner, we could use this previously reported effect size for our sample size estimate. Essentially, this approach relies on using past findings to predict future results.

While this is certainly a reasonable approach, it can often be challenging to find previous research that's comparable enough to extrapolate from, especially when a proposed study is very novel in its approach or topic. We must often make generalizations based on studies that are comparable to, but not exactly the same as, our proposed study. For instance, consider our fictitious balance training study. In this case, we made the assumption that individuals with multiple sclerosis would respond in a similar manner to older adults without multiple sclerosis. This may be true, but we can't really be sure. In the end, it's a bit of a judgment call regarding whether previous research is close enough to produce a reasonable effect size estimate.

Estimating an effect size based on results from a pilot study

Another option is to conduct a preliminary 'pilot study' with a relatively small number of subjects and then used the observed effect size from this sample as an estimate of the effect size for the main study. While this is a great approach, it requires investigators to devote time, effort, and resources to conducting a pilot study, which may not be feasible in some cases.

Using an effect size that's considered meaningful or reasonable to expect

When data isn't available from previous research or from a pilot study, investigators may simply elect to use an effect size that's considered meaningful in some way and/or an effect size that they deem reasonable to expect based on their intuition. In many cases, investigators will consult available guidelines for standardized effect size measures (note: some common guidelines are provided in Chapter 13). For example, if an investigator anticipates that a new type of intervention will have a large effect on their dependent variable of interest, they may consult generic guidelines to determine what effect size corresponds with a 'large effect' and then use this effect size to derive their sample size estimate. It's important to note that the values considered 'small', 'moderate', 'large', and so on vary among different effect size metrics. Therefore, it's important to understand what effect size metric is most relevant to the intended analysis.

Of the three approaches described, this is certainly the easiest to implement, since it doesn't require the effort associated with identifying an effect size from previous research or collecting preliminary pilot data; however, it's generally considered the weakest approach, since it isn't based on empirical evidence. In general, it's probably best to start by examining previous research related to your topic to determine if there's a comparable study that can be used to generate an effect size. If not, then consider conducting a pilot study. And, finally, resort to selecting an effect size you generally think is meaningful or reasonable to expect if these other options aren't feasible.

Regardless of the approach used, it's important to come up with a reasonable effect size estimate. While overestimating the effect size could result in a study being underpowered, underestimating the effect size potentially wastes valuable time and resources and may place an unnecessary number of individuals at risk if there's the potential for study participants to experience an adverse event.

Resources for sample size estimation

There are tables referred to as 'Power Tables' available that can be used for sample size estimation; Cohen (1988) includes these types of tables. In addition, many statistical analysis software packages, such as SPSS, have the capability of generating a sample size estimate.

Another software package that's commonly used for sample size estimation is G*Power (Faul et al., 2007, 2009). G*Power is freely available for download and offers a high level of functionality. It's also fairly user-friendly, as long as you have a solid understanding of basic concepts such as effect size, power, and alpha/beta levels, which you should at this point. I'll use G*Power as part of my example in the next section to give you a general idea of how it works and the user interface. If you're planning to conduct your own research, I recommend downloading and trying it out. The user manual is also very comprehensive and generally easy to follow.

Example

Now, let's walk through an example. Let's say that I'm planning to conduct a study to examine the effects of a home-based abdominal muscle retraining program on inter-recti distance (i.e. the distance between the right and left rectus abdominis muscles) in women exhibiting persistent diastasis recti following childbirth. Diastasis recti is a condition where there's an atypically large degree of separation between the rectus abdominis muscles. It's fairly common among women following childbirth.

My plan is to examine the change in inter-recti distance from baseline to post-training using a paired *t*-test (discussed in Chapter 5). Through a literature search, I find a previous study by Deering et al. (2020) which examined the effects of a clinic-based abdominal muscle retraining program on inter-recti distance in postpartum women. Although this previous study had participants train in the clinic, I think it's reasonable to expect similar results with a home-based training program; therefore, I decide to use the results reported by these authors to estimate an effect size for my study. Based on the means and standard deviations reported by Deering et al. (2020), I calculate a Cohen's *d* effect size statistic of 0.67 (Cohen's $d = \dfrac{1.8 - 1.2}{0.9} = 0.67$), which is generally considered a 'moderate-large' effect based on proposed guidelines (Cohen, 1988). This observed effect size can then serve as an estimate of the effect size for my sample size estimate. Again, this is merely an educated guess about how my study will turn out.

Now that I have an estimate of the effect size (Cohen's $d = 0.67$), I can determine the minimum number of subjects needed to reach my desired level of statistical power of 0.80, given an alpha level of 0.05. In this case, G*Power indicates that a sample size of 20 subjects is needed in order to be adequately powered to detect the estimated effect (Figure 14.1). Essentially, what this indicates is that if I observe the anticipated effect (Cohen's $d = 0.67$), my results will likely be statistically significant, as long as my sample includes at least 20 subjects. Basically, what I'm attempting to do is set myself up for a successful outcome, as long as my results turn out as expected. Since a sample of 20 represents the minimum sample size needed to reach my desired level of statistical power, I would likely enroll a few additional subjects in my actual study.

While what I've presented is a fairly simple example, it should help you appreciate the general process involved in sample size estimation. As you can see, the main obstacle is coming up with a reasonable effect size estimate.

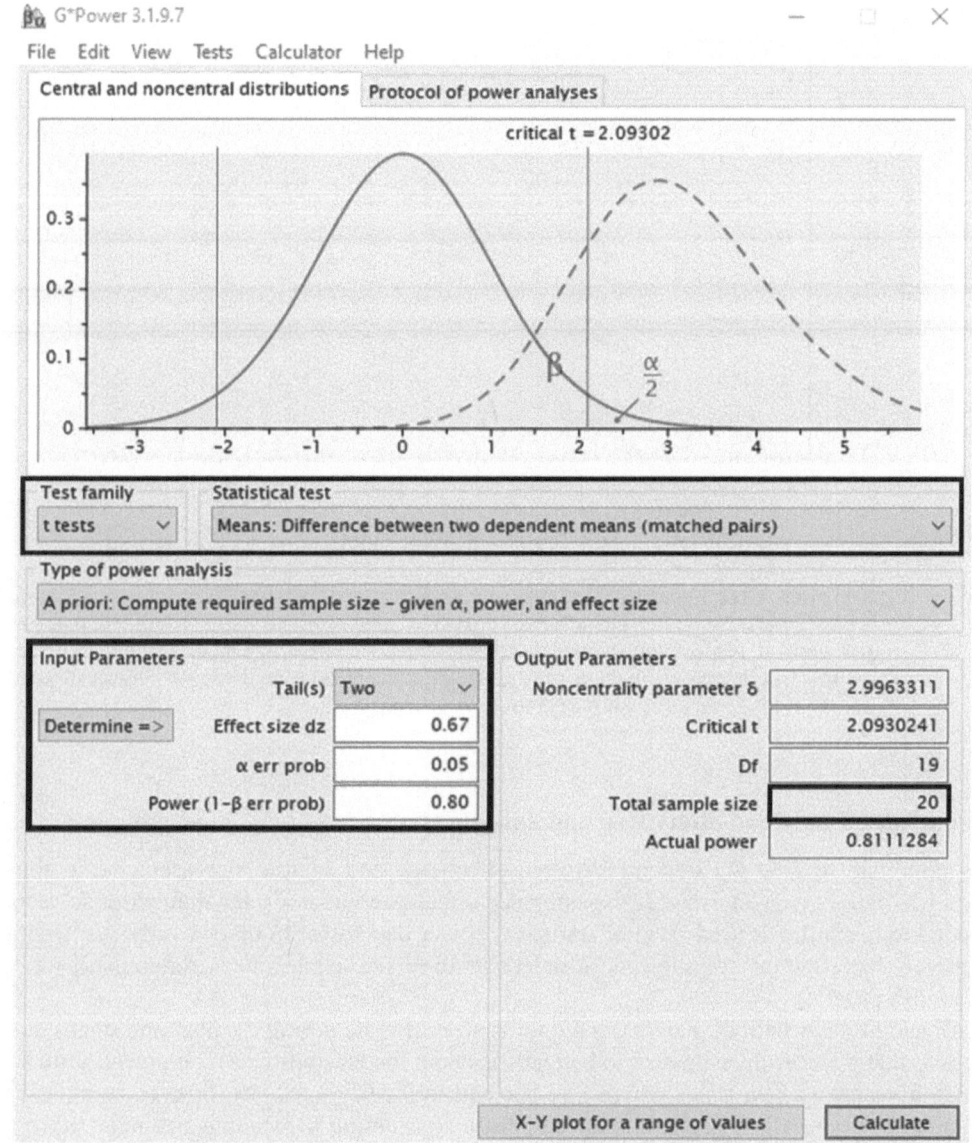

Figure 14.1 Example of the G*Power user interface with pertinent areas outlined. Notice that for our abdominal muscle retraining example, the 'Test family' is 't tests' and the 'Statistical test' is 'Means: Difference between two dependent means (matched pairs)', since we're planning to conduct a paired *t*-test. The input parameters are the estimated effects size ('Effect size dz' = 0.67), the alpha level ('α err prob' = 0.05), and the desired level of statistical power ['Power (1 − β err prob)' = 0.80]. In this case, we also need to indicate whether we plan to conduct a one- or two-tailed test ['Tail(s)' = two], since this will also influence statistical power. The output parameters include the minimum sample size ('Total sample size' = 20). Note: G*Power can be used to generate a sample size estimate for a wide range of analyses, including any of those discussed in this book. The G*Power user manual includes instructions for how to compute the required sample size for different types of analyses. It's worth exploring if you're planning to conduct your own research.

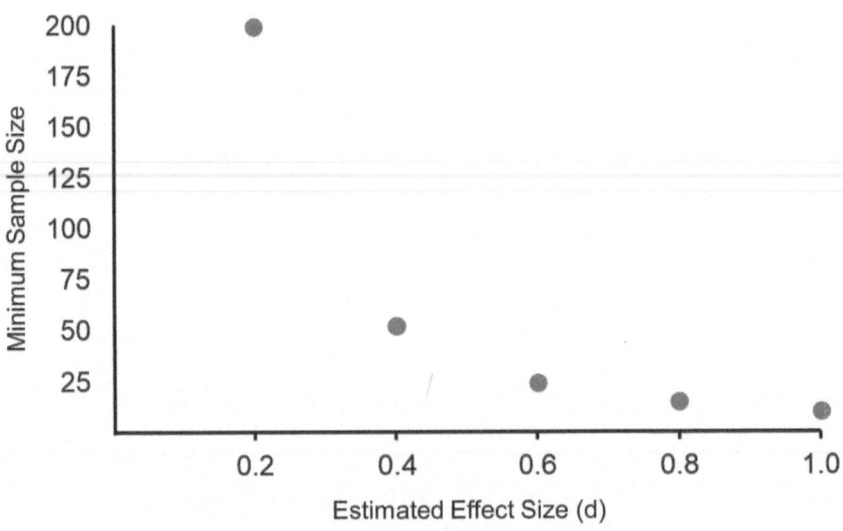

Figure 14.2 The minimum sample size needed to achieve a statistical power of 0.80 when conducting a paired *t*-test (two-tails, alpha level = 0.05) for Cohen's *d* effect sizes (*d*) of 0.2, 0.4, 0.6, 0.8, and 1.0, respectively. Notice that as the estimated effect size increases, the necessary sample size decreases. In other words, the larger the effect size, the fewer subjects needed for the study to be adequately powered.

The tradeoff between effect size and sample size

It's important to note the tradeoff between effect size and sample size (depicted in Figure 14.2). For a given analysis, as the estimated effect size increases, the number of subjects needed to reach the desired level of statistical power decreases. In other words, we need a relatively large number of subjects to detect small effects (small mean differences, weak relationships, etc.).

An additional benefit of generating a sample size estimate during the planning stages of a study is that it forces investigators to be realistic about the feasibility of their potential study. There have been a few times where I've decided to modify a project, or even completely abandon it, because I've realized it isn't realistic considering the sample size required. It's always best to come to these realizations during the planning stages of a study, before you've invested too much time and too many resources on a project that's not realistic.

Final thoughts

What I've presented in this chapter is a very general overview of the procedures involved in sample size estimation. There's certainly more to learn on this important topic. That said, this chapter should give you a general idea of the purpose of, and general processes involved in, sample size estimation. That's a great start, especially if your goal is simply to be a more informed consumer of scientific literature.

15 Analysis of covariance

Chapter Objectives

The objectives of this chapter are to . . .

1) define what a covariate is and provide examples of covariates
2) introduce the conceptual basis for analysis of covariance
3) highlight key advantages of analysis of covariance
4) discuss how analysis of covariance is used with pretest-posttest study designs
5) provide examples of research questions that have been addressed using analysis of covariance

Introduction

Analysis of covariance (ANCOVA) is an extension of analysis of variance, which was first discussed in Chapter 6. In general, ANCOVA involves adjustments to the sample means for the dependent variable of interest. These adjustments account for the influence of an extraneous variable referred to as a *covariate*. A covariate is a continuous variable that's linearly related to the dependent variable. The effect of this covariate can be accounted for by including it as a variable in the ANCOVA model. Aside from the inclusion of a covariate (or covariates in some instances), ANCOVA is conceptually the same as ANOVA, as it involves an F-test for each of the study factors.

ANCOVA has two key advantages over ANOVA. First, ANCOVA accounts for the influence of the covariate so that the effects of the independent variable(s) of interest can be isolated. This helps to prevent the covariate from distorting the true relationship between the independent variable(s) and dependent variable. In addition, ANCOVA generally has greater statistical power, since the variance associated with the covariate is partitioned out in the analysis. Remember that ANOVA involves examining the variance associated with the independent variable(s) relative to the total variance in the dependent variable. Partitioning out the variance associated with the covariate essentially reduces the error variance ('noise'), making ANCOVA more sensitive to the effects attributed to the independent variable(s) of interest. I like to think of this as 'trimming the fat' from the analysis so we can focus on the crux of the matter.

One-way ANCOVA example

As an example, let's consider a study I conducted with some of my former students (Stricker et al., 2021). As part of our study, we compared the step lengths of individuals with Parkinson's disease who were classified as 'fallers' or 'non-fallers'. Participants were classified as

DOI: 10.4324/9781003179757-15

fallers if they had experienced at least one fall in the past 12 months or as non-fallers if they hadn't fallen in the past 12 months. On average, the fallers exhibited a shorter step length than the non-fallers, suggesting that the independent variable, 'fall history', was related to the dependent variable, step length. However, the fallers also tended to be shorter in stature than the non-fallers, and therefore, it's possible that the observed difference in step length was due, at least partially, to the group differences in height, since shorter individuals tend to take shorter steps.

To account for the height difference, we used one-way ANCOVA to compare the groups (fallers vs. non-fallers), with height included as the covariate. This allowed us to address the question of whether there was a significant difference in step length between the fallers and non-fallers while accounting for the effects of height (i.e. the covariate) on step length. Note that in this case, our statistical analysis included three variables: 1) the dependent variable: step length, 2) the independent variable: 'group' (fallers, non-fallers), and 3) the covariate: height.

The null hypothesis associated with our ANCOVA test was that there is no difference in the adjusted mean step lengths of the fallers and non-fallers, with the means adjusted based on height. An F-test for the factor 'group' resulted in a p-value of 0.01 ($p = 0.01$), which was less than our predefined alpha level of 0.05. This indicated that, after accounting for height, the difference in step length between the fallers and non-fallers was statistically significant. In other words, fallers took shorter steps, even after accounting for the height difference between the groups. Another way to conceptualize this is to consider that if we had groups of fallers and non-fallers of equivalent height, fallers would tend to take shorter steps compared to non-fallers.

Using baseline scores as a covariate

One common application of ANCOVA is to control for baseline group differences in pretest-posttest study designs, where performance is examined before (baseline) and after treatment (posttest). In this case, posttest scores are compared for the different groups of interest (e.g. treatment, control), while subjects' baseline scores serve as the covariate. This allows us to examine whether there are between-group differences in posttest performance while accounting for differences in baseline performance. Note that baseline scores can often serve as a covariate, since they tend to be linearly related to posttest scores. In other words, individuals who perform relatively poorly at baseline also tend to perform relatively poorly during posttesting, while individuals who perform relatively well at baseline also tend to perform relatively well during posttesting.

Let's consider an example. A group of collaborators and I conducted a study to examine the effects of a neuromuscular training program on knee proprioception in athletes who had undergone anterior cruciate ligament reconstruction (Ghaderi et al., 2020). As part of the study, a group of 24 male athletes who had undergone ACL reconstruction and completed rehabilitation were randomly allocated to either an experimental group that participated in an 8-week neuromuscular training program ($n = 12$) or to a control group ($n = 12$) that simply continued their typical training routine.

All athletes completed testing to assess their knee position sense before (baseline) and after (posttest) the 8-week period. During testing, athletes began in a sitting position with their ACL-reconstructed knee flexed to 90°. Then their knee was passively extended via an isokinetic dynamometer. The athletes were asked to press a button when they perceived that their knee had reached a target angle of 45° of flexion. Any deviation from this target angle was reported as an 'error', with greater errors reflecting poorer knee proprioception.

In this case, our dependent variable of interest was the posttest knee position sense errors for the athletes' ACL-reconstructed knees. The ANCOVA model included the independent variable 'group' (experimental, control) and athletes' baseline knee position sense errors as a covariate. Our results indicated that after adjusting for baseline differences in knee position sense, the experimental group demonstrated significantly lower knee position sense errors compared to the control group ($p < 0.001$; p-value based on an F-test for the factor 'group'), which suggests that participation in the neuromuscular training program promoted better knee proprioception. In this case, including baseline knee position sense errors as a covariate helped us account for differences in baseline performance. This can be important, since randomization doesn't always produce equivalent groups, especially when dealing with small samples. Remember, randomization isn't perfect.

It's important to note that this is just one way to analyze data for these types of pretest-posttest designs. Other methods include mixed-model ANOVA and comparison of change scores via independent t-tests or one-way ANOVA. There are quite a few papers comparing these different approaches (e.g. O'Connell et al., 2017; Van Breukelen, 2006). It may be worth exploring this topic in greater detail if you're planning to conduct a study which involves a pretest-posttest design.

A word of caution

Whenever possible, it's best to attempt to control for the effects of confounding variables with your study design instead of attempting to account for them statistically. ANCOVA shouldn't be seen as a 'band-aid' to deal with a carelessly designed study. It's still critical to carefully consider ways to minimize the effects of confounding factors when establishing your eligibility criteria, sampling methods, and randomization procedures. In general, ANCOVA should only be used in cases where it's not possible to control for a covariate through a study's design.

Final thoughts

The focus of this chapter was on the most basic applications of ANCOVA, since the goal was to simply introduce you to the topic. However, there's much more to learn about ANCOVA. If you're planning to use ANCOVA for your own research, you'll want to consult more advanced resources that go into greater detail about how to deal with covariates and the assumptions that underlie ANCOVA. Regardless, this chapter should serve as a good starting point, especially if your goal is to better understand the use of ANCOVA when reading the literature.

16 Multivariate analysis of variance

Chapter Objectives

The objectives of this chapter are to . . .

1) introduce the conceptual basis for multivariate analysis of variance
2) provide an example of the type of research questions that can be addressed using multi-variate analysis of variance
3) highlight some potential advantages of multivariate analysis of variance
4) introduce multivariate analysis of covariance

Introduction

Chapters 6 and 7 discussed analysis of variance, which is a family of statistical analyses that can be used to compare means across two or more groups, time points, or conditions for a single dependent variable. Multivariate analysis of variance (MANOVA) is an extension of ANOVA, which can be used to examine multiple interrelated dependent variables simultaneously.*

MANOVA involves combining the dependent variables into a new composite variable (often referred to as a 'supervariable') and then comparing the means for this composite variable instead of the means for the individual dependent variables. With MANOVA, the dependent variables are combined in a manner that maximizes the differences between the groups, time points, or conditions.

Like ANOVA, MANOVA can be applied in cases where there's a single independent variable or multiple independent variables (e.g. one-way MANOVA, two-way MANOVA). When there are multiple independent variables, both the interaction effect(s) and main effects can be examined. Again, MANOVA is conceptually the same as ANOVA, except for the fact that MANOVA is based on a linear combination of multiple dependent variables instead of a single dependent variable.

* **Note:** MANOVA is considered a *multivariate test*, since it incorporates *multiple* dependent variables. *t*-tests and ANOVA are generally considered *univariate* tests, since they only examine a single dependent variable.

One-way MANOVA example

In my mind, the best way to begin to conceptualize MANOVA is to consider an example. Imagine that we conduct a study to examine how concussion history influences neurocognitive

DOI: 10.4324/9781003179757-16

functioning in athletes. Our study includes three distinct groups of athletes: 1) athletes with no history of concussion ('control group'), 2) athletes with a history of 1–2 concussions ('1–2 group') and 3) athletes with a history of 3+ concussions ('3+ group'). Let's say that all athletes complete a battery of neuropsychological tests, which produce scores related to their reaction time, cortical processing speed, and working memory. In this case, we have three dependent variables (reaction time, cortical processing speed, and working memory), which all represent different aspects of the more general construct 'neurocognitive functioning'.

One way to analyze this data would be to conduct separate one-way ANOVA tests to compare the group means for the individual dependent variables. However, we could also use one-way MANOVA to combine the variables (reaction time, cortical processing speed, working memory) into a composite variable that represents a more global measure of general neurocognitive functioning. In this case, the variables would be combined in a manner that results in the greatest separation among the groups (control group, 1–2 group, 3+ group). In other words, the variables would be weighted so that the group means for the composite variable differed as much as possible.

Like ANOVA, the MANOVA test would produce a *p*-value that we would compare to our predefined alpha level (typically 0.05). If this *p*-value were less than our alpha level, we would conclude that there's a statistically significant difference in neurocognitive functioning among the groups. Notice that our results don't tell us about whether the groups differed with respect to their reaction time, cortical processing speed, or working memory, since the test was based on the composite variable which incorporated all three variables.

This example is the type of scenario where MANOVA may be particularly useful. While the variables reaction time, cortical processing speed, and working memory are unique, they're all related to some extent, since they're aspects of the more general construct 'neurocognitive functioning'. Therefore, if our objective was to examine how concussion history influences general neurocognitive functioning, it may make sense to consider the variables together instead of conducting univariate tests for each individual variable.

Note: in general, the dependent variables should have some logical relationship to one another if they're going to be combined and analyzed together using MANOVA.

Potential advantages of MANOVA

One potential advantage of MANOVA, when compared to ANOVA, is that combining the variables may result in greater statistical power (at least in some cases). In other words, by combining the variables, we may be able to detect differences that aren't evident when the variables are considered individually. Consider our concussion history example. It's possible that we wouldn't observe any statistically significant differences among the groups if the variables were assessed individually (i.e. separate univariate tests comparing reaction time, cortical processing speed, and working memory) but that we would observe a statistically significant difference if the variables were examined together using MANOVA.

In some instances, MANOVA can also provide protection against familywise error since it may eliminate the need to conduct multiple univariate tests. For instance, in our concussion history example, we would limit the number of statistical tests, and thus the familywise error rate, by using MANOVA to compare the groups instead of conducting separate univariate tests for each of the individual variables (i.e. three separate univariate tests for the reaction time, cortical processing speed, and working memory variables, each with its own risk of Type I error).

It's important to note that while MANOVA has some distinct advantages over ANOVA, it's not the best option in all circumstances. Investigators need to carefully consider a number of factors when deciding between MANOVA and ANOVA. It's certainly not as simple as throwing all the variables into the statistical model and seeing what happens.

MANOVA as a precursor to univariate tests?

MANOVA is often conducted as a preliminary analysis before performing multiple univariate tests as a follow-up. When used in this manner, investigators will typically only conduct follow-up univariate tests (ANOVA, *t*-tests) if the MANOVA test is statistically significant. The idea is that if there's no difference when the variables are combined, there's no need to examine the variables individually.

The general premise behind this use of MANOVA is that it helps to reduce the risk of Type I error, since investigators avoid running unnecessary univariate tests unless the MANOVA test suggests that some type of difference exists. While this is a commonly cited reason for using MANOVA, this approach appears to provide little protection against Type I error and is generally unfounded. A paper by Huberty and Morris (1989) provides a strong argument against this use of MANOVA (full reference provided in the references section). It's certainly worth reading if you're considering using MANOVA for your own research.

MANCOVA

MANOVA can also be extended to include a covariate (or covariates), which is generally referred to as *multivariate analysis of covariance* (MANCOVA). In this case, the statistical model incorporates a covariate (or covariates) along with the independent variable(s) and dependent variables of interest. Remember that a covariate is a continuous variable that's related to the dependent variables but isn't an independent variable of interest in the study. By incorporating a covariate in the MANCOVA model, we can account for the influence of this extraneous variable and essentially remove its effect from the analysis.

Chapter 15 ('Analysis of Covariance') discusses methods for accounting for covariates; therefore, we won't discuss MANCOVA in detail here. Just realize that covariates can be incorporated into a multivariate model (MANCOVA), in much the same way that they can be incorporated into a univariate model (ANCOVA).

Final thoughts

This chapter presents a very superficial introduction to MANOVA and multivariate statistics in general. My goal is to simply make you aware of what MANOVA is, when it may be useful, and how it generally functions. There are certainly more details to consider regarding how the optimal combination of variables is determined, specific instances where MANOVA may work well, key assumptions, and so on.

If you're interested in learning more about MANOVA and/or multivariate statistics in general, I recommend Tabachnick and Fidell's textbook, *Using Multivariate Statistics* (2019; full reference included in the references section). It's a tremendous book that covers a wide array of multivariate techniques, including MANOVA, in greater detail.

Data Sets

Loading	BMD
2.05	1.14
2.12	1.16
2.33	1.23
2.60	1.40
2.43	1.19
2.60	1.13
2.66	1.00
2.49	1.06
2.54	0.91
2.48	0.87
2.43	0.97
2.43	0.84
2.43	0.81
2.39	0.70
2.39	0.96
2.38	1.01
2.39	0.95
2.02	1.02
2.08	1.03
2.11	0.99
2.16	0.92
2.26	1.01
2.28	0.95
2.33	0.95
2.33	0.92
2.34	0.83
1.99	0.95
2.02	0.93
2.07	0.89
2.07	0.88
2.11	0.89
2.14	0.88
2.16	0.88
1.95	0.89

Loading	BMD
2.03	0.87
2.03	0.86
2.03	0.84
2.05	0.81
2.10	0.81
2.09	0.79
2.01	0.79
2.00	0.78
1.95	0.76
1.98	0.74
1.95	0.70
1.98	0.69
2.03	0.68
2.07	0.62
2.09	0.69
2.17	0.69
2.07	0.75
2.25	0.70
2.28	0.72
2.25	0.91
2.25	0.89
2.29	0.88
2.31	0.88
2.23	0.76
2.24	0.80
2.18	0.79
2.17	0.86
2.17	0.83
2.20	0.83
2.20	0.87
2.23	0.87
2.24	0.87
2.25	0.84
2.21	0.84

Grip strength	
Cases (Kg)	*Controls (Kg)*
13	22
20	25
12	25
17	20
30	37
33	26
33	37
30	30
30	38
25	30
35	40
46	35
22	28
32	35
42	46
40	40
20	28
25	30
18	27
35	36
35	35
22	23
23	29
20	30
10	25
15	23
18	22
12	23
15	22
19	25
10	15

Hip extension strength		
Group	*Pre*	*Post*
1	48.3	45.2
1	43.8	42.5
1	37.1	36.4
1	32.9	32.4
1	38.6	38.9
1	29.8	30.6
1	34.8	38.4
1	41	45
1	51.8	56.4
1	26.9	33
1	31.1	39.8
1	41	51.7
1	29.6	40.9
1	27.6	39.8
2	38.1	37.6

(Continued)

Hip extension strength		
Group	Pre	Post
2	33.7	33.9
2	37.6	37.9
2	32.6	33.8
2	35.7	38.1
2	48	51.6
2	27.8	31.8
2	40.9	45
2	36.7	42
2	38.3	44
2	20.4	26.3
2	33.3	43
2	27.7	37.6
2	36	46.1
2	28.3	41
2	35.6	52.8

Leg stiffness (N/kg/m)			
Subject	Base	IF	EF
1	72.932	72.331	75.175
2	101.607	72.421	83.069
3	85.191	68.741	45.456
4	83.671	70.405	70.105
5	83.708	62.154	60.854
6	95.082	71.955	61.049
7	232.641	220.879	114.801
8	118.894	61.830	60.564
9	88.339	68.309	41.054
10	99.209	67.467	60.529
11	78.245	95.288	74.548
12	100.731	67.770	63.407
13	136.116	86.882	71.775
14	125.277	92.128	96.448
15	121.895	94.889	70.264
16	142.847	70.857	62.930

Sex	Age	Diabetes	Exercise	Sarcopenia
0	55	0	1	0
0	55	0	1	0
0	55	0	1	0
0	55	1	1	0
0	56	0	1	0
0	57	1	1	0
0	57	0	1	0
0	57	1	1	0

(*Continued*)

Sex	Age	Diabetes	Exercise	Sarcopenia
0	58	1	1	0
0	59	0	1	0
0	59	0	1	0
0	60	0	1	0
0	60	0	1	0
0	61	1	0	0
0	62	0	1	0
0	63	0	1	0
0	63	0	1	0
0	64	0	1	0
0	65	1	1	0
0	65	0	1	0
0	66	0	0	0
0	66	0	1	0
0	66	1	1	0
0	67	0	1	0
0	69	1	1	0
0	71	1	1	0
0	71	0	1	0
0	72	0	1	0
0	79	0	1	0
0	80	0	1	0
0	89	0	1	0
1	55	1	1	0
1	55	0	0	0
1	55	0	1	0
1	56	0	1	0
1	56	0	1	0
1	56	0	0	0
1	56	0	1	0
1	57	0	1	0
1	58	0	1	0
1	58	0	1	0
1	58	0	1	0
1	58	0	0	0
1	58	0	1	0
1	58	0	1	0
1	59	1	0	0
1	59	0	1	0
1	59	1	1	0
1	60	0	1	0
1	60	0	0	0
1	60	0	1	0
1	60	1	1	0
1	60	0	1	0
1	60	1	1	0
1	60	0	1	0
1	61	1	1	0
1	61	0	1	0
1	62	1	1	0
1	62	0	1	0
1	62	0	0	0
1	62	0	1	0
1	62	1	1	0
1	62	1	1	0

(*Continued*)

Sex	Age	Diabetes	Exercise	Sarcopenia
1	62	0	1	0
1	62	0	1	0
1	63	0	1	0
1	63	0	1	0
1	64	0	1	0
1	64	0	0	0
1	64	0	1	0
1	66	0	0	0
1	66	1	1	0
1	66	0	0	0
1	66	1	0	0
1	66	1	1	0
1	66	0	1	0
1	67	1	0	0
1	67	1	1	0
1	68	0	0	0
1	68	0	0	0
1	70	0	0	0
1	70	0	1	0
1	72	0	1	0
1	73	0	1	0
1	73	0	1	0
1	73	0	1	0
1	74	0	1	0
1	75	0	1	0
1	75	0	1	0
1	77	0	0	0
1	78	0	1	0
1	90	1	1	0
0	55	1	1	1
0	59	0	1	1
0	59	1	0	1
0	59	1	0	1
0	60	1	0	1
0	60	1	1	1
0	62	0	1	1
0	64	0	0	1
0	67	1	0	1
0	67	1	0	1
0	68	0	0	1
0	69	1	1	1
0	69	0	1	1
0	71	1	1	1
0	71	0	1	1
0	72	0	1	1
0	80	0	0	1
0	82	0	1	1
0	85	1	1	1
0	87	0	0	1
0	88	1	1	1
1	55	1	1	1
1	57	0	1	1
1	59	1	0	1
1	59	1	0	1
1	60	0	0	1

(*Continued*)

Sex	Age	Diabetes	Exercise	Sarcopenia
1	61	1	0	1
1	63	0	1	1
1	63	1	1	1
1	63	0	1	1
1	64	0	0	1
1	66	1	1	1
1	67	0	0	1
1	69	0	0	1
1	71	0	0	1
1	71	1	1	1
1	72	0	1	1
1	75	1	0	1
1	76	0	1	1
1	77	1	1	1
1	79	1	0	1
1	80	1	0	1
1	85	0	1	1
1	86	0	0	1
1	88	1	1	1

STS test times (s)		
Younger	Older	OA
6.6	10.8	8.1
7.2	11.0	12.3
8.0	10.8	11.5
9.0	12.9	14.6
8.3	8.1	9.0
9.4	13.5	11.3
11.8	11.6	15.6
9.6	8.6	13.4
7.7	8.5	13.2
7.1	11.4	14.6
6.9	11.3	16.9
7.3	10.7	15.9
7.0	11.3	11.5
8.2	8.8	12.8

Sex	Age	Strength	Knee_motion	Pain	Gait_speed
1	81	12	90	2.0	0.90
1	58	15	120	3.5	1.22
1	71	13	130	0.0	1.36
0	55	11	125	5.5	1.23
0	73	1	140	1.0	1.56
1	68	8	125	1.0	0.97
1	69	12	125	3.0	1.49
0	74	18	130	4.0	1.43

(*Continued*)

Sex	Age	Strength	Knee_motion	Pain	Gait_speed
0	78	9	130	4.0	0.67
0	85	14	125	0.0	1.39
1	66	15	110	0.0	1.44
0	77	18	110	2.5	1.24
1	68	15	115	0.0	1.00
1	70	11	140	2.0	0.81
0	53	16	150	3.0	1.48
1	68	15	115	0.0	0.83
1	64	15	125	0.0	1.58
1	78	17	135	2.0	1.22
0	70	15	115	0.0	1.29
1	77	2	130	1.0	0.93
1	66	17	120	0.0	1.35
1	75	9	125	5.0	1.22
0	64	10	120	1.0	1.52
1	67	9	120	2.0	1.00
1	71	11	110	0.0	0.97
1	83	9	110	5.0	0.52
0	77	10	120	1.0	1.29
1	61	7	115	2.0	0.73
1	66	19	130	6.0	1.52
1	74	18	115	1.0	1.18
1	61	6	125	9.0	0.70
1	68	5	110	5.0	0.56
0	69	7	105	3.0	1.00
1	72	5	110	2.0	0.60
1	71	15	115	1.0	1.28
1	71	12	125	3.0	1.13
0	69	15	135	2.0	1.63
1	78	7	125	2.0	0.82
1	86	10	130	2.0	1.04
1	62	4	115	8.0	0.61
1	79	11	125	5.0	1.01
0	71	10	125	5.0	1.45
1	72	6	120	7.0	0.49
1	71	10	130	3.0	0.95
1	84	10	130	0.0	0.87
0	72	5	135	6.0	1.01
1	73	12	125	0.0	1.60
1	55	0	105	8.0	0.55
0	63	14	115	1.0	1.51
1	68	14	130	1.0	1.48
0	60	5	105	6.0	1.07
1	72	11	110	1.0	1.02
0	63	7	110	2.0	1.04
0	62	9	130	5.0	1.07
0	79	8	120	8.0	1.12
1	74	9	125	4.0	0.70
1	71	2	140	2.0	1.08
1	64	10	135	4.0	1.16
1	75	12	105	6.5	1.06

PPT	Morphine
147	29
181	32
219	34
222	30
217	29
224	26
214	25
187	24
241	21
253	22
237	23
212	21
196	21
188	21
188	19
193	13
228	16
224	18
249	16
262	16
264	18
277	15
303	16
303	18
310	20
299	19
309	21
302	24
276	26
344	20
350	20
339	19
330	17
332	16
341	16
356	14
373	16
388	17
430	11
360	9

Subject	RT
1	288.7
2	289.4
3	342.9
4	307.8
5	253.0
6	295.1
7	295.0
8	315.4
9	264.8
10	262.5

(Continued)

Subject	RT
11	252.7
12	256.9
13	268.7
14	268.5
15	317.7
16	270.0
17	275.1
18	299.8
19	254.2
20	308.8
21	257.2
22	282.2
23	268.8
24	272.0
25	246.1
26	256.4
27	290.8
28	271.9
29	258.2
30	246.9

Vastus lateralis – CSA (cm^2)	
Pre	*Post*
13.50	12.12
22.17	18.91
15.47	15.38
17.88	16.18
14.98	14.33
17.13	16.75
13.37	13.54
18.64	12.65
14.02	15.14
19.77	16.97
20.24	20.61
14.04	14.36
16.03	15.90

Appendixes

Appendix A Assessing normality

Introduction

Many parametric statistical procedures assume that the dependent variable is normally distributed. While minor violations of this assumption tend to have little influence on the results of most analyses, more substantial deviations can affect statistical validity. Therefore, it's important to check the assumption of normality when indicated. This supplementary chapter introduces some commonly used methods for checking the assumption of normality.

Approaches used to assess normality can generally be categorized as *graphical methods* or *normality tests*. Graphical methods involve visually examining plots that display how the data is distributed or how the observed distribution differs in comparison to the normal distribution. While graphical methods can be helpful in getting a general impression of whether the data is normally distributed, they're purely qualitative. Therefore, it's common to supplement these graphical methods with more quantitative methods, including formal normality tests. Normality tests are null hypothesis significance tests that essentially test whether the sample data differs significantly from the normal distribution.

Graphical methods

Histograms

A good starting point for assessing normality is to examine a histogram. Remember that a histogram is a graphical display of a frequency distribution (note: histograms were introduced in Chapter 2). If a histogram appears to approximate the shape of the normal distribution curve ('bell curve'), it suggests that the assumption of normality is met. Figure A.1, subplot A, includes an example of a histogram. You'll see that the normal distribution curve has been superimposed over this histogram to aid in visual analysis.

While histograms are a good starting point, they can often be misleading, since the apparent shape of a histogram depends on the width of the intervals used to group the data ('bin width'). Therefore, it's best not to rely solely on visual analysis of a histogram for checking the assumption of normality.

Note: stem-and-leaf plots can also be used to visualize the shape of a frequency distribution in much the same way as a histogram (remember that a stem-and-leaf plot is essentially a histogram turned onto its side). Stem-and-leaf plots were also introduced in Chapter 2.

Box plots

Box plots can also be examined to get an impression of whether a variable is normally distributed (note: box plots were introduced in Chapter 2). Remember that in a box plot, the first

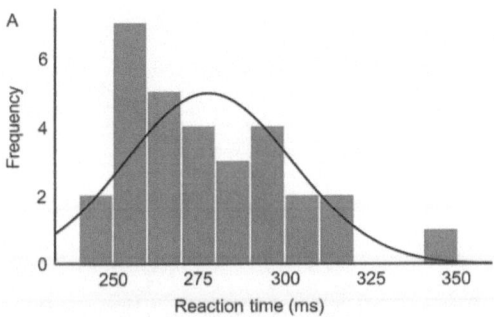 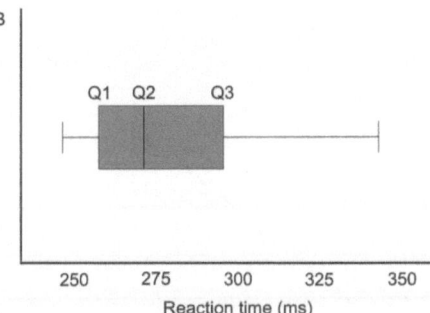

Figure A.1 Histogram (subplot A – left) and box plot (subplot B – right) based on a set of reaction time data. Subplot A: notice that the right/upper tail extends beyond where most values tend to cluster, indicating that the distribution is positively skewed. Note: the normal distribution curve has been superimposed over the histogram in subplot A; this can be helpful when assessing normality based on visual inspection of a histogram. Subplot B: notice that the third quartile (Q3) and upper whisker extend out farther from the median (Q2) than the first quartile (Q1) and lower whisker, which is also a sign of a positively skewed distribution.

quartile (Q1) and third quartile (Q3) make up the outer boundaries of the box, while the median (seconds quartile – Q2) is represented by a line that splits the box in half. If the halves of the box are roughly evenly split and the whiskers are comparable length, it suggests that the data is normally distributed. Marked asymmetry in the upper and lower halves of the box plot indicates that the distribution is skewed. Figure A.1, subplot B, includes an example of a box plot.

Quantile-quantile plots

Quantile-quantile (Q-Q) plots are also useful for assessing the assumption of normality. The general logic behind a Q-Q plot is to compare the observed values to what would be expected if the data were normally distributed. If the variable of interest is normally distributed, then there should be agreement between the observed values and the expected values.

In a Q-Q plot, the observed values are plotted along one axis, while the values expected for the normal distribution are plotted along the other axis.* If the variable is normally distributed, the points on the plot will form a straight diagonal line (Figure A.2; subplot A). If the variable isn't normally distributed, the points on the plot will deviate from a straight diagonal line (Figure A.2; subplot B). This may be due to issues of skewness, kurtosis, or both. Minor deviations are expected, since variables will rarely follow the normal distribution exactly; however, marked deviations indicate that the variable differs substantially from the normal distribution (i.e. the assumption of normality isn't met).

* Note: it's actually quantiles that are plotted against each other, not the actual values, hence the term 'quantile-quantile plot'. Quantiles are essentially values that divide a distribution into equal intervals. For example, the median is a quantile, since it divides a distribution in half.

Probability-probability plots

Probability-probability (P-P) plots are similar to Q-Q plots, except instead of quantiles, P-P plots plot the cumulative probabilities associated with the observed distribution against that

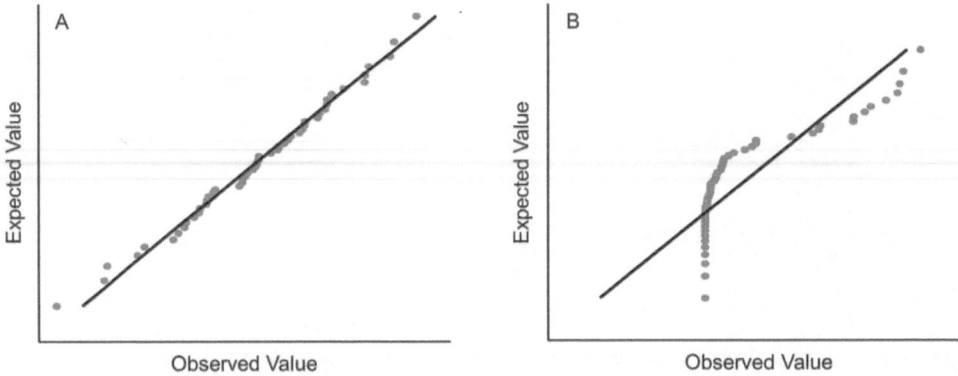

Figure A.2 Subplot A (left) and subplot B (right) include examples of Q-Q plots. The observed values are plotted along the horizontal axes ('Observed Value'), while the theoretical values based on the normal distribution are plotted along the vertical axes ('Expected Value'). The values for subplot A (left) were taken from a set of random numbers that were normally distributed, while the values for subplot B (right) were taken from a set of random numbers that were positively skewed. Notice that in subplot A, most of the points fall close to the diagonal reference line, indicating that the data is normally distributed. In contrast, in subplot B, the points on the plot deviate markedly from the diagonal reference line, indicating that the data isn't normally distributed.

of the normal distribution. Essentially, a P-P plot compares the areas under the curve for the observed distribution to the areas under the curve for the normal distribution (remember, we can consider the areas of a distribution in terms of probabilities). Like Q-Q plots, when the points on a P-P plot deviate from a diagonal reference line, it indicates that the observed distribution differs from the normal distribution. As an example, Figure A.3 includes a Q-Q plot and P-P plot for a set of reaction time data.

Q-Q plots tend to be used more often than P-P plots, since they're more sensitive to deviations in the tails of the distribution; however, most statistical analysis software packages allow you to generate both Q-Q plots and P-P plots.

Note: what I've presented here is a very general introduction to Q-Q plots and P-P plots. There's certainly more to consider. My goal in this supplementary chapter is simply to introduce the conceptual basis for these plots and begin to explain what they represent. While they can be very informative, it takes some experience to be able to make correct judgments based on visual analysis of Q-Q plots and P-P plots.

Normality tests

Normality tests are null hypothesis significance tests that are used to formally test the assumption of normality. While normality tests differ in their approach, they generally test whether the data follows the shape of the normal distribution. When the p-value associated with a normality test is less than the alpha level (typically 0.05), it indicates that the observed data differs significantly from the normal distribution (i.e. the assumption of normality is violated). This is a bit counterintuitive, since in most cases, we're actually hoping to observe a non-significant finding ($p \geq$ alpha) for these normality tests, since this indicates that our data satisfies the assumption of normality.

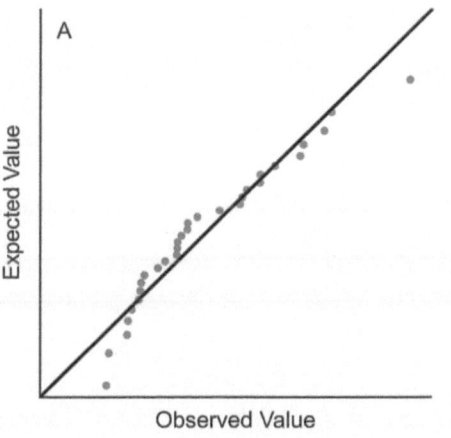
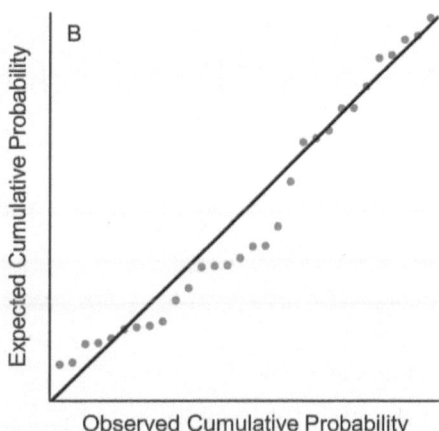

Figure A.3 Q-Q plot (subplot A – left) and P-P plot (subplot B – right) based on a set of reaction time data. For subplot A, the observed values are plotted along the horizontal axis ('Observed Value'), while the theoretical values based on the normal distribution are plotted along the vertical axis ('Expected Value'). Subplot B is laid out in the same manner, except the axes represent cumulative probabilities (observed vs. expected) instead of quantiles.

As with any significance test, sample size has an effect on the statistical power of normality tests. With a large sample, minor deviations from normality may be statistically significant, whereas with a small sample, large deviations from normality may not be statistically significant. It's important to keep this in mind when conducting these types of normality tests.

Two commonly used normality tests are the Shapiro-Wilk test and the Kolmogorov-Smirnov test. While there isn't a consensus regarding which normality test is best, the Shapiro-Wilk test has been found to be particularly sensitive to slight deviations from normality, while the Kolmogorov-Smirnov test appears to have poor sensitivity (Razali & Wah, 2011).

Note: you can also examine the skewness and kurtosis statistics to quantitatively assess normality. Ghasemi and Zahediasl (2012) describe this approach in their guide to assessing normality.

Combining methods

As I mentioned earlier in the chapter, it's best to use a combination of qualitative and quantitative methods when assessing normality. I typically start by examining a histogram to get a general impression of how my data is distributed and a Q-Q plot to see if there are marked deviations from normality. If it appears that the assumption of normality may have been violated, I'll conduct a normality test and/or examine sample statistics, such as the skewness statistic, as a follow-up. I consider this all part of 'getting to know my data', which is a critical preliminary step in any analysis.

Appendix B Data transformation

General overview

Most of the inferential statistical procedures covered in this book make certain assumptions regarding normality, homogeneity of variance, and/or linearity. Many times, our data doesn't meet these assumptions. For example, we may have a skewed distribution, there may be large differences in variance between groups, or there may be a nonlinear relationship between variables. One way to address these types of problems is to transform our data.

Data transformation involves applying a mathematical function to replace the original data values with transformed values. Once transformed, the data may better meet the assumptions associated with the statistical procedure we plan to conduct. Some commonly used transformations are log $[X' = \log(X)]$, square root $[X' = \sqrt{X}]$, square $[X' = X^2]$, and reciprocal $[X' = \frac{1}{X}]$ transformations (note: X' represents the transformed version of the variable X). These various transformations can help to address different issues. For instance, log transformations are useful for reducing skew in a distribution, while square root transformation can help to equalize variances between groups. Many times, investigators will try different transformations in order to find the one that best meets their objectives. Then they'll proceed with their analysis using the transformed data.

As an example, consider the data displayed Figure B.1. The histogram in subplot A is based on the original data for the variable X. Notice that this distribution is positively skewed. The

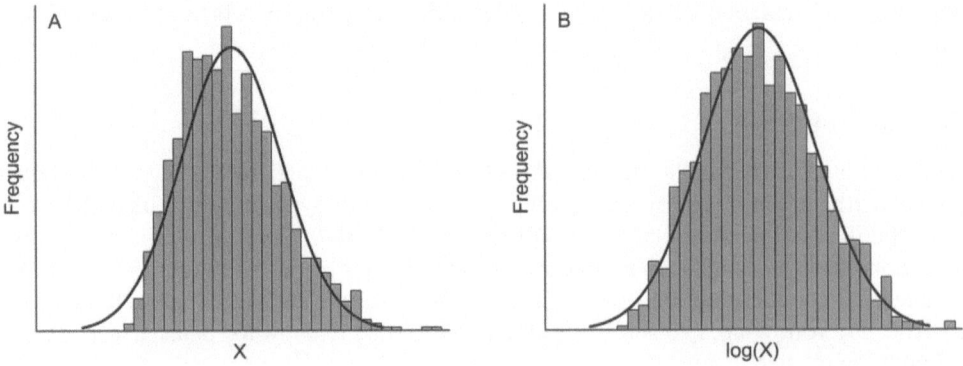

Figure B.1 Subplot A (left) includes a histogram based on the original data for variable X, while subplot B (right) includes a histogram based on the same data which has been log transformed [$\log(X)$]. Notice that log transforming the data helped to reduce the positive skew in the distribution.

histogram in subplot B is based on the same data that has been log transformed [$\log(X)$]. Notice that once transformed, the data is more normally distributed (i.e. less skew). As you can see, this log transformation was effective in reducing the skew in the distribution.

Final thoughts

The purpose of this supplementary chapter was simply to introduce the general purpose and process of data transformation. There's certainly more to consider. If you're preparing to conduct your own analysis and your data fails to meet assumptions related to normality, homogeneity of variance, or linearity, it's worth exploring data transformation procedures in greater detail.

Appendix C Standard normal (z) distribution table.

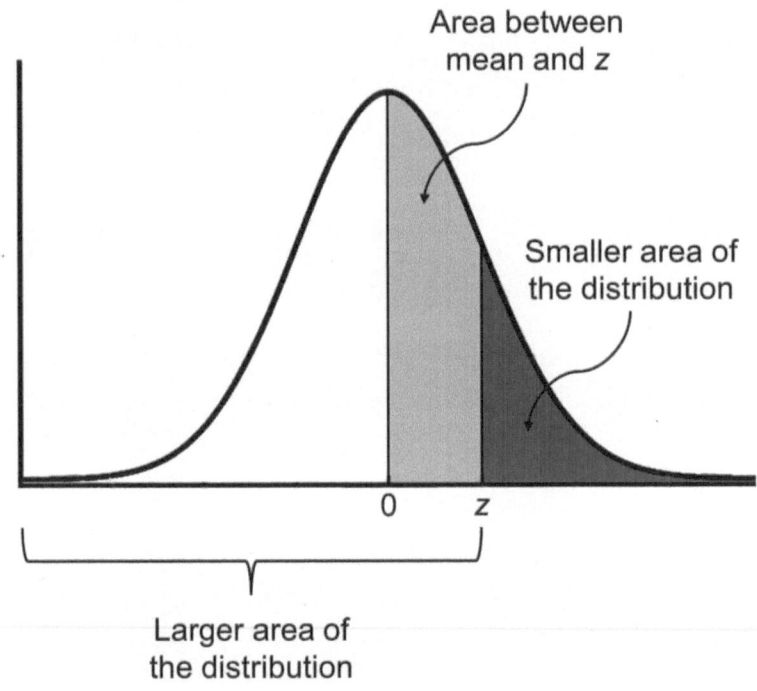

Area between mean and z

Smaller area of the distribution

Larger area of the distribution

z (±)	Area between mean and z	Larger area of the distribution	Smaller area of the distribution
0.00	0.0000	0.5000	0.5000
0.01	0.0040	0.5040	0.4960
0.02	0.0080	0.5080	0.4920
0.03	0.0120	0.5120	0.4880
0.04	0.0160	0.5160	0.4840
0.05	0.0199	0.5199	0.4801
0.06	0.0239	05239	0.4761
0.07	0.0279	0.5279	0.4721
0.08	0.0319	0.5319	0.4681
0.09	0.0359	0.5359	0.4641
0.10	0.0398	0.5398	0.4602

(Continued)

z (±)	Area between mean and z	Larger area of the distribution	Smaller area of the distribution
0.11	0.0438	0.5438	0.4562
0.12	0.0478	0.5478	0.4522
0.13	0.0517	0.5517	0.4483
0.14	0.0557	0.5557	0.4443
0.15	0.0596	0.5596	0.4404
0.16	0.0636	0.5636	0.4364
0.17	0.0675	0.5675	0.4325
0.18	0.0714	0.5714	0.4286
0.19	0.0753	0.5753	0.4247
0.20	0.0793	0.5793	0.4207
0.21	0.0832	0.5832	0.4168
0.22	0.0871	0.5871	0.4129
0.23	0.0910	0.5910	0.4090
0.24	0.0948	0.5948	0.4052
0.25	0.0987	0.5987	0.4013
0.26	0.1026	0.6026	0.3974
0.27	0.1064	0.6064	0.3936
0.28	0.1103	0.6103	0.3897
0.29	0.1141	0.6141	0.3859
0.30	0.1179	0.6179	0.3821
0.31	0.1217	0.6217	0.3783
0.32	0.1255	0.6255	0.3745
0.33	0.1293	0.6293	0.3707
0.34	0.1331	0.6331	0.3669
0.35	0.1368	0.6368	0.3632
0.36	0.1406	0.6406	0.3594
0.37	0.1443	0.6443	0.3557
0.38	0.1480	0.6480	0.3520
0.39	0.1517	0.6517	0.3483
0.40	0.1554	0.6554	0.3446
0.41	0.1591	0.6591	0.3409
0.42	0.1628	0.6628	0.3372
0.43	0.1664	0.6664	0.3336
0.44	0.1700	0.6700	0.3300
0.45	0.1736	0.6736	0.3264
0.46	0.1772	0.6772	0.3228
0.47	0.1808	0.6808	0.3192
0.48	0.1844	0.6844	0.3156
0.49	0.1879	0.6879	0.3121
0.50	0.1915	0.6915	0.3085
0.51	0.1950	0.6950	0.3050
0.52	0.1985	0.6985	0.3015
0.53	0.2019	0.7019	0.2981
0.54	0.2054	0.7054	0.2946
0.55	0.2088	0.7088	0.2912
0.56	0.2123	0.7123	0.2877
0.57	0.2157	0.7157	0.2843
0.58	0.2190	0.7190	0.2810
0.59	0.2224	0.7224	0.2776
0.60	0.2257	0.7257	0.2743
0.61	0.2291	0.7291	0.2709
0.62	0.2324	0.7324	0.2676
0.63	0.2357	0.7357	0.2643
0.64	0.2389	0.7389	0.2611

(Continued)

z (±)	Area between mean and z	Larger area of the distribution	Smaller area of the distribution
0.65	0.2422	0.7422	0.2578
0.66	0.2454	0.7454	0.2546
0.67	0.2486	0.7486	0.2514
0.68	0.2517	0.7517	0.2483
0.69	0.2549	0.7549	0.2451
0.70	0.2580	0.7580	0.2420
0.71	0.2611	0.7611	0.2389
0.72	0.2642	0.7642	0.2358
0.73	0.2673	0.7673	0.2327
0.74	0.2704	0.7704	0.2296
0.75	0.2734	0.7734	0.2266
0.76	0.2764	0.7764	0.2236
0.77	0.2794	0.7794	0.2206
0.78	0.2823	0.7823	0.2177
0.79	0.2852	0.7852	0.2148
0.80	0.2881	0.7881	0.2119
0.81	0.2910	0.7910	0.2090
0.82	0.2939	0.7939	0.2061
0.83	0.2967	0.7967	0.2033
0.84	0.2995	0.7995	0.2005
0.85	0.3023	0.8023	0.1977
0.86	0.3051	0.8051	0.1949
0.87	0.3078	0.8078	0.1922
0.88	0.3106	0.8106	0.1894
0.89	0.3133	0.8133	0.1867
0.90	0.3159	0.8159	0.1841
0.91	0.3186	0.8186	0.1814
0.92	0.3212	0.8212	0.1788
0.93	0.3238	0.8238	0.1762
0.94	0.3264	0.8264	0.1736
0.95	0.3289	0.8289	0.1711
0.96	0.3315	0.8315	0.1685
0.97	0.3340	0.8340	0.1660
0.98	0.3365	0.8365	0.1635
0.99	0.3389	0.8389	0.1611
1.00	0.3413	0.8413	0.1587
1.01	0.3438	0.8438	0.1562
1.02	0.3461	0.8461	0.1539
1.03	0.3485	0.8485	0.1515
1.04	0.3508	0.8508	0.1492
1.05	0.3531	0.8531	0.1469
1.06	0.3554	0.8554	0.1446
1.07	0.3577	0.8577	0.1423
1.08	0.3599	0.8599	0.1401
1.09	0.3621	0.8621	0.1379
1.10	0.3643	0.8643	0.1357
1.11	0.3665	0.8665	0.1335
1.12	0.3686	0.8686	0.1314
1.13	0.3708	0.8708	0.1292
1.14	0.3729	0.8729	0.1271
1.15	0.3749	0.8749	0.1251
1.16	0.3770	0.8770	0.1230
1.17	0.3790	0.8790	0.1210
1.18	0.3810	0.8810	0.1190

(Continued)

z (±)	Area between mean and z	Larger area of the distribution	Smaller area of the distribution
1.19	0.3830	0.8830	0.1170
1.20	0.3849	0.8849	0.1151
1.21	0.3869	0.8869	0.1131
1.22	0.3888	0.8888	0.1112
1.23	0.3907	0.8907	0.1093
1.24	0.3925	0.8925	0.1075
1.25	0.3944	0.8944	0.1056
1.26	0.3962	0.8962	0.1038
1.27	0.3980	0.8980	0.1020
1.28	0.3997	0.8997	0.1003
1.29	0.4015	0.9015	0.0985
1.30	0.4032	0.9032	0.0968
1.31	0.4049	0.9049	0.0951
1.32	0.4066	0.9066	0.0934
1.33	0.4082	0.9082	0.0918
1.34	0.4090	0.9099	0.0901
1.35	0.4115	0.9115	0.0885
1.36	0.4131	0.9131	0.0869
1.37	0.4147	0.9147	0.0853
1.38	0.4162	0.9162	0.0838
1.39	0.4177	0.9177	0.0823
1.40	0.4192	0.9192	0.0808
1.41	0.4207	0.9207	0.0793
1.42	0.4222	0.9222	0.0778
1.43	0.4236	0.9236	0.0764
1.44	0.4251	0.9251	0.0749
1.45	0.4265	0.9265	0.0735
1.46	0.4279	0.9279	0.0721
1.47	0.4292	0.9292	0.0708
1.48	0.4306	0.9306	0.0694
1.49	0.4319	0.9319	0.0681
1.50	0.4332	0.9332	0.0668
1.51	0.4345	0.9345	0.0655
1.52	0.4357	0.9357	0.0643
1.53	0.4370	0.9370	0.0630
1.54	0.4382	0.9382	0.0618
1.55	0.4394	0.9394	0.0606
1.56	0.4406	0.9406	0.0594
1.57	0.4418	0.9418	0.0582
1.58	0.4429	0.9429	0.0571
1.59	0.4441	0.9441	0.0559
1.60	0.4452	0.9452	0.0548
1.61	0.4463	0.9463	0.0537
1.62	0.4474	0.9474	0.0526
1.63	0.4484	0.9484	0.0516
1.64	0.4495	0.9495	0.0505
1.645	**0.4500**	**0.9500**	**0.0500**
1.65	0.4505	0.9505	0.0495
1.66	0.4515	0.9515	0.0485
1.67	0.4525	0.9525	0.0475
1.68	0.4535	0.9535	0.0465
1.69	0.4545	0.9545	0.0455
1.70	0.4554	0.9554	0.0446
1.71	0.4564	0.9564	0.0436

(Continued)

z (±)	Area between mean and z	Larger area of the distribution	Smaller area of the distribution
1.72	0.4573	0.9573	0.0427
1.73	0.4582	0.9582	0.0418
1.74	0.4591	0.9591	0.0409
1.75	0.4599	0.9599	0.0401
1.76	0.4608	0.9608	0.0392
1.77	0.4616	0.9616	0.0384
1.78	0.4625	0.9625	0.0375
1.79	0.4633	0.9633	0.0367
1.80	0.4641	0.9641	0.0359
1.81	0.4649	0.9649	0.0351
1.82	0.4656	0.9656	0.0344
1.83	0.4664	0.9664	0.0336
1.84	0.4671	0.9671	0.0329
1.85	0.4678	0.9678	0.0322
1.86	0.4686	0.9686	0.0314
1.87	0.4693	0.9693	0.0307
1.88	0.4699	0.9699	0.0301
1.89	0.4706	0.9706	0.0294
1.90	0.4713	0.9713	0.0287
1.91	0.4719	0.9719	0.0281
1.92	0.4726	0.9726	0.0274
1.93	0.4732	0.9732	0.0268
1.94	0.4738	0.9738	0.0262
1.95	0.4744	0.9744	0.0256
1.96	**0.4750**	**0.9750**	**0.0250**
1.97	0.4756	0.9756	0.0244
1.98	0.4761	0.9761	0.0239
1.99	0.4767	0.9767	0.0233
2.00	0.4772	0.9772	0.0228
2.01	0.4778	0.9778	0.0222
2.02	0.4783	0.9783	0.0217
2.03	0.4788	0.9788	0.0212
2.04	0.4793	0.9793	0.0207
2.05	0.4798	0.9798	0.0202
2.06	0.4803	0.9803	0.0197
2.07	0.4808	0.9808	0.0192
2.08	0.4812	0.9812	0.0188
2.09	0.4817	0.9817	0.0183
2.10	0.4821	0.9821	0.0179
2.11	0.4826	0.9826	0.0174
2.12	0.4830	0.9830	0.0170
2.13	0.4834	0.9834	0.0166
2.14	0.4838	0.9838	0.0162
2.15	0.4842	0.9842	0.0158
2.16	0.4846	0.9846	0.0154
2.17	0.4850	0.9850	0.0150
2.18	0.4854	0.9854	0.0146
2.19	0.4857	0.9857	0.0143
2.20	0.4861	0.9861	0.0139
2.21	0.4864	0.9864	0.0136
2.22	0.4868	0.9868	0.0132
2.23	0.4871	0.9871	0.0129
2.24	0.4875	0.9875	0.0125
2.25	0.4878	0.9878	0.0122

(Continued)

z (±)	Area between mean and z	Larger area of the distribution	Smaller area of the distribution
2.26	0.4881	0.9881	0.0119
2.27	0.4884	0.9884	0.0116
2.28	0.4887	0.9887	0.0113
2.29	0.4890	0.9890	0.0110
2.30	0.4893	0.9893	0.0107
2.31	0.4896	0.9896	0.0104
2.32	0.4898	0.9898	0.0102
2.33	0.4901	0.9901	0.0099
2.34	0.4904	0.9904	0.0096
2.35	0.4906	0.9906	0.0094
2.36	0.4909	0.9909	0.0091
2.37	0.4911	0.9911	0.0089
2.38	0.4913	0.9913	0.0087
2.39	0.4916	0.9916	0.0084
2.40	0.4918	0.9918	0.0082
2.41	0.4920	0.9920	0.0080
2.42	0.4922	0.9922	0.0078
2.43	0.4925	0.9925	0.0075
2.44	0.4927	0.9927	0.0073
2.45	0.4929	0.9929	0.0071
2.46	0.4931	0.9931	0.0069
2.47	0.4932	0.9932	0.0068
2.48	0.4934	0.9934	0.0066
2.49	0.4936	0.9936	0.0064
2.50	0.4938	0.9938	0.0062
2.51	0.4940	0.9940	0.0060
2.52	0.4941	0.9941	0.0059
2.53	0.4943	0.9943	0.0057
2.54	0.4945	0.9945	0.0055
2.55	0.4946	0.9946	0.0054
2.56	0.4948	0.9948	0.0052
2.57	0.4949	0.9949	0.0051
2.576	**0.4950**	**0.9950**	**0.0050**
2.58	0.4951	0.9951	0.0049
2.59	0.4952	0.9952	0.0048
2.60	0.4953	0.9953	0.0047
2.61	0.4955	0.9955	0.0045
2.62	0.4956	0.9956	0.0044
2.63	0.4957	0.9957	0.0043
2.64	0.4959	0.9959	0.0041
2.65	0.4960	0.9960	0.0040
2.66	0.4961	0.9961	0.0039
2.67	0.4962	0.9962	0.0038
2.68	0.4963	0.9963	0.0037
2.69	0.4964	0.9964	0.0036
2.70	0.4965	0.9965	0.0035
2.71	0.4966	0.9966	0.0034
2.72	0.4967	0.9967	0.0033
2.73	0.4968	0.9968	0.0032
2.74	0.4969	0.9969	0.0031
2.75	0.4970	0.9970	0.0030
2.76	0.4971	0.9971	0.0029
2.77	0.4972	0.9972	0.0028
2.78	0.4973	0.9973	0.0027

(Continued)

z (±)	Area between mean and z	Larger area of the distribution	Smaller area of the distribution
2.79	0.4974	0.9974	0.0026
2.80	0.4974	0.9974	0.0026
2.81	0.4975	0.9975	0.0025
2.82	0.4976	0.9976	0.0024
2.83	0.4977	0.9977	0.0023
2.84	0.4977	0.9977	0.0023
2.85	0.4978	0.9978	0.0022
2.86	0.4979	0.9979	0.0021
2.87	0.4979	0.9979	0.0021
2.88	0.4980	0.9980	0.0020
2.89	0.4981	0.9981	0.0019
2.90	0.4981	0.9981	0.0019
2.91	0.4982	0.9982	0.0018
2.92	0.4982	0.9982	0.0018
2.93	0.4983	0.9983	0.0017
2.94	0.4984	0.9984	0.0016
2.95	0.4984	0.9984	0.0016
2.96	0.4985	0.9985	0.0015
2.97	0.4985	0.9985	0.0015
2.98	0.4986	0.9986	0.0014
2.99	0.4986	0.9986	0.0014
3.00	0.4987	0.9987	0.0013
…	…	…	…
3.25	0.4994	0.9994	0.0006
…	…	…	…
3.50	0.4998	0.9998	0.0002
…	…	…	…

Bolded z values correspond with 90% (1.645), 95% (1.96), and 99% (2.576) confidence intervals

Appendix D Critical values of t

Degrees of freedom	Alpha level – one-tailed test				
	0.10	0.05	0.025	0.01	0.005
	Alpha level – two-tailed test				
	0.20	0.10	0.05	0.02	0.01
1	3.078	6.314	12.706	31.821	63.657
2	1.886	2.920	4.303	6.965	9.925
3	1.638	2.353	3.182	4.541	5.841
4	1.533	2.132	2.776	3.747	4.604
5	1.476	2.015	2.571	3.365	4.032
6	1.440	1.943	2.447	3.143	3.707
7	1.415	1.895	2.365	2.998	3.499
8	1.397	1.860	2.306	2.896	3.355
9	1.383	1.833	2.262	2.821	3.250
10	1.372	1.812	2.228	2.764	3.169
11	1.363	1.796	2.201	2.718	3.106
12	1.356	1.782	2.179	2.681	3.055
13	1.350	1.771	2.160	2.650	3.012
14	1.345	1.761	2.145	2.624	2.977
15	1.341	1.753	2.131	2.602	2.947
16	1.337	1.746	2.120	2.583	2.921
17	1.333	1.740	2.110	2.567	2.898
18	1.330	1.734	2.101	2.552	2.878
19	1.328	1.729	2.093	2.539	2.861
20	1.325	1.725	2.086	2.528	2.845
21	1.323	1.721	2.080	2.518	2.831
22	1.321	1.717	2.074	2.508	2.819
23	1.319	1.714	2.069	2.500	2.807
24	1.318	1.711	2.064	2.492	2.797
25	1.316	1.708	2.060	2.485	2.787
26	1.315	1.706	2.056	2.479	2.779
27	1.314	1.703	2.052	2.473	2.771
28	1.313	1.701	2.048	2.467	2.763
29	1.311	1.699	2.045	2.462	2.756
30	1.310	1.697	2.042	2.457	2.750
…	…	…	…	…	…
40	1.303	1.684	2.021	2.423	2.704
…	…	…	…	…	…
50	1.299	1.676	2.009	2.403	2.678
…	…	…	…	…	…

(Continued)

Degrees of freedom	Alpha level – one-tailed test				
	0.10	0.05	0.025	0.01	0.005
	Alpha level – two-tailed test				
	0.20	0.10	0.05	0.02	0.01
60	1.296	1.671	2.000	2.390	2.660
…	…	…	…	…	…
70	1.294	1.667	1.994	2.381	2.648
…	…	…	…	…	…
80	1.292	1.664	1.990	2.374	2.639
…	…	…	…	…	…
90	1.291	1.662	1.987	2.368	2.632
…	…	…	…	…	…
100	1.290	1.660	1.984	2.364	2.626

Note: the null hypothesis is rejected when the t-statistic exceeds the t critical value

Appendix E Critical values of F (alpha level = 0.05)

Degrees of freedom in the denominator	Degrees of freedom in the numerator									
	1	2	3	4	5	6	7	8	9	10
1	161.45	199.50	215.71	224.58	230.16	233.99	236.77	238.88	240.54	241.88
2	18.51	19.00	19.16	19.24	19.30	19.33	19.35	19.37	19.38	19.40
3	10.13	9.55	9.28	9.12	9.01	8.94	8.89	8.85	8.81	8.79
4	7.71	6.94	6.59	6.39	6.26	6.16	6.09	6.04	6.00	5.96
5	6.61	5.79	5.41	5.19	5.05	4.95	4.88	4.82	4.77	4.74
6	5.99	5.14	4.76	4.53	4.39	4.28	4.21	4.15	4.10	4.06
7	5.59	4.74	4.35	4.12	3.97	3.87	3.79	3.73	3.68	3.64
8	5.32	4.46	4.07	3.84	3.69	3.58	3.50	3.44	3.39	3.35
9	5.12	4.26	3.86	3.63	3.48	3.37	3.29	3.23	3.18	3.14
10	4.96	4.10	3.71	3.48	3.33	3.22	3.14	3.07	3.02	2.98
11	4.84	3.98	3.59	3.36	3.20	3.09	3.01	2.95	2.90	2.85
12	4.75	3.89	3.49	3.26	3.11	3.00	2.91	2.85	2.80	2.75
13	4.67	3.81	3.41	3.18	3.03	2.92	2.83	2.77	2.71	2.67
14	4.60	3.74	3.34	3.11	2.96	2.85	2.76	2.70	2.65	2.60
15	4.54	3.68	3.29	3.06	2.90	2.79	2.71	2.64	2.59	2.54
16	4.49	3.63	3.24	3.01	2.85	2.74	2.66	2.59	2.54	2.49
17	4.45	3.59	3.20	2.96	2.81	2.70	2.61	2.55	2.49	2.45
18	4.41	3.55	3.16	2.93	2.77	2.66	2.58	2.51	2.46	2.41
19	4.38	3.52	3.13	2.90	2.74	2.63	2.54	2.48	2.42	2.38
20	4.35	3.49	3.10	2.87	2.71	2.60	2.51	2.45	2.39	2.35
...	...	...	...	...	...	...	...	...	...	...
30	4.17	3.32	2.92	2.69	2.53	2.42	2.33	2.27	2.21	2.16
...	...	...	...	...	...	...	...	...	...	...
40	4.08	3.23	2.84	2.61	2.45	2.34	2.25	2.18	2.12	2.08
...	...	...	...	...	...	...	...	...	...	...
50	4.03	3.18	2.79	2.56	2.40	2.29	2.20	2.13	2.07	2.03
...	...	...	...	...	...	...	...	...	...	...
60	4.00	3.15	2.76	2.53	2.37	2.25	2.17	2.10	2.04	1.99
...	...	...	...	...	...	...	...	...	...	...
70	3.98	3.13	2.74	2.50	2.35	2.23	2.14	2.07	2.02	1.97
...	...	...	...	...	...	...	...	...	...	...
80	3.96	3.11	2.72	2.49	2.33	2.21	2.13	2.06	2.00	1.95
...	...	...	...	...	...	...	...	...	...	...
90	3.95	3.10	2.71	2.47	2.32	2.20	2.11	2.04	1.99	1.94
...	...	...	...	...	...	...	...	...	...	...
100	3.94	3.09	2.70	2.46	2.31	2.19	2.10	2.03	1.97	1.93

Note: the null hypothesis is rejected when the F-statistic exceeds the F critical value

Appendix F Critical values of chi-square

Degrees of freedom	Alpha level				
	0.10	0.05	0.025	0.01	0.005
1	2.706	3.841	5.024	6.635	7.879
2	4.605	5.991	7.378	9.210	10.597
3	6.251	7.815	9.348	11.345	12.838
4	7.779	9.488	11.143	13.277	14.860
5	9.236	11.071	12.833	15.086	16.750
6	10.645	12.592	14.449	16.812	18.548
7	12.017	14.067	16.013	18.475	20.278
8	13.362	15.507	17.535	20.090	21.955
9	14.684	16.919	19.023	21.666	23.589
10	15.987	18.307	20.483	23.209	25.188
11	17.275	19.675	21.920	24.725	26.757
12	18.549	21.026	23.337	26.217	28.299
13	19.812	22.362	24.736	27.688	29.819
14	21.064	23.685	26.119	29.141	31.319
15	22.307	24.996	27.488	30.578	32.801
16	23.542	26.296	28.845	32.000	34.267
17	24.769	27.587	30.191	33.409	35.718
18	25.989	28.869	31.526	34.805	37.156
19	27.204	30.144	32.852	36.191	38.582
20	28.412	31.410	34.170	37.566	39.997
21	29.615	32.671	35.479	38.932	41.401
22	30.813	33.924	36.781	40.289	42.796
23	32.007	35.172	38.076	41.638	44.181
24	33.196	36.415	39.364	42.980	45.559
25	34.382	37.652	40.646	44.314	46.928
26	35.563	38.885	41.923	45.642	48.290
27	36.741	40.113	43.194	46.963	49.645
28	37.916	41.337	44.461	48.278	50.993
29	39.087	42.557	45.722	49.588	52.336
30	40.256	43.773	46.979	50.892	53.672
...	...	...	...	...	...
40	51.805	55.758	59.342	63.691	66.766
...	...	...	...	...	...
50	63.167	67.505	71.420	76.154	79.490
...	...	...	...	...	...
60	74.397	79.082	83.298	88.379	91.952
...	...	...	...	...	...
70	85.527	90.531	95.023	100.425	104.215
...	...	...	...	...	...

(Continued)

Degrees of freedom	Alpha level				
	0.10	*0.05*	*0.025*	*0.01*	*0.005*
80	96.578	101.879	106.629	112.329	116.321
…	…	…	…	…	…
90	107.565	113.145	118.136	124.116	128.299
…	…	…	…	…	…
100	118.498	124.342	129.561	135.807	140.169

Note: the null hypothesis is rejected when the chi-square statistic exceeds the chi-square critical value

References

Almonroeder TG, Jayawickrema J, Richardson CT, Mercker KL. The influence of attentional focus on landing stiffness in female athletes: a cross-sectional study. *Int J Sports Phys Ther*. 2020;15(4): 510–518.

American Thoracic Society, Committee on Proficiency Standard for Clinical Pulmonary Function Laboratories. ATS statement: guidelines for the six-minute walk test. *Am J Respir Crit Care Med*. 2002;166(1):111–117.

Berg K, Wood-Dauphinee S, Williams JI, Gayton D. Measuring balance in the elderly: preliminary development of an instrument. *Physiotherapy Canada*. 1989;41(6):304–311.

Biering-Sorensen F. Physical measurements as risk indicators for low-back trouble over a one-year period. *Spine*. 1984;9(2):1106–119.

Bologna M, Leodori G, Stirpe P, Paparella G, Colella D, Belvisi D, Fasano A, Fabbrini G, Berardelli A. Bradykinesia in early and advanced Parkinson's disease. *J Neurol Sci*. 2016;369:286–291.

Butland RJ, Pang J, Gross ER, Woodcock AA, Geddes DM. Two-, six-, and 12-minute walking tests in respiratory disease. *Br Med J*. 1982;284(6329):1607–1608.

Carville SF, Perry MC, Rutherford OM, Smith ICH, Newham DJ. Steadiness of quadriceps contractions in young and older adults with and without a history of falling. *Eur J Appl Physiol*. 2007;100(5);527–533.

Chen Y-S, Cai Y-X, Kang X-R, Zhou Z-H, Qi X, Ying C-T, Zhang Y-P, Tao J. Predicting the risk of sarcopenia in elderly patients with patellar fracture: development and assessment of a new predictive nomogram. *PeerJ*. 2020;8:e8793.

Cheung RTH, Sze LKY, Mok NW, Ng GYF. Intrinsic foot muscle volume in experienced runners with and without chronic plantar fasciitis. *J Sci Med Sport*. 2016;19(9):713–715.

Cholewicki J, Reeves NP, Everding VQ, Morrisette DC. Lumbosacral orthoses reduce trunk muscle activity in a postural control task. *J Biomech*. 2007;40(8):1731–1736.

Cohen J. *Statistical Power Analysis for the Behavioral Sciences*. 2nd edition. Hillsdale, NJ: Lawrence Erlbaum Associates; 1988.

Cohen J. The earth is round (*p* < .05). *Am Psychol*. 1994;49(12):997–1003.

Cox DR, Snell DJ. *The Analysis of Binary Data*. London: Chapman & Hall; 1989.

Deering RE, Chumanov ES, Stiffler-Joachim MR, Heiderscheit BC. Exercise program reduces inter-recti distance in female runners up to 2 years postpartum. *J Women's Health Physical Therapy*. 2020;44(1):9–18.

Delmore B, Lebovits S, Suggs B, Rolnitzky L, Ayello EA. Risk factors associated with heel pressure ulcers in hospitalized patients. *J Wound Ostomy Continence Nurs*. 2015;42(3):242–248.

Eitzen I, Fernandes L, Nordsletten L, Risberg MA. Sagittal plane gait characteristics in hip osteoarthritis patients with mild to moderate symptoms compared to health controls: a cross-sectional study. *BMC Musculoskelet Disord*. 2012;13:258.

Eken MM, Dallmeijer AJ, Buizer AI, Hogervorst S, van Hutten K, Piening M, van der Krogt M, Houdijk H. Intraobserver reliability and construct validity of the squat test in children with cerebral palsy. *Pediatr Phys Ther*. 2020;32(4):399–403.

Eken MM, Harlaar J, Dallmeijer AJ, de Waard E, van Bennekom CAM, Houdijk H. Squat test performance and execution in children with and without cerebral palsy. *Clin Biomech.* 2017;41:98–105.

Falvo MJ, Earhart GM. Six-minute walk distances in persons with Parkinson disease: a hierarchical regression model. *Arch Phys Med Rehabil.* 2009;90(6):1004–1008.

Faul F, Erdfelder E, Buchner A, Lang A-G. Statistical power analyses using G*Power 3.1: tests for correlation and regression analyses. *Behav Res Methods.* 2009;41(4):1149–1160.

Faul F, Erdfelder, Lang A-G, Buchner A. G*Power 3: a flexible statistical power analysis program for the social, behavioral, and biomedical sciences. *Behav Res Methods.* 2007;39(2):175–191.

Freire APCF, Elkins MR, Ramos EMC, Moseley AM. Use of 95% confidence intervals in the reporting of between-group differences in randomized controlled trials: analysis of a representative sample of 200 physical therapy trials. *Braz J Phys Ther.* 2019;23(4):302–310.

Fryar CD, Carroll MD, Gu Q, Afful J, Ogden CL. Anthropometric reference data for children and adults: United States, 2015–2018. *Vital Health Stat 3.* 2021;36:1:44.

Garcia-Pinillos F, Carton-Llorente A, Jaen-Carrillo D, Delgado-Floody P, Carrasco-Alarcon V, Martinez C, Roche-Seruendo LE. Does fatigue alter step characteristics and stiffness during running? *Gait Posture.* 2020;76:259–263.

Ghaderi M, Letafatkar A, Almonroeder TG, Keyhani S. Neuromuscular training improves knee proprioception in athletes with a history of anterior cruciate ligament reconstruction: a randomized controlled trial. *Clin Biomech.* 2020;80:105157.

Ghasemi A, Zahediasl S. Normality tests for statistical analysis: a guide for non-statisticians. *Int J Endocrinol Metab.* 2012;10(2):486–489.

Granger CV, Hamilton BB, Keith RA, Zielezny M, Sherwin FS. Advances in functional assessment for medical rehabilitation. *Top Geriatr Rehabil.* 1986;1(3):59–74.

Green SB. How many subjects does it take to do a regression analysis? *Multivariate Behav Res.* 1991;26(3):499–510.

Grenier JG, Peyrot N, Castells J, Oullion R, Messonnier L, Morin J-B. Energy cost and mechanical work of walking during load carriage in soldiers. *Med Sci Sports Exerc.* 2012;44(6):1131–1140.

Hannigan JJ, Pollard CD. Differences in running biomechanics between a maximal, traditional, and minimal running shoe. *J Sci Med Sport.* 2020;23(1):15–19.

Hobara H, Sakata H, Hashizume S, Kobayashi Y. Leg stiffness in unilateral transfemoral amputees across a range of running speeds. *J Biomech.* 2019;84:67–72.

Hollman JH, Kovash FM, Kubik JJ, Linbo RA. Age-related differences in spatiotemporal markers of gait stability during dual task walking. *Gait Posture.* 2007;26(1):113–119.

Holm B, Kristensen MT, Bencke J, Husted H, Kehlet H, Bandholm T. Loss of knee-extension strength is related to knee swelling after total knee arthroplasty. *Arch Phys Med Rehabil.* 2010;91(11): 1770–1776.

Hosseinzadeh S, Kiapour AM. Age-related changes in ACL morphology during skeletal growth and maturation are different between females and males. *J Orthop Res.* 2021;39(4):841–849.

Hsu Y-W, Somma J, Hung Y-C, Tsai P-S, Yang C-H, Chen C-C. Predicting postoperative pain by preoperative pressure pain assessment. *Anesthesiology.* 2005;103(3):613–618.

Huberty CJ, Morris JD. Multivariate analysis versus multiple univariate analyses. *Phsycol Bull.* 1989;105(2):302–308.

Ireland ML, Willson JD, Ballantyne BT, Davis IM. Hip strength in females with and without patellofemoral pain. *J Orthop Sports Phys Ther.* 2003;33(11):671–676.

Jerez-Mayorga D, Rios LJC, Reyes A, Delgado-Floody P, Payer RM, Requena IMG. Muscle quality index and isometric strength in older adults with hip osteoarthritis. *PeerJ.* 2019;7:e7471.

Jewell DV. *Guide to Evidence-Based Physical Therapy Practice.* Burlington, MA: Jones & Bartlett Learning; 2018.

Kaji A, Sasagawa S, Kubo T, Kanehisa H. Transient effect of core stability exercises on postural sway during quiet standing. *J Strength Cond Res.* 2010;24(2):382–388.

Kamper SJ. Confidence intervals: linking evidence to practice. *J Orthop Sports Phys Ther.* 2019;49(10):763–764.

Kennedy-Shaffer L. Before $p < 0.05$ to beyond $p < 0.05$: using history to contextualize p-values and significance testing. *Am Stat*. 2019;73:82–90.

Khalaj N, Osman NAA, Mokhtar AH, Mehdikhani M, Abas WABW. Balance and risk of fall in individuals with bilateral mild and moderate knee osteoarthritis. *PLoS One*. 2014;9(3):e92270.

Kim PS, Mayhew JL, Peterson DF. A modified YMCA bench press test as a predictor of 1 repetition maximum bench press strength. *J Strength Cond Rest*. 2002;16(3):440–445.

Kobayashi Y, Hobara H, Matsushita S, Mochimaru M. Key joint kinematic characteristics of the gait of fallers identified by principal component analysis. *J Biomech*. 2014;47(1):2424–2429.

Koontz AM, Cooper RA, Boninger ML, Souza AL, Fay BT. Shoulder kinematics and kinetics during two speeds of wheelchair propulsion. *J Rehabil Res Dev*. 2002;39(6):635–649.

Kwan MM-S, Lin S-I, Chen C-H, Close JCT, Lord SR. Sensorimotor function, balance abilities and pain influence Timed Up and Go performance in older community-living people. *Aging Clin Exp Res*. 2011;23(3):196–201.

Lakens D. Calculating and reporting effect sizes to facilitate cumulative science: a practical primer for t-tests and ANOVAs. *Front Psychol*. 2013;4:863.

Lariviere C, Gagnon DH, Mecheri H. Trunk postural control in unstable sitting: effect of sex and low back pain status. *Clin Biomech*. 2015;30(9):933–939.

Lehecka BJ, Turley J, Stapleton A, Waits K, Zirkle J. The effects of gluteal squeezes compared to bilateral bridges on gluteal strength, power, endurance, and girth. *PeerJ*. 2019;7:e7287.

Llamas-Ramos R, Pecos-Martin D, Gallego-Izquierdo T, Llamas-Ramos I, Plaza-Manzano G, Ortega-Santiago R, Cleland J, Fernandez-de-Las-Penas C. Comparison of the short-term outcomes between trigger point dry needling and trigger point manual therapy for the management of chronic mechanical neck pain: a randomized clinical trial. *J Orthop Sports Phys Ther*. 2014;44(11):852–861.

MacLennan RJ, Sahebi M, Becker N, Davis E, Garcia JM, Stock MS. Declines in skeletal muscle quality vs. size following two weeks of knee joint immobilization. *PeerJ*. 2020;8:e8224.

Madansingh SI, Ngufor CG, Fortune E. Quality over quantity: skeletal loading intensity plays a key role in understanding the relationship between physical activity and bone density in postmenopausal women. *Menopause*. 2020;27(4):444–449.

Magadle R, McConnell AK, Beckerman M, Weiner P. Inspiratory muscle training in pulmonary rehabilitation program in COPD patients. *Respir Med*. 2007;101(7):1500–1505.

Mangione KK, Craik RL, Lopopolo R, Tomlinson JD, Brenneman SK. Predictors of gait speed in patients after hip fracture. *Physiother Can*. 2008;60(1):10–18.

Mathiowetz V, Weber K, Kashman N, Volland G. Adult norms for the nine hole peg test for finger dexterity. *OTJR*. 1985;5(1):24–38.

McShane BB, Gal D, Gelman A, Robert C, Tackett JL. Abandon statistical significance. *Am Stat*. 2019;73:235–245.

Mistry S, Ali T, Qasheesh M, Beg RA, Shaphe MA, Ahmad F, Kashoo FZ, Shalaby AS. Assessment of hand function in women with lymphadenopathy after radical mastectomy. *PeerJ*. 2021;9:e11252.

Nagelkerke NJD. A note on a general definition of the coefficient of determination. *Biometrika*. 1991;78:691–692.

O'Connell N, Dai L, Jiang Y, Speiser JL, Ward R, Wie W, Carroll R, Gebregziabher M. Methods for analysis of pre-post data in clinical research: a comparison of five common methods. *J Biom Biostat*. 2017;8(1):1–8.

Parker JC, Frank RG, Beck NC, Smarr KL, Buescher KL, Phillips LR, Smith EI, Anderson SK, Walker SE. Pain management in rheumatoid arthritis patients. A cognitive-behavioral approach. *Arthritis Rheum*. 1988;31(5):593–601.

Paterno MV, Schmitt LC, Ford KR, Rauh MJ, Myer GD, Hewett TE. Effects of sex on compensatory landing strategies upon return to sport after anterior cruciate ligament reconstruction. *J Orthop Sports Phys Ther*. 2011;41(8):553–559.

Pereira S, Foley N, Salter K, McClure JA, Meyer M, Brown J, Speechley M, Teasell R. Discharge destination of individuals with severe stroke undergoing rehabilitation: a predictive model. *Disabil Rehabil*. 2014;36(9):727–731.

Podsiadlo D, Richardson S. The timed "Up & Go": a test of basic functional mobility for frail elderly persons. *J Am Geriatr Soc*. 1991;39(2):142–148.

Portney LG. *Foundations of Clinical Research: Applications to Evidence-Based Practice*. Philadelphia, PA: F. A. Davis Company; 2020.

Razali NM, Wah YB. Power comparisons of Shapiro-Wilk, Kolmogorov-Smirnov, Lilliefors and Anderson-Darling tests. *J Stat Modeling and Analytics*. 2011;2(1):21–33.

Reinold MM, Wilk KE, Fleisig GS, Zheng N, Barrentine SW, Chmielewski T, Cody RC, Jameson GG, Andrews JR. Electromyographic analysis of the rotator cuff and deltoid musculature during common shoulder external rotation exercises. *J Orthop Sports Phys Ther*. 2004;34(7):385–394.

Reinold MM, Wilk KE, Macrina LC, Sheheane C, Dun S, Flesig GS, Crenshaw K, Andrews JR. Changes in shoulder and elbow passive range of motion after pitching in professional baseball players. *Am J Sports Med*. 2008;36(3):523–527.

Roberts LA, Nosaka K, Coombes JS, Peake JM. Cold water immersion enhances recovery of submaximal muscle function after resistance exercise. *Am J Physiol Regul Integr Comp Physiol*. 2014;307(8):R998–R1008.

Rosnow RL, Rosenthal R. Statistical procedures and the justification of knowledge in psychological science. *Am Psychol*. 1989;44(10):1276–1284.

Sarzynski MA, Rankinen T, Earnest CP, Leon AS, Rao DC, Skinner JS, Bouchard C. Measured maximal heart rates compared to commonly used age-based prediction equations in the Heritage Family Study. *Am J Hum Biol*. 2013;25(5):695–701.

Schucker L, Hagemann N, Strauss B, Volker K. The effect of attentional focus on running economy. *J Sports Sci*. 2009;27(12):1241–1248.

Schwartz SJ, Sturr M, Goldberg G. Statistical methods in rehabilitation literature: a survey of recent publications. *Arch Phys Med Rehabil*. 1996;77(5):497–500.

Shimoyama Y, Sawai T, Tatsumi S, Nakahira J, Oka M, Nakajima M, Jotoku T, Minami T. Perioperative risk factors for deep vein thrombosis after total hip arthroplasty or total knee arthroplasty. *J Clin Anesth*. 2012;24(7):531–536.

Son D-H, Yoo J-W, Cho M-R, Lee Y-J. Relationship between handgrip strength and pulmonary function in apparently healthy older women. *J Am Geriatr Soc*. 2018;66(7):1367–1371.

Stevens SS. On the theory of scales of measurement. *Science*. 1946;103(2684):677–680.

Streiner DL, Norman GR. Correction for multiple testing: is there a resolution? *Chest*. 2011;140(1):16–18.

Stricker M, Hinde D, Rolland A, Salzman N, Watson A, Almonroeder TG. Quantifying step length using two-dimensional video in individuals with Parkinson's disease. *Physiother Theory Pract*. 2021;37(1):252–255.

Student. The probable error of a mean. *Biometrika*. 1908;6:1–25.

Tabachnick BG, Fidell LS. *Using Multivariate Statistics*. Hoboken, NJ: Pearson; 2019.

Tanaka H, Monahan KD, Seals DR. Age-predicted maximal heart rate revisited. *J Am Coll Cardio*. 2001;37(1):153–156.

Terradas-Monllor M, Ochandorena-Acha M, Salinas-Chesa J, Ramirez S, Beltran-Alacreu H. Assessment of postoperative health functioning after knee arthroplasty in relation to pain catastrophizing: a 6-month follow-up cohort study. *PeerJ*. 2020;8:e9903.

Thompson B. Significance, effect sizes, stepwise methods, and other issues: strong arguments move the field. *J Exp Educ*. 2001;70(1):80–93.

Tiedemann A, Shimada H, Sherrington C, Murray S, Lord S. The comparative ability of eight functional mobility tests for predicting falls in community-dwelling older adults. *Age Ageing*. 2008;37(4):430–435.

Tsang YL, Mak MK. Sit-and-reach test can predict mobility of patients recovering from acute stroke. *Arch Phys Med Rehabil*. 2004;85(1):94–98.

Vacek PM, Slauterbeck JR, Tourville TW, Sturnick DR, Holterman L-A, Smith HC, Schultz SJ, Johnson RJ, Tourville KJ, Beynnon BD. Multivariate analysis of the risk factors for first-time noncontact ACL injury in high school and college athletes. *Am J Sports Med*. 2016;44(6):1492–1501.

Van Breukelen GJP. ANCOVA versus change from baseline: more power in randomized studies, more bias in nonrandomized studies. *J Clin Epidemiol.* 2006;59(9):920–925.

Wainner RS, Fritz JM, Irrgang JJ, Boninger ML, Delitto A, Allison S. Reliability and diagnostic accuracy of the clinical examination and patient self-report measures for cervical radiculopathy. *Spine.* 2003;28(1):52–62.

Wee JYM, Hopman WM. Stroke impairment predictors of discharge function, length of stay, and discharge destination in stroke rehabilitation. *A J Phys Med Rehabil.* 2005;84(8):604–612.

Wisloff U, Castagna C, Helgerud J, Jones R, Hoff J. Strong correlation of maximal squat strength with sprint performance and vertical jump height in elite soccer players. *Br J Sports Med.* 2004;38(3):285–288.

Wright DB, London K. *First (and Second) Steps in Statistics.* Thousand Oaks, CA: SAGE Publications Inc.; 2009.

Yalamanchi SV, Stewart KJ, Ji N, Golden SH, Dobs A, Becker DM, Vaidya D, Kral BG, Kalyani RR. The relationship of fasting hyperglycemia to changes in fat and muscle mass after exercise training in type 2 diabetes. *Diabetes Res Clin Pract.* 2016;122:154–161.

Yavuz HU, Erdag D, Amca AM, Aritan S. Kinematics and EMG activities during front and back squat variations in maximum loads. *J Sports Sci.* 2015;33(10):1058–1066.

Yavuzer G, Selles R, Sezer N, Sutbeyaz S, Bussmann JB, Koseoglu F, Atay MB, Stam HJ. Mirror therapy improves hand function in subacute stroke: a randomized controlled trial. *Arch Phys Med Rehabil.* 2008;89(3):393–398.

Zaffagnini S, Marcacci M, Presti ML, Giordano G, Iacono F, Neri MP. Prospective and randomized evaluation of ACL reconstruction with three techniques: a clinical and radiographic evaluation at 5 years follow-up. *Knee Surg Sports Traumatol Arthrosc.* 2006;14(11):1060–1069.

Index

Page numbers in italics indicate a figure and page numbers in bold indicate a table on the corresponding page.